## CENTIMETER CONVERSION TO FEET AND INCHES

| CM. | FT. | IN. | CM. | FT. | IN. | CM. | FT. | IN. |
|---|---|---|---|---|---|---|---|---|
| 132.1 | 4 | 4 | 157.5 | 5 | 2 | 182.9 | 6 | 0 |
| 133.4 | 4 | 4½ | 158.8 | 5 | 2½ | 184.2 | 6 | ½ |
| 134.6 | 4 | 5 | 160.0 | 5 | 3 | 185.4 | 6 | 1 |
| 135.9 | 4 | 5½ | 161.3 | 5 | 3½ | 186.7 | 6 | 1½ |
| 137.2 | 4 | 6 | 162.6 | 5 | 4 | 188.0 | 6 | 2 |
| 138.4 | 4 | 6½ | 163.8 | 5 | 4½ | 189.2 | 6 | 2½ |
| 139.7 | 4 | 7 | 165.1 | 5 | 5 | 190.5 | 6 | 3 |
| 141.0 | 4 | 7½ | 166.4 | 5 | 5½ | 191.8 | 6 | 3½ |
| 142.2 | 4 | 8 | 167.6 | 5 | 6 | 193.0 | 6 | 4 |
| 143.5 | 4 | 8½ | 168.9 | 5 | 6½ | 194.3 | 6 | 4½ |
| 144.8 | 4 | 9 | 170.2 | 5 | 7 | 195.6 | 6 | 5 |
| 146.1 | 4 | 9½ | 171.5 | 5 | 7½ | 196.9 | 6 | 5½ |
| 147.3 | 4 | 10 | 172.7 | 5 | 8 | 198.1 | 6 | 6 |
| 148.6 | 4 | 10½ | 174.0 | 5 | 8½ | 199.4 | 6 | 6½ |
| 149.9 | 4 | 11 | 175.3 | 5 | 9 | 200.7 | 6 | 7 |
| 151.1 | 4 | 11½ | 176.5 | 5 | 9½ | 201.9 | 6 | 7½ |
| 152.4 | 5 | 0 | 177.8 | 5 | 10 | 203.2 | 6 | 8 |
| 153.7 | 5 | ½ | 179.1 | 5 | 10 | 204.5 | 6 | 8½ |
| 154.9 | 5 | 1 | 180.3 | 5 | 11 | 205.7 | 6 | 9 |
| 156.2 | 5 | 1½ | 181.6 | 5 | 11½ | | | |

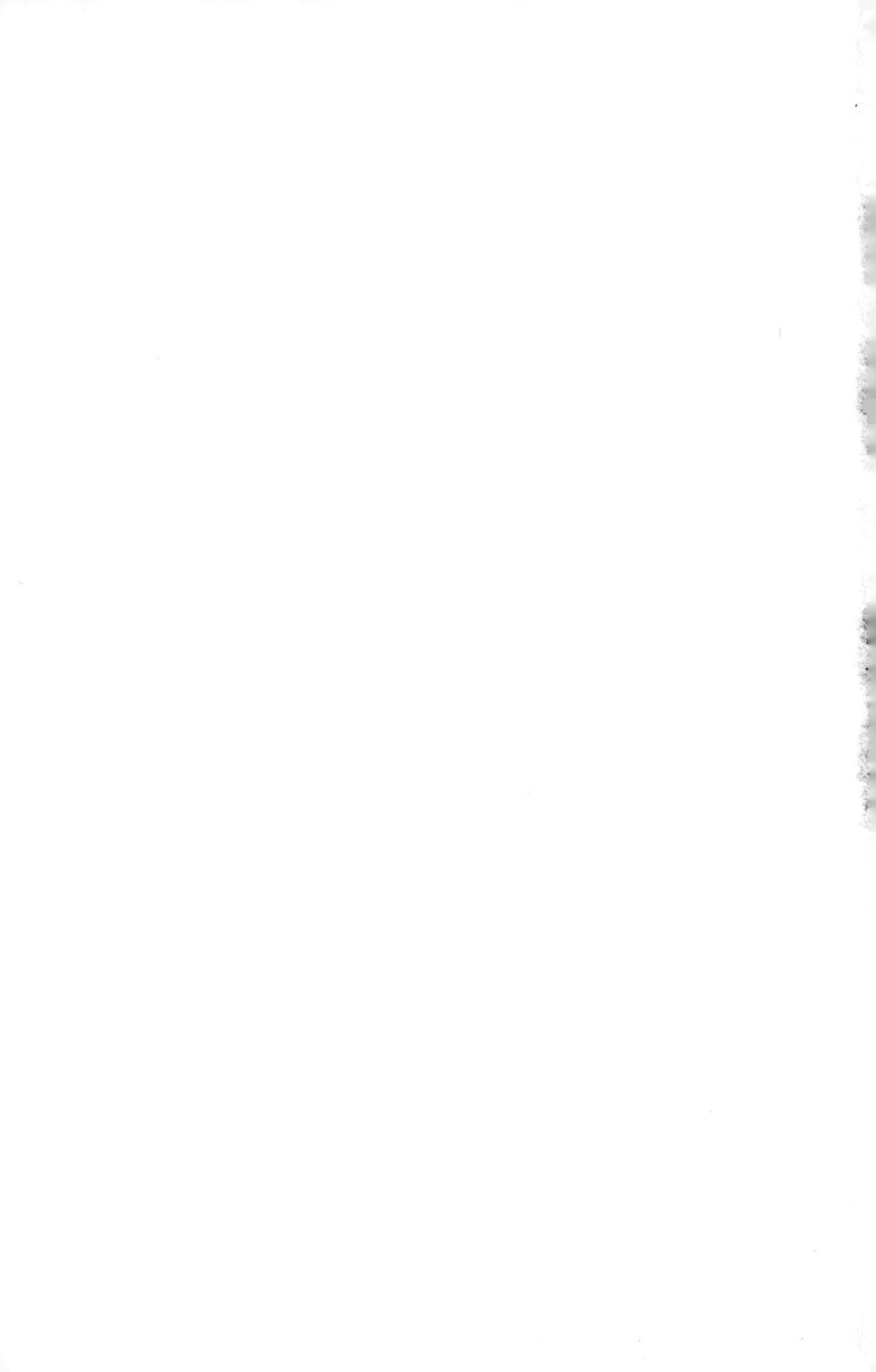

# The Practitioner's Handbook of Ambulatory Ob/Gyn

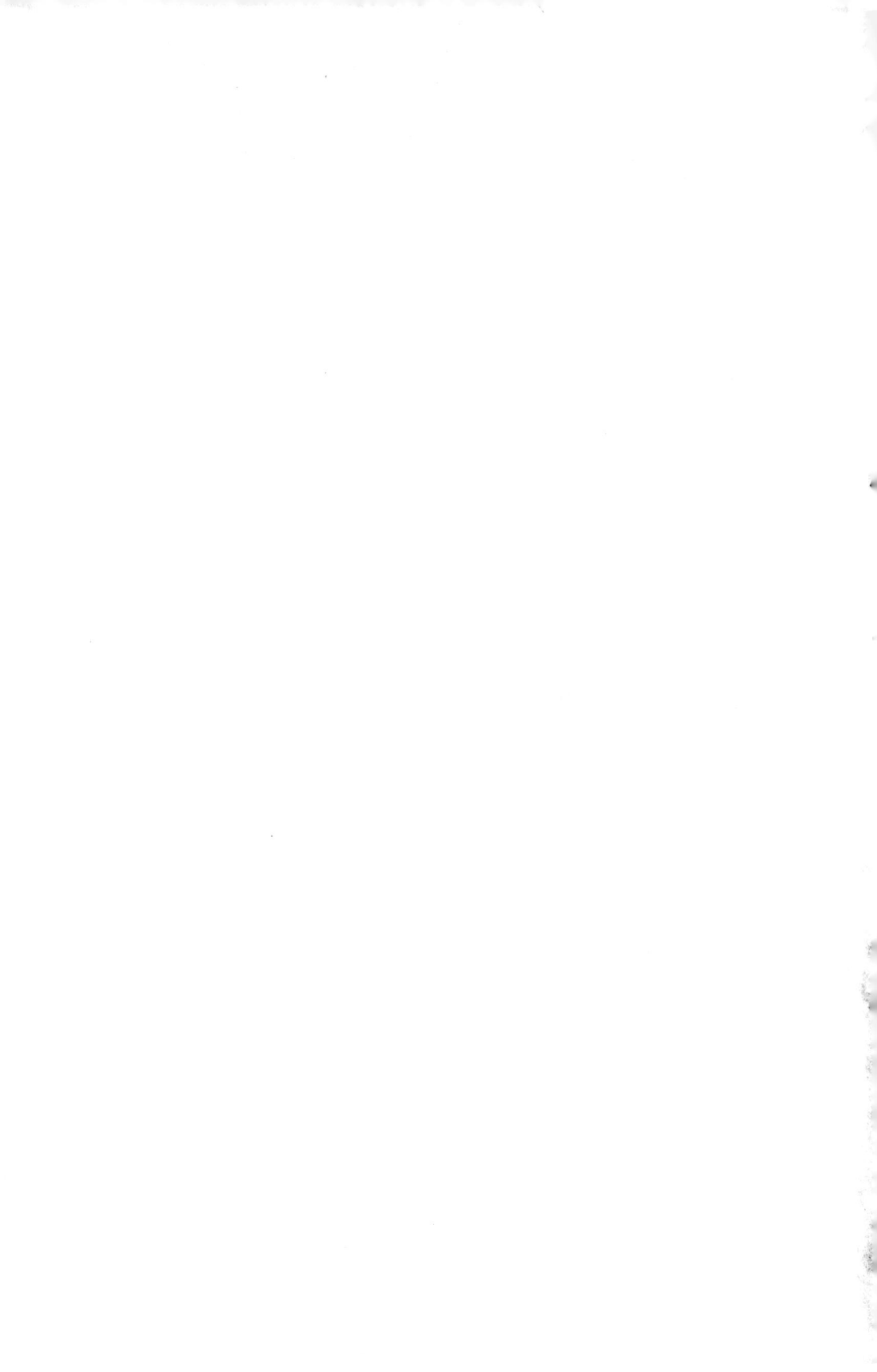

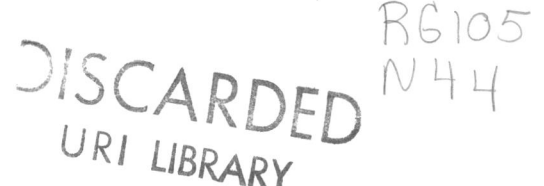

# The Practitioner's Handbook of Ambulatory Ob/Gyn

JEAN D. NEESON, R.N., M.S.N.
Ambulatory Women's Health Nurse Practitioner
Assistant Clinical Professor
University of California School of Nursing
San Francisco, California

CONNIE R. STOCKDALE, R.N., M.N., C.N.M.
Formerly Faculty Member
Nurse Midwifery Education Program
University of California
San Francisco, California

A WILEY MEDICAL PUBLICATION
JOHN WILEY & SONS
New York • Chichester • Brisbane • Toronto

Copyright © 1981 by John Wiley & Sons, Inc.

All rights reserved. Published simultaneously in Canada.

Reproduction or translation of any part of this
work beyond that permitted by Sections 107 or 108
of the 1976 United States Copyright Act without the
permission of the copyright owner is unlawful. Requests
for permission or further information should be addressed
to the Permissions Department, John Wiley & Sons, Inc.

**Library of Congress Cataloging in Publication Data:**

Neeson, Jean D
  The Practitioner's Handbook of Ambulatory Ob/Gyn

  Includes index.
  1. Gynecologic nursing. 2. Generative organs,
Female–Diseases. 3. Obstetrical nursing. 4. Pregnancy, Complications of. 5. Ambulatory medical care.
I. Stockdale, Connie R., joint author. II. Title.
RG105.N44     618     80-26151
ISBN 0-471-05670-7

Printed in the United States of America

10 9 8 7 6 5 4 3 2 1

*To Vince, Stan, and Jonathan*

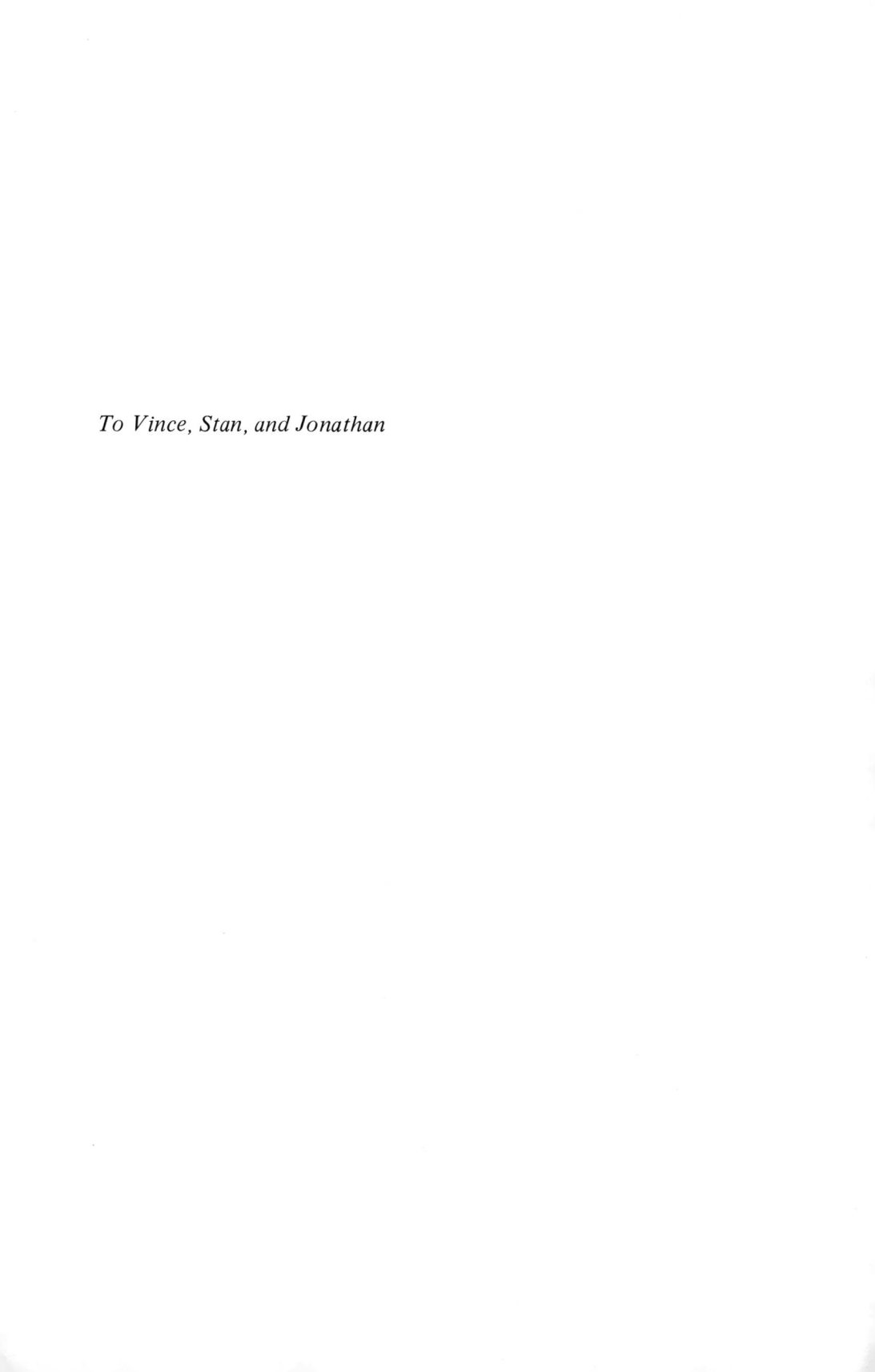

# Foreword

A significant portion of patient care in obstetrics and gynecology is "routine"—ambulatory care for basic health maintenance, screening, and treatment of common problems. This type of care is increasing as the emphasis in medicine shifts toward prevention and patient education. Much of the impetus in women's health care has come from the women's movement of the past decade. The female consumer desires a participatory, informed role in her own health care and actively seeks medical attention that is safe and sensitive to her needs. It has been amply demonstrated in different practice settings that such health care can be provided by specialty trained nurse practitioners and nurse midwives. These specialty nurses are in a particularly favorable position to bring about many of the changes women desire in their health care.

This book has been written by two highly regarded and skilled nurses, one a practitioner and one a midwife, who have a wealth of clinical and educational expertise in the health care of women. Their knowledge of the natural history and management of health care problems is combined with skill in teaching, counseling, and interpersonal dynamics. This work is a response to recent developments in health care and to the evolution of the role of the nurse in the medical care system. It should be helpful not only to practitioners and midwives but also to many others involved in the ambulatory health care of women—family practitioners, residents, interns, medical students, and nursing students.

*Donald L Snyder, M.D.*
Assistant Clinical Professor
Department of Ob-Gyn
University of California
San Francisco, California

# Preface

Women are more likely than men to seek attention for illness and health maintenance and, therefore, comprise the majority of the ambulatory health care population. The increased demands of women for sensitive, informed medical care have made health professionals more aware of women's special needs. This book is intended as an aid to meeting these special needs and is directed not only to nurse practitioners and midwives but to all professionals providing primary health care in ambulatory obstetric and gynecologic settings. Included are the most common health problems peculiar to women, their identification, assessment, management, and guidelines for patient teaching. A wide range of possible symptoms, treatments, and complications are discussed to offer the practitioner alternatives for decision making.

The format of this volume is a modified outline, which affords ready accessibility of pertinent information dealing with diagnosis and management. While this data may be found in other sources, the outline form provides the reader with a synthesis of current medical information in a concise, logical sequence.

The book is divided into three major sections—Problems in Ambulatory Obstetrics, Problems in Ambulatory Gynecology, and Diagnostic Procedures and Laboratory Values in Obstetrics and Gynecology. The obstetric section deals specifically with problems in the maternity cycle, and where gynecologic problems are incident, a cross reference to the gynecologic section is provided. Descriptions of procedures and laboratory values are reserved for the third section in order to eliminate repetition between sections and to provide substantive information in a single location. Not included in this book are complications that are usually judged to be solely in the realm of physician diagnosis and management even though they may arise as complications of the reproductive cycle. Also excluded is family planning theory and management since this topic is lengthy and has been adequately covered in other sources dealing solely with contraception.

We would like to thank Dr. Donald Snyder for his knowledgeable and painstaking review of our text. His thoughtful suggestions were essential to the accuracy of the medical content in this book. We would also like to acknowledge the efforts of Patrick Arbore in the organization and typing of the manuscript.

*Jean D. Neeson*
*Connie R. Stockdale*

# Contents

### SECTION I
### PROBLEMS IN AMBULATORY OBSTETRICS

1. Physiologic Changes and Common Discomforts    3
2. Bleeding Disorders    28
3. Hypertensive Disorders    59
4. Common Anemias    75
5. Urinary Tract Infection    85
6. Variations in Uterine Growth Patterns    90
7. Other Complications of Pregnancy    105
8. Common Postpartum Problems    118

### SECTION II
### PROBLEMS IN AMBULATORY GYNECOLOGY

9. Gynecologic Infections    129
10. Menstrual Disorders    212
11. Endometriosis    235
12. Benign Breast Disease    242
13. Urinary Tract Infection    256

14. Benign Pelvic Masses   267
15. Pelvic Relaxation   303
16. Problems During Menopause   323

## SECTION III
## DIAGNOSTIC PROCEDURES AND LABORATORY VALUES

17. Diagnostic Procedures and Laboratory Values in Obstetrics and Gynecology   349

INDEX   383

# The Practitioner's Handbook of Ambulatory Ob/Gyn

# Section I

## Problems in Ambulatory Obstetrics

# 1
# Physiologic Changes and Common Discomforts

The most frequently encountered problems of pregnancy are considered in this chapter (except vaginal infections, which are presented in Chapter 9). These are the so-called "common discomforts" of pregnancy. Although these problems do not usually constitute serious complications, explanation of their etiology and appropriate counseling/treatment help to relieve patient fears and discomfort and to enhance enjoyment of the pregnancy experience.

These common complaints with brief discussions of causation and management are presented in the last section of the chapter. For a more complete reference, the chapter begins with description of the basic hormonal influences of gestation and the organ system effects of pregnancy.

## HORMONAL INFLUENCES IN PREGNANCY

| Hormone | Site of Production | Actions | Clinical Implications |
|---|---|---|---|
| Estrogen<br>Three most common:<br>Estrone $E_1$ (menopause)<br>Estradiol $E_2$ Most potent in nonpregnant state<br>Estriol $E_3$ Estrogen of pregnancy; increased 1,000-fold in pregnancy | Ovary<br>Adrenal cortex<br>Fetoplacental unit<br>(After the seventh week of gestation, a 50% increase in secretion is ascribed to the placenta.)<br>Secreted with precursors from the fetal liver and adrenals | • Controls growth and function of the uterus<br>Hypertrophy of the musculature<br>Proliferation of the endometrium<br>Increased blood supply to the uteroplacental unit (estriol)<br>• Breast development; ducts, alveoli, nipples<br>• Enlargement of external genitalia<br>• Increased pliability of connective tissue (becomes hygroscopic and softer)<br>Relaxation of pelvic joints and ligaments<br>Stretching capacity of the cervix (?)<br>• Decreased gastric secretion of hydrochloric acid and pepsin<br>• Increased pigmentation of skin (increased melanocyte-stimulating hormone to pituitary) | • Measurement of etriol in urine or amniotic fluid serves as an index of fetal well being.<br>*Decreased*: ancephaly; Addison's disease in mother; fetal demise; drug use such as ampicillin, stilbesterol, meprobamate; or glucose in urine<br>*Increased*: twins, erythroblastosis<br>• Increased breast size and tenderness<br>• Lordosis, backache<br>• Tenderness of the symphysis pubis<br>• Cervical dilatation<br>• Indigestion, nausea, heartburn, decreased absorption of fat<br>• Hyperpigmentation: chloasma, darkened genitalia, areola, linea nigra |

| | | |
|---|---|---|
| | | • Sodium and water retention
• Vascular changes: 50% increase in clotting potential of blood fribrinogen (Factor I)
• Increased production of estriol in the late third trimester
• Psychologic changes | • Edema: increased plasma volume (physiologic anemia)
• Increased sedimentation rate
• Palmar erythema, vascular spiders, angiomata
• Enhances rhythmic uterine contractions and increased vascularity and responsiveness to oxytocin stimulation; may stimulate prostaglandin production
• Emotional lability, and libido changes (?) |
| Progesterone (increased 10-fold in pregnancy) | Corpus luteum of the ovary for the first seven weeks of pregnancy; then by the maternal/fetal unit | • Development of decidual cells in the enometrium
• A possible role in suppression of the maternal immunologic response to the fetus
• Decreases contractility of gravid uterus
• Development of lobule-alveolar system of the breasts (secretory character) | • Meets early nutritional needs of the embryo by deposition of glycogen
• Prevention of premature labor
• Breast tenderness |

## HORMONAL INFLUENCES IN PREGNANCY (continued)

| Hormone | Site of Production | Actions | Clinical Implications |
|---|---|---|---|
| | These three hypothalamic centers appear to be reset by pregnancy. | • Extensive fat depot storage | • Average body fat stored is 4 kg (8.8#).; energy stores for protection of mother and fetus during starvation or hard physical exertion |
| | | • Stimulation of the respiratory center; inducing hyperventilation (decreases $P_{CO_2}$ in the plasma) | • Decreased alveolar and arterial $P_{CO_2}$ of mother to facilitate easy transfer of $CO_2$ from fetal to maternal blood |
| | | • Increased basal body temperature by 0.5°C until midpregnancy, it then becomes normal | • Sensations of being overly warm by pregnant women, increased perspiration |
| | | • Stimulates natriuresis | • Stimulates secretion of aldosterone (sodium saver) to maintain water and electrolyte balance |
| | | • Relaxation of smooth muscle Decreased stomach motility Decreased colonic activity | • Nausea, reflex esophagitis, indigestion |
| | | | • Delayed emptying with readsorption of water from the bowel resulting in constipation and hemorrhoids |
| | | Decreased tone of bladder and ureter (dilatation throughout the system) | • Stasis of urine, urinary tract infections |

| | | |
|---|---|---|
| | Decreased vascular tone | • Reduced diastolic blood pressure, venous dilatation with stasis in lower limbs—dependent edema, varicosities |
| | Decreased motility and distention of the ducts of the gallbladder | • Slow gallbladder emptying with thickening of the bile—possible predisposition to gallstones and gallbladder symptoms |
| Oxytocin<br><br>Hypothalamus to pituitary for release | • Stimulates milk let-down and ejection<br>• Stimulates uterine contractions—is not responsible for initial labor, but increases the intensity of the contractions<br>• Ferguson's reflex—release of oxytocin by cervical and vaginal distention during labor | • Lactation<br>• Uterine involution<br>• Role in onset of labor unknown |
| Human chorionic gonadotropin (hCG)<br><br>Placenta by the syncytiotrophoblasts | • Maintains the function of the corpus luteum in early pregnancy<br>• Appears as early as eight days post conception<br>• Peaks at 60–90 days when corpus luteum function is no longer essential to maintain the pregnancy<br>• Peak secretion is 500,000–1,000,000 IU/liter day, then falls rapidly to 25,000–50,000 IU/liter after four months' gestation<br>• May function to regulate steroid production in the fetus | • Nausea (relationship uncertain)<br>• Basis of pregnancy testing (negative test after 16–20 weeks)<br>• Amount increased in multiple pregnancies<br>• Amount decreased in threatened abortion<br>• Greatest value in diagnosis of trophoblastic disease (measured by the subunit hCG radioimmuno-assay—no cross reaction with LH) |

## HORMONAL INFLUENCES IN PREGNANCY (continued)

| Hormone | Site of Production | Actions | Clinical Implications |
|---|---|---|---|
| Prostaglandin | Widely distributed in all cells of the body; produced by the maternal/placental/fetal unit | • Its role in pregnancy is uncertain<br>• Found in amniotic fluid, decidua, and maternal venous blood before labor ($PGF_2$)<br>• Anti-inflammatory drugs such as aspirin and indomethacin inhibit the synthesis of prostaglandins | • May exert an oxytoxic effect on the uterine muscle<br>• Presently used IV, vaginally, or in amniocentesis for second trimester abortions<br>• Possible future use in labor induction<br>• May increase length of gestation<br>• Use of indomethacin to halt premature labor is now under study. |
| Thyroxine | Produced in the thyroid gland with stimulation from the adenohypophysis | • Thyroid enlargement with a 20% increase in function (from tissue hyperplasia and increased vascularity)<br>• $T_3$ decreases until the end of the first trimester, then stabilizes; returns to normal 12–13 weeks post partum<br>• $T_4$ increased during pregnancy | • BMR increased 25% resulting from metabolic activity of the fetoplacental unit<br>• Protein bound iodine (PBI) increases from 3.6–8.8 to 10–12 units/dl during pregnancy.<br>• Palpitations, tachycardia, emotional lability, heat intolerance, fatigue, perspiration |

| | | |
|---|---|---|
| Prolactin | Pituitary secretion and possibly by the fetal pituitary gland or trophoblastic tissue | • Elevated blood levels appear at eight weeks' gestation and reach a peak of 200 ng/ml at term | • Sustains milk protein, casein, fatty acids, lactose and volume of milk secretion during lactation |
| Human placental lactogen (HPL) OR Human chorionic somatomammotropin | Placenta, syncytiotrophoblasts<br><br>Detected in the serum of pregnant women at six weeks' gestation and reaches 6,000 ng/ml at term | • Growth hormonelike action in pregnancy<br>Anti-insulin effect<br>Sparer of glucose and protein in the mother<br>• Maintains adequate supply of nutrients for the fetus when the mother is fasting<br>• Amount of HPL secreted correlates with fetal and placental weight<br>• May effect the increased incorporation of iron into erythrocytes (currently under study)<br>• Stimulates breast development, casein synthesis and promotes milk production<br>• Blood levels relate to placental function, which may provide basis of screening for potential fetal complications | • More glucose is available for fetal use<br>• Increased protein synthesis<br>• Increased circulating fatty acids for increased metabolic needs (conservation of glucose and amino acids for use by the fetus)<br>• Inadequate maternal glucose intake results in ketosis, which may impair fetal brain development<br>• High levels of HPL are found in association with multiple pregnancies<br>• Serial HPL levels used to assess: Suspected small gestational age Post-term pregnancies 42 weeks Chronic hypertension |

# CARDIOVASCULAR CHANGES IN PREGNANCY

| Physiologic Changes | Clinical Importance |
|---|---|
| Mechanical changes<br>• Cardiac volume increased by 10% (75 ml)<br>• Elevation of diaphragm from pressure of the uterus displaces the heart to the left and upward | • Increased size of cardiac silhouette on x-ray films<br>• Changes (murmurs) in cardiac sounds that would be considered abnormal in the nonpregnant state:<br>    Pulmonic systolic murmurs common<br>    Apical systolic murmurs are heard in 50% of pregnant women |
| • Lowered blood viscosity and torsion of the great vessels by displacement from the enlarged uterus | • Exaggerated splitting of first heart sound, loud third sound<br>• Diastolic murmurs are abnormal (18% of women have soft, transient murmurs) |
| Blood volume changes<br>• Increased plasma volume by 50% (1,250 ml)<br>    Peaks at 30-34 weeks<br>    Decreased total plasma albumin<br>        Nonpregnant value: 4.0-4.5 g/dl<br>        Pregnant value: 3.0-3.5 g/dl | • Significant hydration of maternal tissues<br>• Physiologic anemia from hemodilution<br>• Decreased colloidal pressure of vessels<br>• Increased permeability of vessel walls |
| Cardiac output changes<br>• Heart rate increase<br><br>• Cardiac output increase (nonpregnant heart pumps 5.0-5.5 liters/min and is increased 30-50% by the end of the first trimester) | • Pulse increases 10-15 beats/min, reaching maximum in third trimester.<br>    Increased kidney filtration<br>    Increased oxygen transport<br>    Increased by 10% during last two trimesters when patient is in the lateral recumbent position |

# CARDIOVASCULAR CHANGES IN PREGNANCY (*continued*)

| *Physiologic Changes* | *Clinical Importance* |
|---|---|
| • Distribution of cardiac output<br>    Uterus | • Maternal placental circulation receives 750 ml of blood per minute (is 10% of cardiac output and a 1,000% increased flow to the uterus). |
|     Factors causing decreased uterine blood flow | • Uterine contractions<br>• Hypertonus, hypertension, hypotension<br>• Severe exercise<br>• Smoking<br>• Pathologic states: anemia, placental problems, infarcts, abruption pre-eclampsia |
|     Factors increasing uterine blood flow | • Bed rest<br>• Lateral recumbent position |
| • Increased red cell volume (erythrocytes) is less than one-third of plasma volume increase | • Fall in packed cell volume (Hct) and hemoglobin values |
| • Accelerated production of red cells | • Increased reticulocyte count |
|     Effects of supplemental iron therapy in pregnancy | |
|       Regular diet without iron supplementation | • Red cell volume increases to 250 ml, or 18% |
|       Therapeutic iron supplementation | • Red cell volume increases to 400–450 ml, or 30% |
|       Oral supplementation of 60–80 mg of elemental iron per day from early pregnancy allows near maximum red cell volume expansion but does not maintain or restore iron stores | • Women with iron stores should receive 30–60 mg of elemental iron per day<br>• Women without iron stores should receive therapeutic amount of 120–240 mg of elemental iron per day |
|       Fifty percent of the red blood cells added to the maternal circulation are lost during delivery and postpartum (about 600 ml) | • A total of 800 mg of iron is needed during pregnancy to meet maternal and fetal demands (200 mg is excreted during the pregnancy) |

## CARDIOVASCULAR CHANGES IN PREGNANCY (*continued*)

| *Physiologic Changes* | *Clinical Importance* |
|---|---|
| Peripheral circulatory changes<br>• Decreased total peripheral resistance<br>    Uteroplacental circulation is a low-resistance system that works as an A-V shunt—decreases total body vascular resistance by bypassing systemic circulation | • Increased venous return to the heart |
| • Stagnation of blood in lower extremities | • Pressure of uterus on pelvic veins and inferior vena cava |
| • Increased blood flow to skin | • Dissipation of fetal heat—feelings of warmth in mother<br>• Vascular dilatation of nasal mucous membranes—nose bleeds<br>• Increased blood flow to skin of hands—erythema |
| Blood pressure changes<br>• Systolic and diastolic pressure is decreased during first half of pregnancy (5-10 mmHg) then rises to nonpregnant level<br>    Brachial artery BP is:<br>      Highest: sitting<br>      Intermediate: supine<br>      Lowest: lateral recumbent | • Any rise of 30 mmHg systolic or 15 mmHg diastolic pressure above the norm is an abnormal finding |
| • Supine hypotensive syndrome | • Compression of the inferior vena cava and aorta in third trimester pregnant women who lie on their backs may cause decreased cardiac output. Faintness may result from an 8-30% decrease in systolic blood pressure. Bradycardia may ensue and the cardiac output may be decreased by 50%. |

## CARDIOVASCULAR CHANGES IN PREGNANCY (*continued*)

| *Physiologic Changes* | *Clinical Importance* |
|---|---|
|  | Causes decrease in uterine arterial pressure, which may be deleterious to the fetus if it occurs with hemorrhage or conduction anesthesia during delivery |

## URINARY CHANGES IN PREGNANCY

Renal function changes dramatically during pregnancy. The kidneys handle increased maternal blood volume and metabolic products and also act as the primary excretory organ for fetal waste products.

| *Physiologic Changes* | *Clinical Importance* |
|---|---|
| Mechanical changes<br>• Enlarged uterus—compression of the bladder against the pelvis<br>• Enlarged dextro-rotated uterus compresses the ureters as they pass over the pelvic brim, especially on the right side. The sigmoid colon cushions the left ureter<br><br>• Vesicoureteral reflux<br>• Dilatation of the ovarian vein complex over the right ureter<br>• Base of the bladder is pushed forward and upward from the engaged, presenting part during delivery | • Reduced bladder capacity causing frequency of urination<br>• Dilatation of the ureters and renal pelvises<br>   May contain as much as 200 ml of urine (increased stagnation)<br>   Increased susceptibility to urinary tract infection (2% pyelonephritis)<br><br>• May cause changes in 24-hour urine collections (hCG, estriols)<br>• Decreased blood drainage<br>• Increased edema and possible trauma<br>• Increased possibility of infection |

## URINARY CHANGES IN PREGNANCY (*continued*)

| *Physiologic Changes* | *Clinical Importance* |
|---|---|
| Circulatory changes | |
| • Increased renal blood flow up to third trimester | • Glomerular filtration rate increased 50% (increased in lateral recumbent position and decreased when standing or sitting) |
| | • Lowered renal threshold for glucose (tubules reach maximum of readsorption); glucose is spilled in the urine. |
| • Total body water retention is seven to eight liters in late pregnancy | • Includes fetus, placenta, and amniotic fluid<br>    Physiologic edema |
| Hormonal changes | |
| • Progesterone | |
|    Increased size of kidney | |
|    Aldosterone antagonist | • Water and electrolyte loss in the urine (natriuresis) |
|    Balanced by: | |
|    Aldosterone secretion from the adrenals and estrogen secretion from the placenta | • Readsorption of sodium chloride and water by renal tubules |
| | • No increase in volume of urine for secretion |
| | • Decreased urine secretion in late pregnancy (increased fluid retention) |
|    Dilatation of ureters and renal pelvises | |
|    Relaxation of bladder and trigone | • Becomes edematous and easily traumatized |
| Postural effects | |
| • Sitting, standing | • Decrease in renal blood flow and GFR from pooling of blood in pelvis and legs |
| | • Decreased urine volume and secretion |
| | • Decreased cardiac output causes compensatory renal vasoconstriction. (Blood goes to more vital organs, 40% in four hours.) |

## URINARY CHANGES IN PREGNANCY (continued)

| Physiologic Changes | Clinical Importance |
|---|---|
| Water accumulated in the body during the day<br>• Supine: At night the effect of gravity is removed, distributing fluid throughout the body. Secretion of water and NaCl is increased.<br>Nutrient value of urine<br>• Nutrients in pregnant urine high | • Dependent edema<br>• Increased kidney filtration (nocturia)<br><br>• Increased excretion of folates, glucose, lactose, amino acids, vitamin $B_{12}$, and ascorbic acid<br>    Favors rapid growth of urinary bacteria with greater risk of urinary tract infection |

## GASTROINTESTINAL CHANGES IN PREGNANCY

The gastrointestinal system has not been extensively studied in pregnancy. The common causes of complaints in pregnancy are those related to the GI tract. Changes in this system have little direct effect on the fetus, but they are of great importance, and possible discomfort, to the pregnant woman.

| Physiologic Changes | Clinical Importance |
|---|---|
| Mechanical changes<br>• Increased pressure from the enlarging uterus on the stomach and intestines<br><br><br><br><br>• Increased venous pressure below the enlarged uterus | • Displacement of the stomach and intestines, the appendix is moved upward and laterally<br>• Hiatus hernia from partial rupture of the stomach through the diaphram<br>• Constipation<br>• Heartburn (pyrosis)<br>• Hemorrhoids and varicosities |

# GASTROINTESTINAL CHANGES IN PREGNANCY (continued)

| Physiologic Changes | Clinical Importance |
| --- | --- |
| Hormonal changes | |
| • Decreased tone and mobility of the smooth muscle of the GI tract | • Reflux esophagitis<br>• Constipation<br>• Nausea |
| • Decreased gastric emptying time<br>• Increased absorption of water from the colon | • Constipation |
| • Cholestasis | • Pruritis—generalized itching of the skin from increased retention of bile salts (possible jaundice) |
| • Decreased gastric secretion hydrochloric acid and pepsin (usually after the first trimester) | • Indigestion<br>• An 80% improvement of peptic ulcers due to decreased secretory response to histamines |
| • Epulis from estrogen effect on adhesiveness of fibers in collagenous tissue | • Swollen, spongy gums, bleed easily, regress spontaneously after delivery |
| • Pica (etiology unknown) | • Craving for substances that may or may not be foods such as clay, laundry starch, soap, toothpaste, plaster |
| • Ptyalism (etiology unknown) | • Increased saliva production (or some feel that nauseated women find it difficult to swallow saliva making it appear excessive) |
| • Dental caries | • No increase in pregnancy, and dental care is needed during pregnancy |

# RESPIRATORY CHANGES IN PREGNANCY

| Physiologic Changes | Clinical Importance |
|---|---|
| Anatomic changes | |
| • Changes that improve gaseous exchange | |
|     Flaring of lower ribs | • Increases space—occurs long before mechanical pressure occurs<br>    May never recover original position after delivery |
|     Level of the diaphragm rises 4 cm and transverse diameter cm and transverse diameter of the chest increases 2 cm | • Increased movement of tidal air (volume with each breath) |
|     Elevation of the diaphragm | • More complete expiration |
| Hormonal influences | |
| • Estrogen and progesterone | • Decreased pulmonary resistance<br>    Increased pliability of connective tissue (estrogen)<br>    Relaxation of smooth muscle (progesterone) |
| • Progesterone | |
|     Minute ventilation increased 50% | • Hyperventilation |
|     Respiratory center sensitive to progesterone | • Respiratory alkalosis |
|     Progesterone, which maintains low serum $CO_2$ levels | |
|     Fetal plasma $CO_2$ level exceeds that of maternal plasma by 4-8 mmHg | • Easy passage of $CO_2$ from the fetus to maternal circulation |
|     Increased size of vocal cords | • Due to increased circulation—causes deepening of the voice |
| Dyspnea (when the need to breathe becomes conscious) | • Consequence of low $CO_2$ levels<br>• Not necessarily related to exercise (unexplained)<br>• Increased pressure from the uterus with lung compression |

## MUSCULOSKELETAL CHANGES PREGNANCY

| *Physiologic Changes* | *Clinical Importance* |
|---|---|
| Hormonal and mechanical influences<br>• Increased relaxation of the joints (estrogenic effect)<br>• Increased weight of the enlarging uterus | • Increased mobility of sacroiliac, sacrococcygeal, and pubic joints<br>• Round ligament pain<br>• Loss of center of gravity with backache (Woman leans backward to compensate, causing lordosis and back strain)<br>• Spasm of the uterosacral ligaments<br>• Aching or numbness of upper extremities—anterior slumping of the shoulder girdle and chest<br>• Increased pliability of joints during delivery |

## COMMON COMPLAINTS OF PREGNANCY

| Complaint | Causes | Treatment and Counseling |
|---|---|---|
| Nausea and vomiting | • Decreased gastric emptying time (increased progesterone)<br>• Nutritional deficiency<br>• Associated with iron supplementation or other drugs<br>• Emotional ambivalence about pregnancy (rejection conflicts)<br>• Increased levels of human chorionic gonadotropin (hCG)<br>• Acute infection or other illness<br>• Fatigue | • Give reassurance that the nausea will pass with time.<br>• Evaluate the diet for assessment of adequate nutrition<br>• Advise the patient to:<br>  Eliminate greasy, spicy foods from diet<br>  Avoid food odors that predispose to nausea<br>  Eat foods high in carbohydrates (better tolerated)<br>  Increase protein snacks<br>  Eat dry (unsalted) crackers before arising in morning<br>  Eat six small meals a day instead of three large ones (Nausea is more common when the stomach is empty)<br>  Drink fluids between meals—decreases dehydration<br>• Refer the patient to a nutritionist if necessary<br>• Bendectine, 2 tablets at night and 1 in the morning, may be given<br>• Advise patient to take iron and vitamins after meals<br>• Vitamin $B_6$ may reduce nausea |
| Heartburn | • Gastric reflux—relaxation of the cardiac sphincter (progesterone)<br>• Decreased hydrochloric acid and Pepsin secretion in the stomach (estrogen)<br>• Displacement of stomach and duodenum by enlarging uterus<br>• Emotional problems | • Give reassurance that changes in pregnancy are causing the heartburn<br>• Assess the diet, advise the patient to:<br>  Eliminate greasy, spicy foods from diet<br>  Eat small bland meals<br>  Eat six small meals instead of three<br>  Chew gum (sometimes helpful) |

## COMMON COMPLAINTS OF PREGNANCY (continued)

| Complaint | Causes | Treatment and Counseling |
|---|---|---|
| | | Drink hot tea<br>Avoid ingestion of soda bicarbonate<br>Avoid lying down after eating<br>• Advise antacids (without phosphorus) when appropriate<br>   Al(OH)$_3$: Gelusil, Amphojel<br>   Ca(CO)$_3$: Tums<br>   Mg(OH)$_3$: Maalox, Mylanta, Riopan<br>• Advise the patient to wear loose-fitting clothing around the waistline<br>• Explore the patient's mental status (tension, depression) |
| Constipation | • Decreased GI tract motility<br>• Increased absorption of water from the bowel<br>• Pressure of the uterus on the bowel<br>• Decreased physical exercise<br>• Decreased fluid intake<br>• Inadequate roughage food in the diet<br>• Dry stool from iron therapy<br>• Fecal impaction | • Assess the diet and advise the patient to:<br>   Increase exercise and fluid intake (drink warm liquids on arising in the morning)<br>   Increase fiber intake by eating whole grain breads and cereals (bran), raw fruits, and vegetables<br>• Discuss establishment of regular bowel habits<br>• Suggest use of extra bulk, such as Metamucil, 1 tsp daily<br>• Use a stool softener when necessary such as Colace, 150–200 mg/day. A mild laxative, such as Milk of Magnesia, may also be used. (Advise the patient against use of mineral oil since it prevents absorption of fat-soluble vitamins from the gut.) |

| | | |
|---|---|---|
| Flatulence | • Ingestion of gas-forming foods<br>• Decreased exercise<br>• Decreased motility of gut<br>• Compression of the uterus on the gut<br>• Constipation<br>• Fecal impaction | • Advise against eating gas-forming foods or large meals<br>• Encourage increased exercise<br>• Advise frequent change of posture<br>• Advise thorough chewing of food<br>• Advise regular bowel habits |
| Pica | • Craving for substances that may, or may not, be foods, such as clay, laundry starch, plaster, soap, toothpaste, ice (often scraped from freezer section); etiology is unknown | • Assess nutritional status<br>  If nutritional status is adequate and the substance eaten is not harmful, counseling only is necessary.<br>  If pica is interfering with nutritional status, counseling is necessary and iron and vitamin supplementation should be given.<br>  Refer the patient to a social worker for financial aid as necessary<br>  Refer the patient to a nutritionist for counseling |
| Leg cramps | • A diet containing large amounts of milk and milk products may disturb the body's calcium/phosphorus balance (increased phosphorus), predisposing to leg cramps<br>• Fatigue or muscle strain of the extremities<br>• Blood vessel occulsion in the legs<br>• Sudden stretching of the leg and foot (pointing the toes) | • Evaluate the diet<br>  Decrease the amount of phosphorus in the diet. (Antacids (Amphojel) bind the phosphorus, with absorption by the aluminum hydroxide.)<br>  Limit intake of dairy products to four servings per day. Give calcium supplementation if patient intake is inadequate (calcium carbonate, 1-gm chewable tablets, three times a day).<br>• Advise the patient to dorsiflex the foot (point toes toward head) when cramping occurs<br>• Advise the patient to avoid the "toe-pointing" stretch of the legs<br>• Advise local heat for sore leg muscles |

## COMMON COMPLAINTS OF PREGNANCY (continued)

| Complaint | Causes | Treatment and Counseling |
|---|---|---|
| Dyspnea | • Supine hypotensive syndrome—weight of the gravid uterus presses on the vena cava and decreases venous return to the heart, compromising the circulatory status<br>• Increased awareness of breathing<br>• Pressure from uterus on lungs expansion (questionable) | • Reassure the patient that leg cramps occur commonly during pregnancy<br>• Advise the patient to:<br>  Sit up straight and stand up straight<br>  Rest after exercise<br>  Lie on the right side if dyspnea occurs when on back<br>  Prop head on pillows when sleeping<br>  Avoid overexertion |
| Urinary frequency | • The enlarging uterus stretches the base of the bladder producing a sensation of fullness<br>• Bladder capacity is diminished by pressure from the enlarging uterus<br>• Excessive fluid intake by the patient<br>• Increased urine output by the kidney occurs in the supine position (nocturia)<br>• Urinary tract infection | • Advise the patient to maintain hydration during the day, with less fluid intake in the evening to reduce nocturia<br>• Explain the need to void when the urge occurs to avoid bladder distention and urinary stasis<br>• Advise limited intake of caffeine-containing beverages (tea, coffee, soft drinks). Alcoholic beverages should not be used.<br>• Stress the need for medical attention if urinary urgency or burning occurs during urination |
| Backache and round ligament pain | • Relaxation of body joints from the hormonal influence of estrogen and relaxin<br>• Muscle strain from increased weight of the growing uterus | • Assess patient's activities at home or on the job<br>• Advise the patient to:<br>  Avoid overexertion and fatigue and to rest frequently in the recumbent position |

- Stretching of the round ligament, which supports the uterus
- Postural changes that occur to compensate for loss of the patient's center of gravity
- Fatigue and muscle tension will cause back pain
- Wearing high-heeled shoes causes postural change
- Exaggerated lordosis may cause aching and numbness of the upper extremities
- Excessive weight gain causes added strain on back muscles

- Wear low-heeled, comfortable shoes, which will reduce strain on the lower back
- Practice the proper lifting technique (demonstrate if necessary)
- Do pelvic rock exercises several times daily for relaxation of the sacroiliac muscles
- Avoid sudden, jerking, or twisting movements, which cause strain to the round ligament (e.g., arise slowly from sitting or recumbent position; turn over in bed in gradual stages)
- Apply local heat to the lower back and round ligaments for symptom reduction
- Perform total body relaxation exercises as learned in childbirth preparation classes

Dizziness

- Sudden standing from a supine or sitting position will cause pooling of blood in the lower extremities
- Supine hypotension caused by compression of the uterus on the vena cava, results in decreased blood flow to the heart and brain.
- Hypoglycemia will cause "lightheadedness"
- Hyperventilation, which causes increased levels of carbon dioxide in the blood, causes dizziness
- Anemia decreases the oxygen-carrying capacity of the red blood cells—less oxygen is supplied to the brain, which causes dizziness

- Explain to the patient the physiologic or emotional factors that may be implicated in dizziness
- Advise the patient to:
  Rise slowly from a sitting position
  Lie on either side rather than on the back when recumbent
  Eat smaller, more frequent meals to prevent hypoglycemia
  Consider assessing factors in her life that may be distressing to her. Counseling sessions may be indicated.
- Assess the patient's hemoglobin. Iron supplementation and diet counseling is necessary if anemia is present. (Ferrous sulfate, 325 mg. two to three times daily, is therapeutic.)

## COMMON COMPLAINTS OF PREGNANCY (continued)

| Complaint | Causes | Treatment and Counseling |
|---|---|---|
| | • Emotional factors may predispose to dizziness | |
| Headache | • Increased circulating blood volume and heart rate<br>• Vascular congestion of nasal turbinates from tissue edema<br>• Emotional tension causing spasm of the sternocleidomastoid muscles of the neck | • Explain the possible mechanisms responsible for headache.<br>• Reassure the patient that the symptoms are temporary and can be relieved by:<br>  Increasing rest and relaxation<br>  Engaging in activities that are relaxing or rewarding<br>  Lying down and performing relaxation exercises when a headache occurs<br>• Explain to the patient that aspirin should not be taken during pregnancy because it may cause blood coagulation problems. If headache is severe, Tylenol (2 tablets) may be taken. |
| Varicosities | • Increased blood volume adds additional pressure on the venous circulation<br>• Increased stasis of blood in the lower limbs from pressure of the enlarged uterus on the venous circulation<br>• Congenital predisposition to weakness in the vascular walls<br>• Inactivity and poor muscle tone decreases optimum blood circulation | • Advise rest in the recumbent position with the legs elevated above the level of the body<br>• Explain the use of support hose—lie flat and raise the legs to drain the veins, roll the stockings on while the legs are still elevated<br>• Advise the patient to:<br>  Refrain from crossing her legs at the knee<br>  Wear loose clothing and avoid using round garters<br>  Get up and move around at least every hour if she is sedentary |

- Prolonged standing causes venous pooling in lower limbs and pelvis
- Obesity places increased pressure on blood circulation

- Wear a pelvic pad supported by a T binder for support of vulvar varicosities
- Try to get outside and walk (not to the point of fatigue) each day

Hemorrhoids

- All the causes under varicosities apply
- Straining at stool predisposes to hemorrhoid formation

- See Varicosities
- Advise the patient to:
  Avoid constipation by increasing fluid intake and eating more fiber-containing foods
  Take warm or cool (whichever is most soothing) sitz baths and if possible, gently replace the hemorrhoid (with the finger) into the anal canal
  Cleanse the anus carefully after defecation
  Place petroleum jelly in the rectum after defecation
  Use witch hazel compresses as needed for comfort
- Advise the use of bulk such as Metamucil, 1 tsp daily. (Anesthetic suppositories to relieve pain such as Nupercainal or Anusol can be used one to four times daily).
- Stress the importance of refraining from straining during defecation since it exacerbates the problem

Edema

- Sodium and water retention from hormonal influences
- Increased venous pressure
- Varicose veins with congestion
- Dietary protein deficiency
- Increased capillary permeability

- Reassure to the patient with physiologic edema of pregnancy that it is a normal process
- Advise the patient to increase her rest, particularly by lying on her left side. Also advise elevation of the legs when sitting.

25

## COMMON COMPLAINTS OF PREGNANCY (continued)

| Complaint | Causes | Treatment and Counseling |
|---|---|---|
| | • Decreased venous return in dependent structures<br>• Increased dietary intake of sodium | • Nutritional assessment and counseling is important. Advise the patient to:<br>Restrict her intake of salty foods such as potato chips, pickles, canned soups, and added table salt<br>Not to use a salt-free diet. Salt may be added for cooking and for table use to taste—elimination of excessively salty foods is adequate. (Diuretics are not to be used in pregnancy.)<br>Increase her intake of protein-containing foods (decreased protein holds fluid in the tissue)<br>Decrease her intake of carbohydrates (especially simple sugars) and fat, since they cause retention of fluid in the tissue<br>Force fluids to two to three liters per day. (In conjunction with resting in a side-lying position, this will aid in diuresis of accumulated fluids.) |
| Increased vaginal discharge | • Increased estrogen secretion of pregnancy causes increased production of cervical mucus—more vaginal discharge becomes evident. | • Reassure patients that the increased discharge is a normal process of pregnancy. Advise good personal hygiene and frequent bathing, and to keep the vulva dry by using cornstarch. Douching *is not* indicated. |
| Insomnia (third trimester) | • Lack of comfortable position from the enlarged abdomen<br>• Excessive concern or worry about the pregnancy | • Reassure the patient that sleeplessness is common in late pregnancy<br>• Explore the patient's concerns and allow her to ventilate |

- A heavy meal late in the evening
- Nocturia, with inability to return to sleep
- Disturbance from fetal movements
- Leg muscle cramps
- Shortness of breath

- Advise the patient to:
  - Use a pillow to prop or between the legs for added comfort
  - Avoid late meals and stimulants such as coffee, tea, and cola drinks before bedtime
  - Decrease fluid intake in the evening but maintain adequate fluid intake during the day
  - Get physical exercise during the day, with a walk in the evening to aid in falling asleep
  - Sleep with a window open

Fatigue

- Influence of increased hormone production in pregnancy
- Lack of exercise
- Malnutrition
- Anemia
- Psychogenic causes
- Incorrect posture
- Excessive weight gain
- Infection

- Reassure the patient that fatigue in early pregnancy is a common symptom due to hormonal changes
- Evaluate the nutritional status of the patient and rule out the presence of anemia
- Evaluate the psychosocial status of the patient giving support if necessary with additional counseling sessions or referral to an appropriate resource
- Advise the patient to:
  - Maintain frequent rest periods and adequate exercise
  - Increase her social stimulation (when appropriate) with family, friends, or groups
  - Decrease activities that may cause overexertion
  - Explore opportunities to participate in activities that she enjoys

27

# 2
# Bleeding Disorders

Ranging in severity from mild to life-threatening, the bleeding disorders of pregnancy present the practitioner with a complex array of possible etiologies. In the majority of cases, the cause of gestational vaginal bleeding is never discovered. However, any amount of bleeding during pregnancy must be viewed seriously and every effort must be made to determine its origin swiftly and safely.

Most known causes of bleeding during pregnancy are presented in this chapter. The sections on cervical polyps (Chap. 14) and cervicitis (Chap. 9) should also be read for information about conditions associated with vaginal bleeding. Since bleeding at any stage of gestation must be viewed as a potentially dire symptom for the pregnancy, a counseling guide for the grief process is given at the end of this chapter.

## SPONTANEOUS ABORTION

### Definition

Spontaneous abortion is the naturally occurring termination of pregnancy before the fetus reaches viability (defined as fetal weight of less than 500 g or gestational age of under 20 weeks). Fetal death usually precedes the expulsion of the products of conception by several weeks. The subdivisions of spontaneous abortion, which may overlap, are:

- Threatened abortion is vaginal bleeding with or without cramping. No cervical effacement or dilatation is present.
- Inevitable abortion is vaginal bleeding with cramps and cervical dilatation. Rupture of the amniotic bag may occur.
- Incomplete abortion occurs when part of the products of conception are expelled, but some tissue (usually placental) is retained. Abortions occurring before the twelfth week of gestation are more likely to be complete; after the twelfth week, placental tissue is often retained.
- Complete abortion is the expulsion of all gestational tissue.
- Missed abortion is the retention of the products of conception for eight weeks or longer after fetal death.
- Habitual abortion is the term applied to three or more successive abortions.
- Early abortion occurs before 12 weeks' gestation.
- Late abortion occurs between 12 and 20 weeks' gestation.

## Etiology

The etiology of spontaneous abortion is unknown in many cases. Following is a list of some of the identified causes:

- Abnormal development: blighted ova, chromosomal aberrations, placental abnormalities, hydatidiform mole
- Maternal factors: diseases and infections (syphilis, influenza, pyelonephritis, pneumonia, rubella, chronic wasting diseases, toxoplasmosis, endocrine abnormalities, peritonitis)
- Uterine factors: incarceration of the uterus, large myomatas, defective uterine environment due to poor hormonal preparation of endometrium, bicornuate uterus, incompetent cervix (see discussion of this condition at end of this section), IUD usage
- Possible but unproven causes: aged or defective sperm, psychogenic factors, trauma, immunologic factors, certain drugs

## Clinical Features

(Lines of demarcation in symptomatology of various classifications are often unclear and overlapping.)

*Symptoms*

- Threatened abortion
    Vaginal bleeding
    Possible uterine cramping (affects the prognosis adversely)
- Inevitable abortion
    Bleeding with cramps
    Possible gush or leakage of clear fluid from vagina
- Incomplete abortion
    Bleeding with cramps
    Gush of clear fluid from vagina
    Possible passage of tissue
- Complete abortion
    History of bleeding with cramps and gush of clear fluid from vagina
    Report of passage of tissue
- Missed abortion
    Possible history of bleeding, sometimes with cramps, earlier in pregnancy
    Regression of breast changes
    Possible loss of weight
    Persistent amenorrhea (may be only symptom when patient is unaware of pregnancy)

*Signs*

- Threatened abortion
    Wide variation in amount of bleeding (may have ceased)
    Cervix closed and uneffaced
    Possible uterine tenderness
    Uterus of normal size and consistency for dates
- Inevitable abortion
    Cervix effaced and dilated
    Variable amount of vaginal bleeding
    Possible presence of nitrazine-positive fluid in vagina
    Possible uterine tenderness
- Incomplete abortion
    Cervix effaced and dilated
    Variable amount of bleeding (may be heavy)

Possible presence of nitrazine-positive fluid in vagina

Possible observation of tissue in cervical canal or tissue saved by the patient after passage (only definitive sign)

Uterine size possibly smaller than expected for dates
- Complete abortion

    Uterus often well contracted

    Minimal or no uterine bleeding

    Possible observation of total products of conception saved by the patient (only definitive sign)
- Missed abortion

    Cessation of uterine growth, then decrease in uterine size

    Failure to hear fetal heart tones by Doptone at appropriate stage of gestation

## Differential Diagnosis

- Cervicitis
- Malignant lesion
- Ectopic pregnancy
- Hydatidiform mole

## Diagnostic Studies as Clinically Indicated

- Sonography (real-time B-scan) can indicate the presence or absence of fetal movement and heart pulsations as early as eight weeks of gestation.
- Urinary or serum hCG level measurements and serial static sonograms are helpful in cases of threatened or possible missed abortion to demonstrate presence or lack of gestational sac growth.

## Management and Treatment as Clinically Indicated

- A careful history should be elicited and should include information on:

    Last menstrual period

    Onset of symptoms

    Amount and character of bleeding

Severity of cramps

Description of any tissue passed

Prior obstetric and pertinent medical history

- Abdominal palpation should be performed to note uterine size, tenderness, and presence or absence of fetal heart tones.
- Speculum examination should be done to verify the source of the bleeding and to rule out other possible causes. The cervix should be checked for abnormalities and for presence of dilatation. The vagina should be inspected for presence of aborted tissue.
- Gentle bimanual examination will reveal the uterine size, consistency, and possible cervical effacement and dilatation. The possibility of ectopic pregnancy should always be considered (see the section on ectopic pregnancy for signs and symptoms).
- In cases of threatened abortion, treatment is expectant, with rest and abstinence from sexual intercourse advised for two weeks after the cessation of bleeding. The woman is advised of the possible progression of the condition and to return promptly in case of progressive symptomotology. Instructions are given about collection of any tissue passed. Frequent office visits (every one to two weeks) are scheduled to assess uterine growth and to observe for signs of missed abortion. Hematocrit or hemoglobin levels should be measured to detect the development of anemia.
- If bleeding from threatened abortion persists for several weeks or becomes profuse, the patient must be referred for physician management. Cases of inevitable, incomplete, complete, or missed abortion also necessitate physician consultation and treatment.
- In cases of fetal death and inevitable or incomplete abortion, immediate evacuation of the uterus is indicated. The method of evacuation depends on the uterine size and amount of bleeding.

    Before 8-10 weeks of gestation, an office or clinic suction curretage may be performed. For longer first trimester gestations, hospitalization and administration of oxytocin in IV fluids, usually followed by curretage, is advisable.

    Second trimester abortions require hospitalization and injection of prostaglandin or dilatation and extraction to evacuate the uterus. Prostaglandin suppositories may also be used to induce labor. Curretage usually is done after these procedures.

    Cervical cultures and sensitivity reports are indicated if signs of infection are present.

    Transfusion may be necessary for treatment of shock or very low hematocrit.

    Any tissue passed or obtained from D&C should be sent to the pathology

department for a report on any abnormalities and on the completeness of the specimen.
- In cases of complete abortion when the uterus is well contracted, the cervix closed, and bleeding minimal, curretage may or may not be done.
- In cases of missed abortion, maternal fibrinogen and platelet levels must be assayed and coagulation studies must be done, since prolonged retention of the conceptus may lead to coagulation defects.
- RhoGAM should be given within 72 hours after abortion to all unsensitized Rh negative women.

## Complications

- Hemorrhage and shock
- Uterine infection
- Coagulation defects in missed abortion
- Uterine lithopedion (calcification of a missed abortion)
- Blood mole (development of a blood clot surrounding the separated conceptus)

## Patient Teaching

- Patient counseling and frequent communication with the practitioner are vital to aid the woman and her family in dealing with the possible or confirmed termination of a pregnancy and their attendant feelings of grief and failure. The fact that the cause of a particular abortion is frequently obscure is difficult for the patient and family to accept. Feelings of guilt are common as the woman searches her memory for possible causes for the event. The practitioner should reassure the woman and family about the normalcy of these feelings as well as provide factual information to ease the guilt feelings.
- If the probable cause of the abortion is known, the woman should be informed about its nature and possible treatment. If no cause is identified, the woman may be told that in many cases, abortion occurs to eliminate a fetus that is defective in some way.
- The patient and family should be reassured that, while about 10 to 15% of all pregnancies end in spontaneous abortion, most women have normal subsequent pregnancies.
- Treatment procedures should be explained fully, and explanations should be repeated as often as necessary since anxiety and grief retard comprehension.
- The patient should be taught about the normal course of recovery from spontaneous abortion and should be told to report any fever, excessive or pro-

longed bleeding, foul-smelling discharge, and/or persistent back or abdominal pain.
- The patient should be provided with appropriate contraceptive counseling and should be advised to delay future conception for four to six months to allow complete recovery.

### Incompetent Cervix

An incompetent cervix is one that is unable to retain and to support a pregnancy to term. The cervix dilates painlessly in the second trimester (usually after the sixteenth week), resulting in a late spontaneous abortion.

Prior cervical trauma (dilatation and curretage, conization, cauterization) is often associated with incompetent cervix. In other cases, developmental abnormalities may be implicated.

Diagnosis of cervical incompetency is based on a clinical history of repeated second trimester abortions with painless cervical dilatation, rupture of membranes, and passage of part or all the products of conception. In the nonpregnant woman with a suggestive history, the easy passage of an 8 mm Hegar cervical dilator adds to the probability of cervical incompetence.

Treatment of incompetent cervix is surgical. When a presumptive diagnosis is made, surgery is usually indicated at about 14 weeks' gestation as long as there is no significant cervical dilatation. The most common surgical procedures are:

- The McDonald operation: This procedure consists of a simple purse-string suture of the cervix, which must be removed near term to allow cervical dilatation in labor.
- The Shirodkar procedure: This operation involves upward dissection of the bladder with incisions of the anterior and posterior vaginal mucosa. A ligature is then placed through the incisions circling the cervix under the mucosa. The ligature may be left in place (for future pregnancies) and a cesarean section may be performed near term, or it may be removed to allow vaginal delivery.

## ECTOPIC PREGNANCY

### Definition

Ectopic pregnancy is the implantation of a blastocyst in a location other than the corpus of the uterus. The ectopic implantation can be intrauterine, as when the zygote nidates in the cervix or the interstitial portion of the tube, or extrauterine, as in ovarian, tubal, abdominal, and ligamentous implantation. Over 95% of ectopic pregnancies occurs in some portion of the fallopian tube, about 60% of tubal pregnancies are in the fimbriated area of the tube, 25% in the tubal isthmus, and 5-10% in the interstitial part, which lies within the myometrium. Because of the comparative rarity of nontubal ectopic implantations, this discussion will deal only with tubal pregnancies, and other types will be mentioned briefly.

The incidence of tubal pregnancy varies from one in 80 pregnancies to one in 230 pregnancies. The variation appears to be dependent on the socioeconomic grouping of the population studied. With a past history of ectopic pregnancy, the incidence rises to one in every five or six pregnancies.

## Etiology

Etiologic factors involved in ectopic pregnancy are those that prevent or delay the transport of the fertilized egg into the cavity of the uterus. These factors include:

- History of endosalpingitis (observed in 25-30% of tubal pregnancies)
- Developmental abnormalities of the tube
- Adhesions around the tube from previous surgery, such as tuboplasty or tubal ligation
- Uterine or adnexal tumors that distort the tube

The progression of an ectopic pregnancy depends on its location. The uterus in general undergoes some of the changes associated with a normal pregnancy, depending on the amount of steriod hormone produced by the chorionic villi. Some increase in uterine size with softening of the cervix is often observed, as is the development of some degree of uterine decidua. Microscopically, the Arias-Stella phenomenon is often seen in cases of ectopic pregnancy. The endometrial cellular changes described by Arias-Stella indicate blighting of the ovum, whether in ectopic pregnancy or intrauterine implantation.

In ampullary tubal pregnancy, the fetus is usually aborted through the fimbriated end of the tube, commonly between the sixth and twelfth weeks of pregnancy. The bleeding due to the abortion may then cease or eventuate in hemorrhage. If the abortion is incomplete, hemorrhage continues and either collects in the retrouterine cul-de-sac or, if the fimbriated end is occluded, causes a hematosalpinx.

In isthmic implantation, intraperitoneal rupture and hemorrhage usually occurs within the first 12 weeks of pregnancy. With an interstitial implantation, rupture may not occur until the third or fourth month. The entire conceptus may or may not be expelled from the tube, but, in either case, profuse, life-threatening hemorrhage occurs after rupture.

Secondary abdominal pregnancy occurs if the fetus survives the tubal rupture and the placenta continues its development. In rare instances, the fetus may continue development between the folds of the broad ligament if the implantation site was near the mesosalpinx. Much more commonly, rupture from this site results in a broad ligament hematoma. Advanced abdominal pregnancy occurs in only about 1 in 3,300 births. The fetus dies in about 90-95% of abdominal pregnancies. If the dead fetus is too large to be resorbed, it undergoes calcification, mummification, or suppuration.

Ovarian pregnancy usually ruptures early in the gestation. Rarely does fetal development continue. Occasionally, degeneration of the products of conception occurs with development of an ovarian tumor.

Cervical implantation is extremely rare and is generally heralded by painless bleeding very early in pregnancy, followed by development of a cervical mass. Treatment is surgical, usually by hysterectomy.

## Clinical Features

(The following signs and symptoms relate to ruptured or aborted tubal pregnancies.)

### Symptoms

- Pain is classically described as stabbing, sharp, and unilateral. However, depending on the location of the rupture and amount of bleeding, the pain may be generalized, bilateral, or upper abdominal. Severity varies from moderate to excruciating.
- Amenorrhea is reported in 75% of the cases. The bleeding, which often occurs in ectopic pregnancy, may be mistaken for a menstrual period.
- Spotting or bleeding occurs when the placental endocrine function stops or becomes inadequate. Bleeding is usually reported as scanty and dark, although in around 45% of the cases, it may be profuse.
- Dizziness and fainting occur in cases of profound blood loss.
- Nauşea and/or vomiting is present in 25-30% of the cases.
- Shoulder pain (usually right-sided) develops due to irritation of the subdiaphragmatic peritoneum by large amounts of hemorrhage into the abdomen.

The practitioner should always give serious consideration to the diagnosis of ectopic pregnancy even if the only symptom is spotting after one missed period, especially if accompanied by lower abdominal pain.

*Signs*

- Hypovolemia is present and develops into shock in those patients in whom hemorrhage is profuse or treatment is delayed.
- Pain on cervical motion or abdominal tenderness is present in about 75% of the cases.
- A pelvic mass is discovered in only about one-half of the cases.
- Anemia occurs in those patients in whom there is slow leakage of blood into the peritoneal cavity. In cases of more active hemorrhage, a drop in the hematocrit during a period of observation is more likely to occur than an initial anemic reading since the body may at first show only a slight reduction in hematocrit levels.
- The cervix is soft and/or blue.
- Displacement of the uterus by the ectopic mass may occur.
- A bluish discoloration of the skin in the umbilical area (from a leakage of blood into the tissue under the skin) is rarely seen.
- Signs of infection may occur secondarily after rupture of an ectopic pregnancy.
- A doughy mass in the posterior cul-de-sac may be palpated in some cases.
- Varying degrees of leukocytosis are present in about 50% of the cases. In the remainder, the leukocyte count is normal.

## Differential Diagnosis

- Acute or chronic salpingitis
- Intrauterine abortion
- Appendicitis
- Rupture of an ovarian cyst
- Torsion of an ovarian cyst
- Pelvic absess or infection

## Diagnostic Studies as Clinically Indicated

- Serum radioimmunoassay pregnancy test: Confirmation of pregnancy aids greatly in differential diagnosis.
- Laparoscopy: Visualization of the ruptured pregnancy is diagnostic but is difficult in cases with profuse hemorrhage.

- Sonography: Although visualization of the extrauterine products of conception may not be possible, a clear demonstration of intrauterine pregnancy makes it unlikely that ectopic pregnancy is also present. Additionally, the clear identification of an empty uterine cavity in the presence of a positive pregnancy test aids in confirming extrauterine pregnancy.
- Culdocentesis: The presence of nonclotting blood in the posterior cul-de-sac is almost diagnostic of intraperitoneal bleeding.
- Colpotomy and coldoscopy: Visualization of the tubes and ovaries may be possible, unless pelvic infection has obliterated the cul-de-sac or tubal adhesions are severe.
- Laparotomy: If there is diagnostic doubt, surgery is preferable to risking a medical catastrophe.

## Management and Treatment as Clinically Indicated

- Consultation with a physician is necessary when the diagnosis of ectopic pregnancy is suggested. A careful menstrual history should be elicited along with a description of pain, its character, location, and onset. The patient should be asked about a possible history of previous ectopic pregnancy, salpingitis, and/or pelvic surgery.
- After the diagnosis is reached, surgery is the only treatment for tubal pregnancy, whether the tube is intact or ruptured.
- Blood transfusion is begun for replacement in cases where hypovolemia and/or anemia is present.
- The usual procedure is salpingectomy with or without ipsilateral oophorectomy. (In some cases, removal of the ovary is necessary because of ovarian involvement and damage during the tubal pregnancy.)
- In some cases where preservation of the patient's fertility is desired, it may be possible to "milk" the conceptus through the end of the tube through a small incision. This treatment is possible, of course, only in cases of tubal pregnancy in which the tube is unruptured or only minimally damaged.
- If the patient's condition is not critical and she desires sterilization, tubal ligation of the other tube or a hysterectomy may be indicated at the time of laparotomy.
- Use of RhoGAM is indicated in the Rh negative patient.

- Oral iron supplementation should be given during and after hospitalization, and the hematocrit should be checked at the postoperative office visit.

## Complications

- Hemorrhage and shock
- Infection
- Death: Nationwide mortality is 1 in 826 ectopic pregnancies. (Among tubal pregnancies, highest mortality is in isthmic implantation.)

## Patient Teaching

- Since diagnosis and treatment of ectopic pregnancy are often done on an emergency basis, emotional support and accurate explanations of procedures, findings, and indicated treatment are basic to adequate care.
- After treatment, the patient not only needs the usual postsurgical teaching but also must be helped to deal with the lost pregnancy and with her feelings of fear, grief, and concern about future reproductive capacity.
- Since the conditions that predispose to tubal pregnancy are often bilateral, the patient should be informed of the apparent condition of her uninvolved tube and ovary when visualized during surgery. Whether or not the other tube appears affected, the woman should be informed that about 50% of all women fail to conceive after ectopic pregnancy (higher percentage if the pregnancy is the first), and that the incidence of recurrence is between 10% and 30%.
- The patient will need encouragement and support in discussing her feelings about her possible future reproductive problems with involvement of significant others in the discussion.
- The woman who desires another pregnancy should be scheduled for tests to determine tubal patency at an appropriate interval after surgery. She should also be told to see a physician promptly should she experience any irregularity of menses, abnormal vaginal bleeding, and/or crampy lower abdominal pain while trying to conceive.
- The Rh negative woman should be informed about the reason for the RhoGAM immunization and should be told that in the future RhoGAM will be given after all births of an Rh positive infant.

# HYDATIDIFORM MOLE

## Definition

Hydatidiform mole is a developmental placental abnormality in which some or all the chorionic villi became edematous and degenerate into grapelike vesicles. The vesicles vary in size and are often clustered together, hanging from thin pedicles of villi. A hydatidiform mole is usually associated with a retained, blighted ovum.

## Etiology

Etiology of hydatidiform mole is unknown. Factors associated with this condition are:

- Age greater than 40: This condition is about ten times as common in women approaching menopause.
- Parity three or greater: Molar pregnancy is 3.5 times more common in this group than in women of lower parity.
- Residence: Incidence is 1/2,000 pregnancies in United States and Europe but much higher in parts of Asia and the South Pacific (1/173 pregnancies in the Philippines; 1/530 pregnancies in Hong Kong).
- Prior molar pregnancy: Incidence is 1/500 pregnancies in women with previous hydatidiform mole.

## Clinical Features

### Symptoms

- Vaginal bleeding, which is usually minimal but persistent, dark-red or brownish, occurring at the end of the first trimester and beginning of the second. Bleeding occurs in 50-90% of the cases
- Severe nausea and vomiting, probably related to the extremely high levels of chorionic gonadatropin (hCG) that are seen with hydatid mole
- Absence of fetal movement reported in those pregnancies that progress to the usual time of quickening
- Passage of grapelike vesicles

*Signs*

- Larger uterus than expected for dates in 50% of the cases; smaller uterine size than expected in 20%
- Anemia, which may be out of proportion to the external loss of blood
- Absence of fetal heart tones and inability to palpate fetal parts
- Signs of toxemia (elevated blood pressure and proteinuria) developing before the twenty-fourth week of pregnancy in 50% of the patients with hydatid mole. Development of toxemia at this stage of pregnancy is virtually diagnostic of a mole.
- Adnexal masses due to ovarian lutein cysts, occurring in about 30% of the cases
- Pulmonary embolism, occurring in rare cases when large amounts of trophoblast are transported to the lungs but do not invade pulmonary tissue. More frequently, trophoblastic tissue in smaller amounts invades pulmonary tissue and is visible on x-ray examination.
- Hyperthyroidism seen in about 8-10% of the patients (resulting from trophoblastic production of a thyrotropin)

## Differential Diagnosis

- Threatened abortion
- Inaccurate pregnancy dating
- Twin pregnancy
- Hyperemesis gravidarum
- Pneumonia (in cases of deportation to the lungs)

## Diagnostic Studies as Clinically Indicated

- Sonography is 98% accurate in the diagnosis of hydatidiform mole and is the best study.
- Amniography (transabdominal injection of radiopaque substance into the uterus) reveals "moth-eaten" molar appearances on x-ray films.
- Measurements of serum hCG after 100 days beyond the last menstrual period show persistently high or rising levels in the patient with molar pregnancy. High levels of hCG suggest, but are not diagnostic of, hydatidiform mole.
- Flat plate roentgenogram of the abdomen fails to show fetal skeleton.

## Management and Treatment as Clinically Indicated

- Consultation with a physician is required for all patients in whom hydatidiform mole is clinically suspected or diagnosed.
- If the patient with molar pregnancy is in labor, oxytocin infusion followed by curretage is indicated.
- If the patient is not in labor, suction curretage with oxytocin infusion is performed with follow-up sharp curretage done one to two weeks after evacuation.
- If patient does not wish to have more children, hysterectomy is the treatment of choice. If the woman is over 40 or has three or more children, hysterectomy is preferred because of the increased risk of malignancy after hydaditiform mole (see below).

### Follow-up

*Note:* Deportation of trophoblastic cells occurs in every case of molar pregnancy. Twenty percent of the women with hydatidiform mole cannot rid themselves of these invasive cells through their immune systems and will develop either choriocarcinoma or invasive mole. Therefore, the follow-up tests and treatment discussed below are of utmost importance in *every* case of hydatidiform mole.

- After termination of molar pregnancy, future pregnancy is prevented for the follow-up period, preferably by the use of oral contraceptives.
- An initial chest x-ray film is obtained to serve as a baseline should further x-ray studies be deemed necessary.
- Patients are followed with weekly 24-hour urine collections for quantitative hCG determinations until titers become negative.
- Then titers of hCG are evaluated weekly by the more sensitive serum radioimmunoassay techniques until hCG levels are undetectable. (This should occur within eight weeks of termination of pregnancy.)
- When serum hCG levels are normal for three consecutive assays, levels are measured monthly for six months.
- When hCG levels have remained normal for six months, follow-up is stopped and pregnancy is permitted.
- If hCG levels plateau for more than two weeks, if the titer rises, or if metastases are detected, chemotherapy is begun.

   hCG levels are assayed weekly during treatment.

Single-agent chemotherapy (usually methotrexate or actinomycin D) is given for five consecutive days.

As many courses are given as are necessary to bring hCG levels to normal.

The first course is given in the hospital; subsequent courses may be given on an outpatient basis.

Subsequent courses are given two to three weeks apart with careful testing of bone marrow and liver function (CBC, platelet count, differential count, SMA 12) and monthly chest x-rays films until hCG levels are normal. If bone marrow suppression or liver malfunction occurs, resumption of chemotherapy is contraindicated.

Pregnancy is delayed until one year after hCG levels are normal for three consecutive weeks.

hCG levels (after three consecutive normal titers) are measured every month for six months, then every other month for six additional months.

- Treatment differs for high-risk patients, including: those who have metastasis to the brain, liver, or bowel; those in whom treatment is not begun within four months of the responsible pregnancy; those in whom initial postevacuation levels of hCG are greater than 100,000 mIU/ml of serum; those who do not respond to single-agent therapy; and those with nongestational choriocarcinoma (not discussed here).

   High-risk patients are treated with three chemotherapeutic agents on an inpatient basis.

   Spacing of triple-agent courses of treatment, lab testing, and follow-up hCG assays are the same as with single-agent therapy.

## Complications

- Malignancy

   Invasive mole occurs in 15-17% of the cases after hydatidiform mole.

   Choriocarcinoma occurs in 3-5% of cases with molar pregnancy.

   *Note:* Choriocarcinoma usually occurs during or after some form of pregnancy. Forty percent of gestational cases happen after abortions, 40% after molar pregnancies, and 20% after normal term pregnancies. Except for cases following molar pregnancy, the first symptom or sign is often subinvolution of the uterus with irregular bleeding during the postpartum period. In other cases, signs arising from metastic lesions may be the first to occur. Health personnel should keep in mind the possibility of choriocarcinoma arising from cases other than hydatidiform mole. Treatment is similar in all cases of choriocarcinoma, but mortality is higher in nonmolar cases because of delay in diagnosis.

Liver malfunction and bone marrow suppression occur in patients receiving chemotherapy.

Cure rate of malignancy after hydatidiform mole is almost 100% except in high-risk patients (identified previously in this section) in whom the cure rate drops to approximately 50%.

## Patient Teaching

- Women with molar pregnancies (and their families) must be helped to comprehend and to deal with:
    Loss of a pregnancy
    Knowledge that the pregnancy was abnormal
    Potential for development of serious complications
    Necessity to postpone another pregnancy
    Importance of follow-up laboratory testing
- Patients should be encouraged to discuss feelings of grief, anger, and fear, which are common in this situation.
- Patients need factual reassurance about favorable statistics for a benign resolution.
- Women with molar pregnancies often need time and repeated information to understand the importance of close physician supervision.
- Patients should be told to notify the physician of the following symptoms, which may indicate malignancy:
    Irregular vaginal bleeding
    Spitting up blood
    Severe, persistent headaches
    Persistent secretion from breasts
- Women who require chemotherapy should be given explicit information about drug(s), planned scheduling of treatment, hoped-for results, and possible side effects of chemotherapy, including stomatitis, skin rash, malaise, anorexia, alopecia, and constipation.
- Patients receiving chemotherapy (and their families) need ongoing emotional support and encouragement to discuss their feelings and concerns.

# PLACENTA PREVIA

## Definition

In placenta previa, the placenta, instead of developing at the usual site well away from the region of the cervical os, attaches and develops in the lower segment of the uterus, over or encroaching on the internal cervical opening. The incidence of placenta previa is about 1 in every 300 deliveries. Four degrees of placenta previa are commonly recognized:

- Total placenta previa: The placenta completely covers the internal cervical os.
- Partial placenta previa: The placenta partially covers the internal os.
- Marginal placenta previa: The edge of the placenta lies at the border of the os.
- Low-lying placenta: The placenta is very near the region of the internal os.

In labor, the classification of previa may change as cervical dilatation progresses.

## Etiology

The etiology of placenta previa is unknown. Following is a list of factors that are often associated with this condition:

- Age greater than 35 and/or high parity are possibly related to the defective vascularization of fundal decidua due to damage from previous pregnancies and/or the aging process.
- A large, thin placenta may develop as a result of low implantation as an attempt to provide adequate placental perfusion. A large placenta may be a causative factor in conditions that normally have larger placentas, such as fetal erythroblastosis and multiple gestations. The lower portion of a normally attached, large placenta may encroach on the area of the internal os.
- Abnormal fetal presentations probably occur due to fetal accommodation to the altered intrauterine space caused by a low placental implantation.
- Placenta accreta results from the thin, poorly developed decidua in the lower uterine segment which leads to implantation of the previa involving deeper uterine musculature.
- Frequency of recurrence of previa suggests an unknown etiologic predisposition.

## Clinical Features

### Symptoms

- Bleeding and passage of tissue early in pregnancy: Many spontaneous abortions probably occur in cases of abnormal placental localizations (see section on spontaneous abortion for symptomatology).
- Painless bleeding: This is the chief initial symptom in pregnancies carried until midterm or later with low placental implantations. The amount of bleeding reported is variable and often ceases for a time after the initial episode. The bleeding may follow intercourse or a vaginal examination, but most often occurs without a precipitating factor. About 90% of patients with placenta previa will have at least one prenatal hemorrhage. Patients with complete previas tend to bleed earlier (before 30 weeks) and more profusely than those with lesser degrees of previa.

### Signs

- Possible vaginal bleeding, usually bright red. The patient's history must be used to document the amount of bleeding if hemorrhage has ceased.
- Soft, nontender uterus
- Unengaged presenting part, even near or at term
- Possible abnormal fetal position
- Possible signs of maternal shock
- Audible, normal fetal heart tones, except in cases of maternal shock when fetal bradycardia/tachycardia may occur

## Differential Diagnosis

- Mild degree of abruptio placenta
- Bleeding from cervicitis, malignancy, or polyps

## Diagnostic Studies as Clinically Indicated

- Sonography is the first choice for accuracy and safety in determining placental localization. If an anterior, normally implanted uterus can be visualized, placenta previa may be ruled out. In other cases, sonography may be

BLEEDING DISORDERS 47

unable to exclude the possibility of previa, especially when implantation is on the posterior aspect of the uterus. When placenta previa can be clearly visualized, the sonogram can frequently determine the degree of previa.

*Note:* Placenta previa may be noted in as many as 5% of all pregnancies ultrasonically scanned in the second trimester. The great majority of these placenta previas are asymptomatic and convert (by an as yet unknown process) to normal implantations by the time of delivery.
- Other tests for placental localization—soft tissue placentography, amniography, or IV injection of radioactive isotopes—may be indicated.

## Management and Treatment as Clinically Indicated

- In nonemergency cases of third trimester bleeding, the clinician (after checking maternal and fetal vital signs) should elicit a careful history of:

    The time of onset of bleeding

    Any precipitating activities

    The approximate amount of bleeding (Patient should be asked if she has blood soaked pads or clothing with her for estimation purposes.)

    The color and character of the bleeding

    Whether or not the bleeding was associated with pain (if so, the location and character of the pain should be determined)

    Any previous bleeding episodes

    Previous history of cervicitis/vaginitis
- The practitioner should review the patient's chart for results of possible prior sonographic studies; notations on possible cervical friability, erosion, or polyps; and Pap smear results.
- An examination of the external genitalia for active bleeding is done, as well as a gentle abdominal examination for fetal position. Vaginal and rectal examinations are *absolutely* contraindicated since such examinations may precipitate uncontollable hemorrhage in cases of placenta previa!
- Physician consultation is mandated in cases of third trimester bleeding.
- Management and treatment of placenta previa usually includes the following:

    Blood is drawn for a CBC with a stat hematocrit and for typing and crossmatching for two units of fresh whole blood. Coagulation studies may be ordered if there is any question about the possibility of placental abruption.

    An IV drip (usually with lactated Ringer's solution) is started.

    In cases of placenta previa when the fetus is premature and uterine bleeding is minimal or has ceased, expectant treatment (careful observation and no vaginal or rectal manipulation) may be tried until the infant is mature or until delivery is forced by heavy hemorrhage. Delivery is by cesarean-section when the infant has reached lung maturity as indicated by the L/S ratio or the shake test performed on amniotic fluid.

In cases when the fetus is within three weeks of term, labor is in progress, or hemorrhage is severe or fails to cease, active intervention is necessary. If the patient is a multipara with a low-lying placenta who had no bleeding until after the onset of labor, vaginal delivery (with careful maternal/fetal monitoring) may be attempted. The membranes are ruptured to permit the fetal head to tamponade the placenta and possibly to control the bleeding. In all other cases, cesarean section is the preferred route of delivery.

- Vaginal examination to determine the cause of hemorrhage or to detect the degree of previa is used only in cases when other diagnostic aids are absent, vaginal hemorrhage is life-threatening, and the physician is willing to deliver the fetus immediately. Vaginal examination is performed in the delivery or operating room with a double setup to permit immediate cesarean-section delivery if necessary.

## Complications

- Maternal
  Shock
  Cesarean-section delivery
  Possible hysterectomy (when bleeding from the placental site cannot be controlled or placenta accreta is present)
  Mortality: almost zero with hospital management
- Fetal
  Possible prematurity
  Anoxia
  Intrauterine growth retardation
  Anemia (about 10% of blood loss is from fetus)
  Mortality: 15-25%

## Patient Teaching

- The patient should be informed about the diagnosis, the possible consequences of the condition, testing procedures, and the plan of care. In nonemergency

cases, the patient (and family) should be taught about the anatomy of placenta previa and about the possible causes of the abnormal implantation.
- Emotional support for the woman and her family is essential in this frightening situation. Reassurance should be given (if appropriate) about the condition of the woman and the baby. Emphasis should be placed on the fact that the woman did not cause the placenta previa and is in no way to blame for this condition. Patients who have had sexual intercourse or who have douched close to the time of hemorrhage are especially in need of this reassurance.
- The woman (and family) should be told promptly of test results and any change in the plan of treatment.
- In some cases where the amount of bleeding was small, bleeding has ceased, the condition of mother and fetus warrants expectant treatment, and the woman lives close to the hospital, discharge from the hospital to await fetal maturity may be indicated. The woman should be given instructions about bed rest, return for prenatal visits, avoidance of vagina intercourse or douching, monitoring of the amount of fetal movement, and prompt return to the hospital if bleeding recurs or fetal movement decreases.
- Patients who require prolonged hospitalization before delivery or who give birth to a premature infant need referral for financial assistance.
- In cases where the infant dies or is premature or hysterectomy is necessary, the woman (and family) need assistance in moving through the stages of grief and grieving (see the grief and grieving guide at the end of this chapter).

## ABRUPTIO PLACENTA

### Definition

Abruptio placenta is the premature (before the birth of the baby) separation from the uterine wall of a portion, or all, of a normally attached placenta. Abruptio placenta occurs in the second half of pregnancy (after 20 weeks' gestation). The condition ranges in severity from mild partial abruption, which is often only diagnosed after delivery, to extensive or total abruption with fetal death and severe maternal complications. The incidence estimates of premature separation of the placenta range from 1 in 59 to 1 in 150 births. This variance is due to difficulty in diagnosis of mild degrees of abruption. Two major classifications of placental abruption are:

- Mild to moderate abruption, which accounts for 85% of all cases, occurs

when 30% or less of the placenta separates from the uterine wall, often close to the placental border. External bleeding is present with little or no concealed hemorrhage trapped behind the placenta.
* Severe abruption occurs when 50% or more of the placenta is prematurely separated. The separation often occurs in the central portion of the placenta with extravasation of blood into the uterine musculature (Couvelaire uterus). External bleeding may or may not be present. Disseminated intravascular coagulation (DIC) is more likely to occur with severe abruption because of a complex change in the normal hemostatic mechanisms that results in depletion of fibrinogen in the general circulation and fibrin deposition in the small vessels of the kidneys, lungs, liver, and brain. Eventually, uncorrected DIC results in vascular collapse.

## Etiology

The primary cause of abruptio placenta is inknown. The condition is believed to result from degenerative changes in the small arteries supplying the intervillous spaces, leading to rupture of these vessels, hemorrhage into the decidua basalis, and clot formation. Factors associated with premature separation of the placenta are:

* Maternal hypertension: pre-eclampsia, chronic hypertension, chronic renal disease
* High parity
* Previous premature placental separation (recurrence rate of 15-20%)
* Circumvallate placenta
* Rare factors: short umbilical cord, abdominal trauma, amniocentesis, or sudden uterine decompression (as in rupture of membranes with polyhyramnios)

## Clinical Features

### Symptoms

* Severe abruptio
    Possible external bleeding (usually dark-red)
    Sudden onset of severe, unremitting abdominal pain
    Possible cessation of fetal movement

- Moderate abruptio
    - Revealed dark-red bleeding (usually)
    - Moderate degree of abdominal pain
- Mild abruptio
    - External bleeding
    - Little or no abdominal pain

*Signs*

- Severe abruptio
    - Rigid, boardlike, unrelaxing uterus
    - Extremely irritable and tender uterus
    - Absent or faint bradycardic/tachycardic fetal heart tones
    - Possible dark-red vaginal bleeding
    - Increase in uterine size (due to concealed hemorrhage)
    - Moderate to profound maternal shock
    - Possible bleeding from maternal mouth and nose (due to DIC)
- Moderate abruptio
    - Failure of uterus to relax or to relax completely between contractions (if present)
    - Irritable, tender uterus on abdominal palpation
    - Possible mild maternal shock
    - Fetal heart tones with tachycardia or bradycardia
    - Usually moderate amount of dark-red vaginal bleeding
    - Possible increase in uterine size
- Mild abruptio
    - Normal uterine tonus, normal relaxation between contractions (if present)
    - Uterine irritability minimal or absent
    - No uterine tenderness
    - Maternal vital signs normal
    - Fetal heart tones present and normal
    - Small to moderate amount of dark-red vaginal bleeding

## Differential Diagnosis

- Bloody show
- Cervicitis, cervical polyps

- Placenta previa
- Rupture of the uterus

## Diagnostic Studies as Clinically Indicated

- Sonography is used to rule out placenta previa and to attempt to visualize the degree of separation. However, in pregnancies with a posterior placenta, the abruption cannot be seen.
- Clot observation test is done to diagnose depletion of clotting factors. If 5 ml of the patient's blood fails to clot in 8-12 minutes, the patient's fibrinogen level is depleted.
- Clotting times are also done for diagnosis of intravascular coagulation. Prothrombin and partial prothrombin times are usually increased in DIC.
- CBC with stat hematocrit is used as a baseline indication of maternal blood loss.

## Management and Treatment as Clinically Indicated

- All patients with third trimester bleeding should be referred to the consulting physician for management.
- If the patient is not in shock, fetal heart tones are normal, and the situation does not appear to be an acute emergency, the practitioner should first:

  Take the patient's vital signs

  Elicit a careful history of the onset and character of pain and/or bleeding

  Review the chart for pertinent information (gestational age, previous episodes of bleeding, possible previous sonogram, signs of hypertension, etc)

  Examine the external genitalia for active bleeding (Do not perform a pelvic or rectal exam even in cases strongly suggestive of abruption since placenta previa may be present.)

  Do a gentle abdominal exam to note the uterine consistency, irritability, and tenderness, as well as fetal position and degree of pelvic engagement

  Mark the top of the fundus as a future reference for measuring concealed hemorrhage

- In all but the mildest cases of placental abruption, management is aimed at correction or prevention of maternal complications (shock, hypovolemia, coagulation defects), followed by rapid delivery.

# BLEEDING DISORDERS

- If there is no fetal or maternal distress and the abruption is mild, expectant therapy may be tried with careful observation and monitoring of fetal and maternal well-being. Blood should be available for possible transfusion. Labor is induced and carefully monitored. In the absence of fetal distress or maternal hemorrhage, vaginal delivery is permitted.
- For cases of moderate to severe abruption, the following measures are indicated:

    Monitoring of fetal and maternal condition is performed by central venous pressure readings, measurement of maternal urine output, frequent determination of maternal blood clotting mechanisms, continuous fetal heart rate monitoring, and measurement of uterine size.

    Shock and clotting deficiencies are treated by means of IV fluids (Ringer's lactate; whole, fresh blood; cryoprecipitate; platelets; or fresh frozen plasma).

    Needling of the fetal membranes to drain amniotic fluid is performed to hasten delivery, to decrease the chance of an amniotic fluid embolism, and to reduce extravasation of blood into the myometrium.

    Delivery is attempted within six hours of the onset of symptoms since most coagulation defect problems are time related.

    If the fetus is alive and in no distress, labor is induced with careful maternal-fetal monitoring and liberal recourse to cesarean section if complications arise or if labor is lengthy.

    If the fetus is alive, but distressed, rapid delivery, usually by cesarian section, is mandated.

    If the fetus is dead or very immature, pitocin induction or stimulation with vaginal delivery is preferred, unless the hemorrhage is so heavy it cannot be managed by replacement or delivery is not anticipated within a reasonable length of time.

    Continued replacement of blood/clotting factors as necessary is carried out postpartum, as well as monitoring of urinary output to detect the possible onset of renal failure.

## Complications

- Maternal

    Hemorrhage and shock
    DIC (20-38% incidence in cases of moderate to severe abruption)
    Renal failure (1.2-3.9% incidence)
    Postpartum Sheehan's syndrome (pituitary necrosis)
    Mortality: 5-5% worldwide

- Fetal
    Hypoxia
    Prematurity
    Birth trauma
    Mortality: 25-50%

## Patient Teaching

- In mild cases of abruption, the woman and her family need complete explanations of the condition, the necessity for careful monitoring, and the plan for care. The pregnant woman should be informed promptly of the results of monitoring procedures and of any change in the degree of abruption. Additionally, emotional support is necessary to help the family to deal with this crisis situation.
- In cases of moderate to severe abruption, explanation of procedures, treatment, and the patient's condition should be as complete as possible. Even when an emergency exists, a few words of explanation and reassurance (if appropriate) can be of great help to the patient and family in coping with a frightening situation.
- If the fetus succumbs, the patient and family need help in moving through the stages of grief and grieving (see the grief and grieving guide at the end of this chapter). If the baby survives, the family may have to adjust to the reality of a premature and/or neurologically damaged infant. Feelings of shock, inadequacy, guilt, and grief are normal in this situation. At times, the family may have begun anticipatory grieving for an infant who survives and must be helped to relate to a live infant.

# GRIEF AND GRIEVING COUNSELING GUIDE

## Definition

Grief is a normal reaction to physical or psychologic loss of a loved person, object, body part, or body function. In the area of obstetrics and gynecology, grief occurs in several contexts:

- The loss or anticipated loss of an embryo, fetus, or baby

- The birth of a premature or defective child
- The failure to conceive or the loss of reproductive capacity
- Abnormality and/or surgical loss of part or all the reproductive system

The practitioner should anticipate the need for grieving in the above situations and should be prepared to help the woman and family to complete sucessfully the stages of grieving as follows:

- The first stage is that of shock and disbelief. The person is stunned by the event and may deny its existence. She may be confused, apathetic, and/or restless, with possible somatic complaints of dizziness, fainting, excessive perspiration, and nausea.
- The second stage is characterized by developing awareness and acute mourning. The person begins to comprehend the reality of the event with subsequent loss of interest in normal activity and preoccupation with thoughts of the loss. Feelings of inadequacy, failure, guilt, loneliness, helplessness, depression, and exhaustion are common in this stage. Anger and blame, inwardly or outwardly projected, comes to the fore. Insomnia, weeping, sighing, and loss of appetite are often present.
- The third stage is that of resolution or acceptance. The person becomes less obsessed with thoughts of the event, breaks the ties with the lost person or object, gradually resumes normal daily life, and forms new relationships.

The usual length of time for completion of the total grieving process is 6-12 months, with the first two stages (acute phase) occupying four to six weeks. Completion of the process varies and can be accelerated or retarded by:

- Lack of support and encouragement to move through the phases
- Extreme feelings of ambivalence about the lost person or object that lead to exaggerated guilt or blame-laying tendencies
- Previous grieving processes that were not successfully completed

The practitioner's ability to help in the grieving process and to recognize unhealthy grieving or inability to grieve is vital to total patient care. Arrest of the grieving process can lead to psychologic and/or physical problems in the future. Assistance in the grieving process may include:

- Encouraging crying, verbalization, or acting out of feelings of shock and loss soon after the event
- Giving permission to grieve
- Expressing one's own feelings of grief or concern about the situation
- Providing time to be with the patient and family
- Giving permission or encouragement to see and touch the lost or impaired infant (when appropriate)

- Providing information about possible somatic and psychologic events in the grieving process
- Validating the normalcy of individual reactions
- Giving any available information on the cause of the loss as well as on possible future treatment or events
- Permitting the expression of anger and hostility

Counseling should be on an ongoing, frequent basis, especially in the first few weeks after a loss. Should the practitioner not be able to provide such access, referral to another counselor should be provided. If the practitioner notes signs of unhealthy grieving (or the inability to grieve), referral to a psychiatrist, psychologist, or psychiatric social worker is necessary. Such abnormal signs may include:

- Lack of weeping or other indications of grief
- Cheerfulness in the acute phase
- Prolonged apathy
- Expression of little or no pain
- Protracted and/or extreme expressions of guilt or hostility
- Immediate diversion of attention toward business or other daily activities
- Nonresolution of the acute grieving phase within six to eight weeks

The practitioner and other personnel should also recognize the presence of grief in themselves when the untoward occurs in the practice of obstetrics and gynecology and should permit its expression and resolution.

## REFERENCES

Baggish M: Gestational trophoblastic neoplasia. *Clin Obstet Gynecol* 17:259, 1974.

Baird AM, Beckly DE, Ross FG: The ultrasound diagnosis of hydatidiform mole. *Clin Radiol* 28:637, 1977.

Ballas S, Gitstein S, Jaffa AJ, et al: Midtrimester placenta previa: Normal or pathologic finding. *Obstet Gynecol* 54:12, 1979.

Ballon SC, Berman ML, Lagasse LD, et al: The unique aspects of gestational trophoblastic disease. *Obstet Gynecol Surv* 32:405, 1977.

Braga C: Lecture notes, University of California, San Francisco, 1978.

Brenner WE, Edelman DA, Hendricks CN: Characteristics of patients with placenta previa and results of "expectant management." *Am J Obstet Gynecol* 132:181, 1978.

Butovsky I, Langer R, Herman A, et al: Conservative surgery for tubal pregnancy. *Obstet Gynecol* 53:709, 1979.

Callen PW, DeMartini WJ, Filly RA: The central uterine cavity echo: A useful anatomic sign in the ultrasonographic evaluation of the female pelvis. *Radiol* 131:187, 1979.

Caplan G: *An Approach to Community Mental Health,* ed 1. New York, Grune & Stratton, 1966, pp 58, 218.

Clausen JP, Flook MH, Ford B: *Maternity Nursing Today,* ed 2. New York, McGraw-Hill Book Company, 1977, p. 674.

Hammond C: Differential diagnosis of gestational trophoblastic diseases. *Contemp Obstet Gynecol* 3(6):59, 1974.

Hibbard LT: Complications of labor and delivery, in Benson RC (ed): *Current Obstetric and Gynecologic Diagnosis and Treatment,* ed 2. Los Altos, Calif, Lange Medical Publications, 1978, p 664.

Jones W: Treatment of chorionic tumors. *Clin Obstet Gynecol* 18:247, 1975.

Kim-Farley RJ, Cates W, Ory HW, et al: Febrile abortion and the IUD. *Contraception* 18:561, 1978.

Kitchen JD, Wein RM, Nunley WC, et al: Ectopic pregnancy: Current clinical trends. *Am J Obstet Gynecol* 134:870, 1979.

Knab DR: Abruptio placenta—an assessment of the time and method of delivery. *Obstet Gynecol* 52:625, 1978.

Kohorn EI: Gestational trophoblastic disease: Diagnosis and management. *Contemp Obstet Gynec* 13:165, 1979.

Kurjak A, Barsic B: Changes of placental site diagnosed by repeated ultrasonic examination. *Acta Obstet Gynecol Scand* 56:161, 1977.

Lauritsen JG: Aetiology of spontaneous abortion. *Acta Obstet Gynecol Scand* 52:1, 1976.

Lindemann E: Symptomatology and management of acute grief, in Parad HJ (ed): *Crisis Intervention: Selected Readings.* New York, Family Service Association of America, 1971, p 7.

Moro R: *Death, Grief and Widowhood: Experiences in Pain and Growth.* Berkeley, Calif, Parallax Press, 1979, p 3.

Naeye RL: Placenta previa: Predisposing factors and effects on the fetus and surviving infants. *Obstet Gynecol* 52:521, 1978.

Niswander K: *Obstetrics: Essentials of Clinical Practice,* ed 1. Boston, Little, Brown and Company, 1976, pp 181, 199, 204, 443–450, 484.

Page EW, Villee CA, Villee DB: *Human Reproduction,* ed 2. Philadelphia, WB Saunders Company, 1976, pp 214–220.

Poland BJ, Miller JR, Jones DC, et al: Reproductive counseling in patients who have had spontaneous abortion. *Am J Obstet Gynecol* 127:68, 1977.

Pritchard JA, MacDonald PC: *Williams Obstetrics,* ed 15. New York, Appleton-Century-Crofts, 1976, pp 406, 416, 431, 453-457, 483.

Sand H: Ultrasonic diagnosis of placenta previa. *Acta Obstet Gynecol Scand* 56:109, 1977.

Sher G: A rational basis for the management of abruptio placenta. *J Reprod Med* 21:123, 1978.

Taber BZ: *Manual of Gynecologic and Obstetric Emergencies,* ed 1. Philadelphia, Saunders Company, 1979, p. 502.

Wald N, Barder S, Cuckle H, et al: Fetal loss after amniocentesis, letter. *Lancet* 2:1093, 1978.

Wexler P, Gottesfeld KR: Early diagnosis of placenta previa. *Obstet Gynecol* 54:231, 1979.

Yaffe H, Navot D, Laufer N: Pitfalls in early detection of ectopic pregnancy, letter. *Lancet* 1:277, 1979.

# 3
# Hypertensive Disorders

Women who are normotensive before pregnancy may have hypertension induced by the pregnant state. Those who are hypertensive before pregnancy may have their hypertension aggravated by gestation. Clinical concern about hypertension in pregnancy is based on the fact that this condition contributes significantly to fetal risk and perinatal morbidity and mortality.

The evaluation of elevated blood pressure in pregnancy is difficult, and differential diagnosis of the hypertensive disorder may only be possible in retrospect. Until recently, even the terminology used in describing hypertension during pregnancy was arbitrary, confusing, and varied from source to source. Since by far the most common causes of persistently elevated blood pressure during pregnancy are essential hypertension and pregnancy-induced hypertension, these conditions are the major focus of this chapter.

## PREGNANCY-INDUCED HYPERTENSION (PRE-ECLAMPSIA)

### Definition

Pregnancy-induced hypertension or pre-eclampsia is the development of significant hypertension, proteinuria, and nondependent edema after the twentieth week of pregnancy. The majority of cases occur after the thirty-second week of pregnancy. In cases of hydatidiform mole, pre-eclampsia usually occurs before the twenty-fourth week, and this early onset is almost diagnostic of molar pregnancy.

Cases of pregnancy-induced hypertension may be divided on the basis of signs and symptoms into classifications of mild and severe preeclampsia. Eclampsia is pre-eclampsia with the addition of one or more tonic-clonic convulsions. The classification is a continuum of severity, and the disease is often progressive. Pre-eclampsia occurs in approximately 5% of all pregnancies in the United States; 5% of pre-eclamptic patients become eclamptic.

There is lack of general agreement about the specific bodily changes caused by pregnancy-induced hypertension. Many complex pathophysiologic alterations are attributed to this disease. The change basic to pre-eclampsia–eclampsia is intermittent vasospasm. Hypoxia, secondary to vasospasm, occurs in many organs and presumably accounts for the changes in organ and system function observed. Some of the changes often seen or inferred in pre-eclampsia–eclampsia are:

- Reduced placental function
- Decreased intravascular volume
- Reduction of kidney function and glomerular filtration with damage to the glomerular capillary endothelium resulting in proteinuria and, perhaps, sodium retention
- Increase in response to circulating vasopressor substances
- Hemoconcentration
- Disseminated intravascular coagulation (DIC) (in some severe cases)
- Ischemic and hemorrhagic lesions in the brain, heart, liver, and lungs (found at autopsy of eclamptic women)

## Etiology

Although pregnancy-induced hypertension has been intensively studied for decades and numerous causative theories have been expounded and discarded, the etiology of this disease is still unknown. Factors known to be associated with an increased incidence of pre-eclampsia are:

- Parity: It occurs almost exclusively in primigravidas, especially those under 17 and over 35 years of age
- Lower socioeconomic grouping
- Family history of pre-eclampsia
- Hydatidiform mole
- Multiple pregnancy
- Vascular abnormalities: It occurs more often in women with essential hypertension, renal diseases, and diabetes mellitus

- Fetal hydrops
- Severe malnutrition

## Clinical Features
(See also Table 1.)

### Symptoms

- Mild pre-eclampsia

    Usually no symptoms

    May report sudden tightness of rings or swelling of face or hands
- Severe pre-eclampsia

    May report increased swelling of face and hands

    May have severe headache

    May complain of visual disturbances such as blurring of vision, "spots before eyes," or "silver lights" (Occasionally, blindness occurs due to retinal detachment.)

    May have epigastric pain and/or nausea and vomiting (usually develops before convulsions)
- Eclampsia

    Report of loss of consciousness (seizure or "fit" described by family), followed by

    Drowsiness, semistupor, or coma

### Signs

- Mild pre-eclampsia

    Blood pressure readings of 140/90 mmHg (or a rise from previous readings of 30 mmHg systolic or 15 mmHg diastolic) occur on two occasions at least six hours apart. (For obese women, use of a thigh cuff is necessary for an accurate reading.)

    Significant proteinuria (more than 0.3 g/l 24 hr or 1–2+ on qualitative examination) is present.

    Sudden, excessive (more than 2 lb/week or 6 lb/month) weight gain may be present even before the development of edema. Weight gain from dietary causes may be difficult to distinguish from that due to fluid retention.

    Generalized edema may be observed.

    Some degree of hyperreflexia may be observed, but is more commonly present in the more severe classifications.

Table 1
Symptomatology of Hypertension

| | Pre-eclampsia[a] | Severe Pre-eclampsia[a] | Eclampsia[a] |
|---|---|---|---|
| Hypertension | + | ++ → 160/110 at bed rest | +++Systolic +60 |
| Systolic pressure +30 | | | Diastolic +30 |
| Diastolic pressure +15 | | | |
| Manifest on two occasions six hours apart | | | |
| Weight gain | + | ++ → 5 kg (11 lb) per week | +++ → 30 kg (66 lb) |
| > 1 kg (2.2 lb)/wk | | | |
| > 2.5 kg (5.5 lb)/mo | | | |
| Common first sign | | | |
| Edema | | | |
| Generalized, orbital, fingers pitting over sacrum, shins (pretibial) | + | ++ | +++ Rapidly massive |
| Pulmonary congestion (terminal) | 0 | 0 | + |
| Proteinuria | + | 5 g or more in 24 hours | +++ |
| 24-hour collection: 300 g/liter | | | |
| Random samples: 1 g/liter (1 to 2) in two or more specimens obtained six hours apart by the clean-catch or catheter method | | | |
| Oliguria: 500 ml or less in 24 hours | + | + | +++ |
| Anuria | 0 | + | + |
| Retinal changes: arteriolar spasm, ischemia, edema; rarely—retinal detachment | + | ++ | ++ |
| Hyperreflexia: cerebral dysrhythmia | 0 | + | ++ |
| Headache: frontal or occipital, constant | 0 → + | ++ | ++ |
| Epigastric pain | 0 | + | ++ |
| Visual disturbance: double, blurred vision | 0 | + | ++ |

| | | |
|---|---|---|
| Convulsions | | |
| Stimulation of motor areas of brain (vasospasm → cerebral ischemia stimuli); epigastric pain or tightening in chest may be premonitory symptom—person is amnesic regarding episode | 0 | + |
| Coma: may result from edema, hypoxia, or biochemical alterations of CNS | 0 | + |
| Pulse: usually strong, bounding | 0 | + |
| Respirations: rapid stertorous during coma → respiratory alkalosis | 0 | + |
| Temperature | 0 | + |
| 38.3° C (101° F) in one-third of patients | | |
| 39.4° C (103° F) serious prognostic sign | | |
| Labor: spontaneous labor not hastened; therefore, elective delivery required (*Exception*: Labor may begin shortly after convulsions start and may be very rapid.) | + | + → +++ |
| Cyanosis, tachycardia, hypotension—terminal stage | 0 | + |
| DIC | | |

[a] Pre-eclampsia: hypertension plus edema and/or proteinuria after twentieth week.
Severe pre-eclampsia: increase in cardinal signs plus headache, epigastric pain, marked visual disturbances, or hyperreflexia.
Eclampsia: pre-eclampsia plus convulsions or come.

SOURCE: Reprinted by permission from Jensen M, Bobak I.: *Handbook of Maternity Care: A Guide for Nursing Practice.* St. Louis, The C.V. Mosby, Company, 1980.

- Severe pre-eclampsia

    Blood pressure readings of 160/110 mmHg (or a rise of 60 mmHg systolic or 30 mmHg diastolic) occur on two occasions at least six hours apart.

    Proteinuria of more than 5 g/24 hr or 3-4+ on qualitative examination is present.

    Urinary output may be less than 500 ml/24 hr.

    Cyanosis or pulmonary edema may be present.

- Eclampsia

    Tonic-clonic convulsions occur.

    Postconvulsive coma ensues for varying lengths of time.

    Respirations, postconvulsion, are rapid, and cyanosis may be observed.

    Urinary output is usually diminished and may be suppressed.

## Differential Diagnosis

- Chronic hypertensive vascular disease may be confused with pre-eclampsia. This is likely to occur if the patient is first seen after the twentieth week of pregnancy or if the normal blood pressure drop of 10-15 mmHg in midpregnancy masks an underlying hypertension. An underlying vascular or renal disease should be suspected when multiparous women develop signs and symptoms of pre-eclampsia. Pre-eclampsia superimposed on chronic hypertensive vascular disease produces a grave prognosis for mother and baby. Chronic hypertension persists beyond three months post partum, unlike pre-eclampsia in which blood pressure readings are usually normal within six weeks after delivery.
- Chronic renal disease may present signs similar to those of pre-eclampsia. A history of repeated urinary tract infections and/or persistent or recurrent infections of the urinary system during pregnancy may help to differentiate hypertension due to primary renal disease from pre-eclampsia. However, the diagnosis is often made through renal function studies.
- Transient pregnancy hypertension occurs in successive pregnancies with normal interpregnancy blood pressure readings. Some authorities think that this condition occurs in women who are destined to develop essential hypertension in later life. In general, this condition is not associated with significant proteinuria.
- Endocrine disorders or connective tissue disease such as pheochromocytoma and lupus erythematosis may produce signs and symptoms similar to those of pre-eclampsia.

- Coarctation of the aorta may be ruled out by checking for bilateral femoral pulses.

## Diagnostic Studies as Clinically Indicated

- 24-Hour urine collection for protein or qualitative protein examination of urine.
- Hematocrit: Hemoconcentration is common in severe pre-eclampsia–eclampsia.
- Uric acid level determinations: Elevated levels may occur, especially in severe pre-eclampsia–eclampsia.
- Hematologic, coagulation, hepatic, and renal function tests: Baseline studies reveal progression and severity of condition, but are not, in themselves, diagnostic.

## Management and Treatment as Clinically Indicated

- Physician consultation is required in all cases of suspected pre-eclampsia.
- In cases of blood pressure levels less than 135/85 mmHg and absence of significant proteinuria, bed rest at home may be tried. The patient should be seen twice a week for blood pressure and urine examination. The regimen of diuretics and sodium restriction often used in the past for treatment of pre-eclampsia is now considered to be of no benefit and potentially dangerous.
- Progression of the condition with an increase in blood pressure and/or significant proteinuria mandates hospitalization. In-hospital evaluation and management may include:

  Blood pressure readings every four hours

  Weight every other day

  Daily urine screening for protein

  Periodic creatinine clearance determination to check kidney function

  Observation and questioning for development of headaches, increased edema, visual disturbances, and epigastric pain

  Frequent evaluation for intrauterine growth (clinical measurement and/or serial sonograms)

  Serial urinary or blood estriol level determinations and/or nonstress tests to evaluate fetal well-being

  Bed rest with or without bathroom privileges

Mild sedation (usually phenobarbital, 60 mg po tid)

Conservative management until spontaneous onset of labor or conditions conducive to induction, followed by careful monitoring in labor with liberal recourse to cesarean-section delivery if complications arise

- More severe or progressive cases of pre-eclampsia necessitate anticonvulsive, possibly antihypertensive, therapy and prompt delivery.

  Magnesium sulfate ($MgSO_4$) is the most commonly used anticonvulsant drug. After an initial loading dose of $MgSO_4$, both IV and IM, therapy is continued either by IM injections every four hours or continuous IV drip until 24 hours after delivery.

  Antihypertensive medication (usually hydralazine) is generally begun in cases with signs of acute renal failure and/or marked elevations in blood pressure.

  In cases where the lecithin/spingomyelin ratio of amniotic fluid is greater than 2.0 (indicating fetal lung maturity) or when pre-eclampsia is compromising fetal well-being, an attempt is made to induce labor. If the induction attempt is not successful or if complications arise, the patient is delivered by cesarean section.

  Postpartum, the hypertension generally improves rapidly. However, since eclampsia may develop up to 24 hours after delivery, the patient is closely observed, and anticonvulsant therapy is continued for this period.

  Postdischarge check of the blood pressure is done two weeks after delivery.

- In patients who develop the convulsions of eclampsia, the maternal and fetal mortality and morbidity are greatly increased. The treatment for eclampsia may include:

  $MgSO_4$, IM and IV, to control and prevent convulsive activity

  Hydralazine or other antihypertensive drugs as needed to lower blood pressure (over 110 mmHg diastolic)

  Diuretics in cases of pulmonary congestion

  Medication as necessary to control agitation after convulsions

  Measures to correct water or electrolyte imbalance by IV infusion

  Hourly monitoring of urinary output through in-dwelling catheter

  Bed rest with side rails up in a darkened room with measures to prevent injury during convulsion

  Laboratory determination of clotting functions, hematocrit, platelet and leukocyte counts, plasma electrolytes, SMA 12, creatine clearance, total urinary protein, and serum creatinine levels

  Delivery by induction (preferred) or by cesarean section (if induction fails or complications arise) after control of convulsions and patient's return to consciousness

Postpartum treatment as outlined above

## Complications

- Maternal
    Retinal detachment
    Cerebral vascular accident
    Renal cortical necrosis
    DIC
    Placental abruption
    Cardiorespiratory failure
    Aspiration pneumonia
    Death (in the United States 2-5% of the patients with eclampsia die; mortality is rare with pre-eclampsia.)
- Fetal
    Prematurity
    Small for gestational age syndrome
    Perinatal mortality and morbidity (20-50% mortality with maternal eclampsia)

## Patient Teaching

- All pregnant women should be taught the symptomatology of pre-eclampsia and the importance of prompt reporting of possible symptoms. Additionally, since an inadequate diet may be a predisposing factor in development of the disease, nutritional counseling must be provided. Education on the importance of adequate prenatal care is also important in the prevention and early detection of pre-eclampsia.
- In cases requiring bed rest at home, the patient and her family should be informed of:
    The importance of adhering to the instruction for bed rest on the left side even though she feels well
    The possibility of progression of the condition with need for hospitalization

## 68     PROBLEMS IN AMBULATORY OBSTETRICS AND GYNECOLOGY

  Symptoms that might indicate increasing severity

  The necessity for frequent blood pressure and urine checks (The woman may need help in finding adequate support systems to permit bed rest, especially if other children are involved.)

- The patient and her family need the opportunity to discuss their concerns about maternal and fetal welfare.
- In cases requiring hospitalization, the woman should be advised of the probable course of treatment and should be kept informed of her progress and the condition of her baby.
- Emotional support and factual reassurance for the woman and family is essential in helping them to cope with this crisis situation.
- Referral to a social worker is often necessary because of the enormous financial burden imposed by extended prenatal hospitalization.
- In the postpartum period, opportunity for discussion of the disease and its treatment should be provided to clear up any misconceptions or fears about future childbearing. (Unless an underlying vascular or renal condition is present, recurrence of pre-eclampsia in subsequent pregnancies is very rare.)
- In cases that become severe or progress to eclampsia, help may be needed to aid the grief process for a fetal demise or to adjust to the birth of a premature and/or small for gestational age infant.
- If the blood pressure has returned to normal by six weeks postpartum, prescription of oral contraception is not contraindicated.

## ESSENTIAL HYPERTENSION

### Definition

Essential or primary hypertension is the presence of chronically elevated blood pressure (over 140/90 mmHg) without an identifiable cause for such elevation (such as renal disease, coarctation of the aorta, pheochromocytoma, lupus erythematosis, or primary aldosteronism). Essential hypertension is the most common type of chronic hypertensive disorder in women of childbearing age, accounting for approximately 85% of such cases. It also accounts for about one-third of all cases of hypertension during pregnancy. The condition varies widely in severity, ranging from blood pressure levels only slightly above normal to markedly elevated readings accompanied by hypertensive vascular disease affecting the kidneys, eyes, heart, and brain. Long-standing and/or severe essential hypertension leads to irreversible changes in the vascular bed (hypertensive vascular disease). Untreated primary hypertension is associated with a much higher risk of premature death and morbidity from cardiovascular causes such as stroke, congestive heart failure, and coronary insufficiency.

## Etiology

The etiology of essential hypertension is unknown. Factors associated with primary hypertension are:

- Age: more common in older age groups (over 35 years)
- Family history of hypertension
- Obesity
- Cigarette smoking
- Diabetes mellitus

## General Considerations in Pregnancy

The increase in cardiac output and blood volume accompanied by a decrease in peripheral vascular resistance, which occurs during pregnancy, acts to lower blood pressure readings during early and midpregnancy. The blood pressure gradually increases to prepregnancy levels near term.

The normal early midpregnancy drop may mask the existence of essential hypertension when the woman is first seen at 16-20 weeks of pregnancy and prepregnancy blood pressure levels are unknown. Even levels of 130/80-85 mmHg and above during midpregnancy have been associated with increased fetal perinatal morbidity and mortality. Abruptio placenta, stillbirth, prematurity, and intrauterine growth retardation are more common in women with primary hypertension. The more severe the hypertension, the greater the risk to mother and fetus. Pregnant women with hypertension develop pre-eclampsia earlier and more frequently than the general population.

It is now known that hypertension, although more common with increasing age, can develop in childhood or young adulthood. Since young women often have their blood pressure taken for the first time during pregnancy, the practitioner frequently may have the responsibility for early detection of primary hypertension and for referral for treatment.

## Clinical Features

### Symptoms

- Usually no symptoms
- Dizziness, fatigue, palpitations and/or persistent occipital headaches in severe hyptertension
- Epistaxis, blurring of vision, and hematuria in hypertensive vascular disease

### Signs

- History of blood pressure readings of 140/90 mmHg or greater before pregnancy
- Blood pressure reading of 130/80-85 mmHg or greater in early to midpregnancy
- Blood pressure readings of 140/85-90 mmHg or greater after the twentieth week of pregnancy, unassociated with other signs and symptoms of pre-eclampsia
- Elevated blood pressure level associated with signs and symptoms of pre-eclampsia that does not return to normal level by three months post partum
- Arteriolar narrowing, arteriovenous nicking, and, perhaps, retinal hemorrhage and wooly exudates on funduscopic examination in hypertensive vascular disease
- Enlargement of the left ventricle on x-ray examination in long-standing severe disease

## Differential Diagnosis

- Pre-eclampsia may be difficult to rule out when the patient is first seen in the third trimester and her blood pressure history is unknown. In general, proteinuria (one of the cardinal signs of pre-eclampsia) is not present in essential hypertension except when vascular disease causes renal incompetence. Additionally, hyperuricemia (often present in pre-eclampsia) is not a sign of essential hypertension.
- Secondary hypertension due to an underlying disease process may be difficult to distinguish from primary hypertension. Symptoms of flushing, diaphoresis, and loss of weight are usually also associated with pheochromocytoma. Urine testing for catechol levels will reveal typical elevation. Clinical history may reveal kidney disease or abnormality (another cause of hypertension). Careful examination should be done to rule out coarctation of the aorta, renal artery stenosis, or polycystic kidneys. Laboratory studies for renal function may be indicated.

## Diagnostic Studies as Clinically Indicated

- Careful funduscopic examination
- Electrocardiogram
- Renal function tests

## Management and Treatment as Clinically Indicated

- All patients with hypertension during pregnancy should be referred to a physician for evaluation and management (or comanagement) after a careful history is taken and a thorough physical examination is done.
- There is lack of general agreement about pharmacologic treatment of essential hypertension during pregnancy. However, in general:

    Women under treatment for essential hypertension before pregnancy should be maintained on medication during pregnancy. An alteration of antihypertensive agents may be necessary since some drugs have negative effects on the fetus and/or maternal blood flow (reduction of cardiac output or renal perfusion).

    Alpha-methyldopa (Aldomet) or hydralazine (Apresoline) are often recommended for use during pregnancy since they do not compromise maternal blood flow nor have proven deleterious fetal effects. Aldomet is the preferred drug.

    The initiation of treatment with thiazide diuretics during pregnancy is controversial. These diuretics, although important in the control of hypertension, cause a transient (two-week) decrease in cardiac output and plasma volume, which may be detrimental to fetal well-being. Women taking thiazides before conception may continue to take them during pregnancy. If these diuretics are to be used in pregnancy, they should be started in early to midpregnancy (before 20 weeks). Potassium supplementation is necessary to prevent hypokalemia from use of thiazides. Hyponatremia may also occur in pregnant women taking thiazide diuretics. Therefore, extreme sodium restriction is not advisable for these patients.

    Since pharmacologic treatment of hypertension during pregnancy has not been proven to improve fetal outcome, indications for initiation of treatment are primarily maternal. Maternal mortality and morbidity are not increased in cases of mild hypertension (diastolic levels under 105 mmHg before pregnancy or in the third trimester; levels under 95 mmHg in first two trimesters). More severe levels of hypertension are usually treated pharmacologically. See the above discussion for preferred agents.

- The patient is urged to rest in bed as frequently as possible on the left side

to increase renal and uterine perfusion. Bed rest is advised (two to three hours per day) after the twenty-eighth week of pregnancy.
- Evaluation of a patient's social situation, dietary patterns, understanding of her condition, and compliance with treatment measures is fundamental to adequate care.
- The patient should be seen frequently (every two weeks from 26–30 weeks' gestation, then every week until delivery) for clinical evaluation of fetal growth and for observation for signs and symptoms of developing pre-eclampsia.
- Extreme sodium restriction during pregnancy is not usually necessary or advisable. A well-balanced, high-protein, "no-added-salt" diet is advised.
- In cases of severe and/or long-standing essential hypertension with vascular disease, monitoring of urinary creatinine levels, and funduscopic examinations aid in the assessment of the maternal condition.
- Fetal well-being may be monitored through serial sonography for total intrauterine volume, biparietal diameters, and breathing movements. Additionally, measurement of blood or urinary estriol levels and placental lactogen levels, nonstress tests, oxytocin challenge tests, and amniocentesis for determination of lung maturity aid in fetal evaluation. The availability of testing techniques determines the choice of monitoring studies. The majority of the tests are begun at 32–34 weeks' gestation in selected cases.
- The spontaneous onset of labor may be awaited if there are no signs of fetal growth retardation or placental insufficiency.
- Hospitalization in the third trimester may be indicated in severe hypertension and/or suspected fetal growth retardation for control of blood pressure, assessment of fetal well-being, and observation for superimposed pre-eclampsia. Delivery at fetal lung maturity may be necessary in cases where the extrauterine environment is judged to be preferable to hostile intrauterine surroundings.
- Development of superimposed pre-eclampsia produces a grave fetal prognosis with increased maternal risk. Maternal blood pressure readings are often disastrously high. Prompt delivery is usually indicated for both maternal and fetal indications.

## Complications

- Stroke, congestive heart failure, coronary insufficiency may result from severe hypertension or hypertensive vascular disease.
- Superimposed pre-eclampsia occurs in about 25–30% of the patients with essential hypertension compared with 1.5–12% in the general population.

- Stillbirths are increased two to four and one-half times the normal rate in severe hypertension.
- Prematurity is increased three to five times over normal occurrence in severe hypertension.
- Intrauterine growth retardation occurs at twice the normal rate with high blood pressure levels.

## Patient Teaching

- Women with mild or controllable hypertension should be reassured that their chances for a normal course of pregnancy and a healthy baby are good.
- Patients must be counseled about the need for lifeling evaluation and treatment of essential hypertension. Since this disease is usually asymptomatic, many patients have difficulty in regarding their condition as potentially serious.
- Patients requiring antihypertensive medication should be taught the possible side effects of therapeutic agents:

    Alpha-methyldopa (Aldomet): lethargy, depression, positive Coombs test, and, rarely, hemolytic anemia

    Hydralazine (Apresoline): flushing, headache, palpitations, tachycardia, nausea, diarrhea, and, rarely, angina pectoris, lupuslike syndrome

    Thiazide diuretics (Hydrochlorothiazide, chlorothiazide, etc): electrolyte depletion, hyperglycemia, and, rarely, gout, thrombocytopenia, hemorrhagic pancreatitis
- The woman and her family should be appraised of maternal and fetal condition at each visit. Indicated laboratory testing should be explained thoroughly, and the patient should be contacted promptly about the results.
- For cases in which hospitalization is necessary, the woman and family should be informed about the purpose of various test procedures and how decisions will be made about possible induction of labor.
- Facilitation of the grief and grieving process of the patient and family is necessary in cases of fetal demise, prematurity, or growth retardation.

## References

Burrow GN, Ferris TF (eds): *Medical Complications During Pregnancy* ed 1. Philadelphia, WB Saunders Company, 1975, pp 63–68.

DeAlvarez RR: Preeclampsia-eclampsia and renal disease in pregnancy. *Clin Obstet Gynecol* 21:881, 1978.

Dukes DC: Hypertension in pregnancy. *Practitioner* 220:285, 1978.

Ferris TF: Toxemia and hypertension, in Burrow GN, Ferris TF (eds): *Medical Complications During Pregnancy.* Philadelphia, WB Saunders Company, 1975, p 88.

Gant NF, Worley RJ, Cunningham FG, et al: Clinical management of pregnancy-induced hypertension. *Clin Obstet Gynecol* 21:397, 1978.

Jagger PI, Braunwald E: Hypertensive vascular disease, in Thron GW, Adam RD, Braunwald E, et al (eds): *Harrison's Principles of Internal Medicine.* New York, McGraw-Hill Book Company, 1977, p 1307.

Jensen MD, Benson RC, Bobak IM: *Maternity Care – The Nurse and the Family,* ed 1. Saint Louis, CV Mosby Company, 1977, pp 247–253.

Kelley JV: Drugs used in the management of toxemia of pregnancy. *Clin Obstet Gynec* 20:395, 1977.

Monroe PR: Hypertension and pregnancy. *Primary Care* 4:31, 1977.

Perkins RP: The conservative management of toxemia. *Obstet Gynecol* 49:498, 1977.

Pritchard JA, Cunningham FG, Mason RA: Coagulation changes in preeclampsia: their frequency and pathogenesis. *Am J Obstet Gynecol* 124:855, 1976.

Pritchard JA, MacDonald PC: *Williams Obstetrics,* ed 15. New York, Appleton-Century-Crofts, 1976, pp 551–579.

Roberts JM: When the hypertensive patient becomes pregnant. *Contemp Obstet Gynec* 13:47–55, 1979.

Roberts JM, Perloff DL: Hypertension and the obstetrician-gynecologist. *Am J Obstet Gynecol* 127:316, 1977.

Welt SI, Crenshaw MC: Concurrent hypertension and pregnancy. *Clin Obstet Gynecol* 21:619, 1978.

# 4
# Common Anemias

Anemia is one of the most frequently encountered complications of pregnancy, occurring in as many as 50-60% of pregnant women in certain populations. Many types of anemia are found in pregnant women, and most of the severe and/or congenital anemias necessitate management by a hematologic/obstetric team. However, the anemia most frequently diagnosed and managed by the practitioner is also the anemia most common in pregnancy—iron-deficiency anemia. This chapter deals primarily with this anemia as well as with another of the microcytic, hypochromic anemias (beta-thalessemia minor) that is often mistaken for the iron-deficiency type.

## IRON-DEFICIENCY ANEMIA

### Definition

Anemia in pregnancy is defined as a hemoglobin level of less than 10.0 g/dl or a hematocrit level of less than 30-31%. The definition of anemia during pregnancy varies, depending on the practitioner, the institution, and the population being served. (The definition of anemia in the nonpregnant woman is a hemoglobin level of less than 12.0 g/dl.) The difference in values is due to the greater expansion of plasma volume compared with the increase in red blood cell volume which occurs in pregnancy. The 50% expansion of plasma volume begins early in pregnancy, reaches a peak at 30-34 weeks, and plateaus thereafter. The usual

17-25% increase in RBC volume begins later and continues steadily until delivery. This results in a normal decrease in hemoglobin and hematocrit levels, which generally reach their lowest point during the second trimester and then stabilize or even slightly increase near term.) Iron-deficiency anemia occurs when the amount of iron required by pregnancy exceeds that which can be provided by the maternal iron stores plus the absorption of iron from the maternal GI tract.

## Etiology

It is estimated that 15-20% of the women of childbearing age have inadequate iron stores, and that 8-10% of these women have iron-deficiency anemia. Many women consume less iron than is needed to replace iron lost during menses and, possibly, during prior pregnancies. The iron demand of a singleton pregnancy (for formation of fetal RBCs, the placenta, and expansion of maternal RBC volume) is about 800 mg. This is more than many women (20-60%) can supply from their body iron stores plus dietary iron absorption. Therefore, iron-deficiency anemia develops, unless iron supplementation is provided. Classically, iron deficiency causes the release of RBCs that are small (microcytic) and, later, are pale from lack of hemoglobin (hypochromic). However, in pregnancy-induced iron-deficiency anemia of short duration, these morphologic changes may not be seen. Factors that add to the likelihood of iron-deficiency anemia are:

- Previous closely spaced pregnancies (can exhaust maternal iron stores)
- Presence of more than one fetus (increases iron requirements)
- Failure to take prescribed iron supplementation
- Poor dietary intake of iron
- Pica (may inhibit iron absorption or deter adequate nutrition)
- Nausea and vomiting

## Clinical Features

### Symptoms

- Usually no symptoms
- Possible fatigue, dizziness, headache, palpitations, mouth soreness

*Signs*

- Usually no signs
- Possible pallor, pale conjunctiva, tachycardia

## Differential Diagnosis

- Beta-thalassemia minor accounts for about 8% of microcytic, hypochromic anemias seen in pregnancy (see the section on beta-thalassemia minor).
- Alpha-thalassemia (see section on beta-thalassemia minor)
- Sideroblastic anemia may be congenital (more common in males) or acquired secondary to chronic illness or ingestion of drugs or toxins (such as antineoplastic agents, chloramphenicol, antitubercular drugs, lead, ethanol). Sideroblastic anemia can usually be ruled out by a negative clinical picture. If bone marrow studies are necessary, "ringed" marrow sideoblasts are found in this anemia.
- Chronic disease may cause hypochromic, microcytic anemia. A history of chronic infection (chronic salpingitis, chronic pyelonephritis, etc) chronic inflammation (rheumatoid arthritis, lupus, etc), and malignancy can usually be elicited. Additionally, laboratory studies reveal normal to increased serum iron levels, decreased iron-binding capacity, and a saturation percentage over 16%.

## Diagnostic Studies as Clinically Indicated

- A complete blood count with a differential count reveals normal WBC, differential, and platelet counts. Hemoglobin level is below 10 g/dl, mean corpuscular volume (MCV) is less than 80 fl (microcytosis), mean corpuscular hemoglobin is less than 28 pg/cell (hypochromia), and mean corpuscular hemoglobin concentration is less than 30 g/dl. (Microcytosis and hypochromia may not be present in iron-deficiency anemia developing during pregnancy).
- Peripheral smear for blood morphology detects the presence of small, pale RBCs, 1-3+ anisocytosis (variability in cell sizes), and 1-3+ poikilocytosis (variability in cell shapes).
- Serum iron level and total iron binding capacity (TIBC) determinations show low serum iron level (below 40 $\mu$g/ml) and an increased TIBC (over 400 $\mu$g/ml) with the serum iron/TIBC ratio of less than 16%. (Serum iron studies should be done after the patient has been off iron medication for at least 24 hours.)

**78** PROBLEMS IN AMBULATORY OBSTETRICS AND GYNECOLOGY

- Reticulocyte count is normal to slightly decreased.
- Bone marrow biopsy (usually not necessary) reveals no demonstrable iron in the marrow.
- Other studies

    If serum iron, TIBC levels, and serum iron/TIBC ratio are normal, hemoglobin electrophoresis with quantitative $A_2$ level should be obtained to check for elevation of hemoglobin $A_2$ indicating beta-thalassemia minor (more common in those of Mediterranean, central African, and Asian ancestry).

    Sickle cell screening should be done as part of the initial lab workup of all black patients.

    Screening for G6PD enzyme deficiency, which can cause hemolytic anemia on ingestion of sulfa drugs, antimalarials, nitrofurantoin, and fava beans, is often done on all patients of Mediterranean or central African origin.

## Management and Treatment as Clinically Indicated

- The patient is assumed to have iron-deficiency anemia when:

    Hemoglobin level is below 10g/dl.

    Microcytosis and hypochromia exist (possibly).

    Serum iron/TIBC ratio is less than 15%.

    There is no history of bleeding, chronic illness, persistent anemia in the patient or family members.

    Hemoglobin electrophoresis with quantitative $A_2$ (when indicated) is normal.

    G6PD screening test results (when indicated) are negative.

- Treatment, in most cases, consists of therapeutic levels of oral iron supplementation (200 mg/day) with one of the following preparations:

    Ferrous sulfate: one 325-mg tablet (contains 60–65 mg of elemental iron) three times a day

    Ferrous gluconate: two 325-mg tablets (each contains 37–39 mg of iron) three times a day

    Ferrous fumarate: one 325-mg tablet (contains 107 mg of iron) twice a day

    (Treatment should be continued for three to six months after correction of anemia to allow for replenishment of maternal stores.)

- If the woman is unable to swallow tablets, liquid iron preparations may be prescribed.

- Hemoglobin and hematocrit levels should rise in response to iron therapy in two to three weeks.
- If the anemia is moderate to severe, reticulocytosis (reticulocyte levels of 2-3%) should occur in 7-10 days.
- If minimal or no response is noted after four weeks of therapy (in a patient compliant with instructions), the anemia should be reevaluated. (In patients with beta-thalassemia minor *and* iron-deficiency anemia, the elevation of $A_2$ characteristic of this thalassemia may be noted only on a hemoglobin electrophoresis repeated after iron therapy.)
- In cases in which the anemia is severe, the patient is not compliant with therapy, and/or rapid replacement of iron is desired, parenteral (IM or IV) injection of iron (Imferon) is indicated. Instructions for dosage and administration are included in package inserts.

## Complications

- Possible hemorrhage, hypovolemia, and shock at time of delivery
- Effects of chronic maternal anemia on the fetus are unknown. It is difficult to separate the effects of severe maternal anemia from the fetal effects of maternal malnutrition.

## Patient Teaching

- Patients with iron-deficiency anemia should be asked to provide a three-day diet history on which to base nutritional counseling. The following questions should be kept in mind when counseling the patient:

    Is pica present? (Excessive ice ingestion or intake of starch, clay, or dirt often accompanies anemia. Intake of certain clays may inhibit iron absorption. Intake of other nonfood items may decrease sensations of hunger and lead to a diet deficient in all nutrients.)

    Who buys the food and does the cooking? (Other members of the household may need instruction as well as the pregnant woman.)

    Are there financial restrictions preventing adequate diet? (Referral to social services for financial assistance or supplementary foods may be necessary.)

    Are there cultural attitudes toward nutrition during pregnancy and lactation affecting the diet?

    What are the woman's attitudes toward weight gain in pregnancy?

    Does the woman follow a special diet (such as vegetarian, macrobiotic)?

What cooking facilities does the woman have access to?

What are the patient's food likes and dislikes?

- Patients should be provided with dietary counseling on an ongoing basis with special attention given to teaching about food sources high in iron:

    The iron in meat is absorbed more efficiently than iron from inorganic sources. Organ meats are especially high in iron content.

    Some iron-fortified cereals provide 18-20 mg of iron per serving.

    Nongreen beans are good sources of iron.

    Fair sources of iron are egg yolk, liverwurst, dark green leafy vegetables, dried fruits (prunes, raisins, dates), and most iron-fortified breads and cereals.

- Anemic women should be told the importance of following orders for prescribed supplementation even though they feel well.
- In cases of moderate to severe anemia, the woman should be advised to take a vitamin C supplement (250-500 mg) with the iron tablet to enhance absorption of iron.
- If the woman experiences GI upset due to iron ingestion, she should be advised to take iron tablets with meals (although absorption is better when the stomach is empty).
- The woman should be informed of possible side effects to iron supplementation:

    GI upset (see above).

    Constipation (Advise high-fiber diet, adequate water and fruit intake, exercise. Stool softeners may be prescribed when constipation persists.)

    Black stools

- The woman should be cautioned to keep iron tablets out of the reach of children since each year many children ingest toxic amounts of prescription drugs. The colorful iron tablets, which resemble candy, are especially tempting to children.

## BETA-THALASSEMIA MINOR

### Definition

The thalassemia disorders are a group of hereditary hemoglobinopathies in which there is reduced or absent production of one or more of the globin chains of hemoglobin causing an impairment in hemoglobin synthesis. The disorders vary widely in severity from lifelong mild anemia to a condition incompatible with extrauterine life. This section will deal with heterozygous beta-thalassemia (beta-thalassemia minor), which usually causes a mild to moderate microcytic, hypochromic anemia often misdiagnosed as iron-deficiency anemia during pregnancy.

In beta-thalassemia minor, the beta-globin chain is inadequately represented, affecting the synthesis of hemoglobin (Hgb) A, which comprises about 96% of normal adult hemoglobin. However, in this heterozygous condition, Hgb A is produced at up to 75% of the normal levels. There is an increase in the level of Hgb $A_2$ and over 50% of the cases also show an elevation of Hgb F levels.

## Etiology

Beta-thalassemia minor is a genetically determined disorder. The incidence is higher in persons of Mediterranean, central African and Asian extraction (although it is found worldwide). The heterozygous state is associated with an increased resistance to malaria, which may account for the preferential evolution of thalassemia minor in these areas.

## Clinical Features

### Symptoms

- Usually no symptoms
- Possible fatigue, dizziness, palpitations, mouth soreness

### Signs

- Usually no signs
- Possible pallor, pale conjunctiva, tachycardia, red tongue

## Differential Diagnosis

- Iron-deficiency anemia accounts for 90-92% of all microcytic hypochromic anemias seen in pregnancy. In contrast to beta-thalassemia minor, iron-deficiency anemia is characterized by low serum iron levels, elevated iron-binding capacity, and normal levels of Hgb $A_2$ on hemoglobin electrophoresis.

- Sideroblastic anemia (see the section on differential diagnosis in the discussion of iron-deficiency anemia)
- Alpha-thalassemia minor may manifest as microcytic, hypochromic anemia. The diagnosis is made by exclusion of other causes of anemia. In alpha-thalassemia minor, hypochromasia, and microcytosis are present, but Hgb $A_2$ levels and serum iron studies are normal.
- Chronic infection, disease, or malignancy (such as salpingitis, chronic pyelonephritis, rheumatoid arthritis, lupus, leukemia) may cause hypochromic, microcytic anemia. However, in these cases, the TIBC is decreased and the levels of Hgb $A_2$ and F are normal.

## Diagnostic Studies as Clinically Indicated

- A complete blood count with a differential count shows normal WBC and differential counts. The hemoglobin level is usually below 10 g/dl. However, beta-thalassemia minor may exist without clinical anemia being present. The mean corpuscular volume (MCV) is less than 80 fl (microcytosis), and the mean corpuscular hemoglobin concentration (MCHC) is usually less than 31.5 g/dl.
- Peripheral blood smear reveals small, pale cells with 1+ variability in cell sizes and shapes. Target cells and basophilic stippling may be present.
- Serum iron level and total iron binding capacity (TIBC) are normal. The serum iron/TIBC ratio is over 16%.
- Hemoglobin electrophoresis (with quantitative $A_2$) shows a Hgb $A_2$ level over 3.5% and a possible elevation of the Hgb F level (in 50% of the cases).

## Management and Treatment as Clinically Indicated

- The management of pregnancy with beta-thalassemia minor is the same as for pregnancies in which no hemoglobinopathy exists.
- The woman is given prenatal genetic counseling and, when possible, the partner is tested for thalassemia trait.

  If the partner is also heterozygous for beta-thalassemia, prenatal fetal diagnosis is now possible. This involves intrauterine aspiration of a fetal blood sample for hemoglobin synthesis studies. This procedure is usually done at 18–20 weeks of gestation. (The chance of conceiving a fetus homozygous with beta-thalassemia is 25% when both parents have the trait).

If analysis reveals homozygous beta-thalassemia in the fetus, the couple must decide whether or not they desire therapeutic abortion. Homozygous beta-thalassemia (thalassemia major or Cooley's anemia) is a condition of severe anemia requiring frequent blood transfusions. Death usually occurs in adolescence or young adulthood.

*Note:* In cases of alpha-thalassemia minor partner evaluation is also performed. When the partner workup reveals microcytosis (MCV less than 80 fl), normal serum iron studies, and normal levels of Hgb $A_2$, intrauterine diagnosis for fetal hemoglobinopathy through amniocentesis is offered. If all four genes for alpha-chains are deleted, the pregnancy will result in a stillborn fetus. If three genes are deleted, the fetus is born with moderately severe hemolytic anemia.

## Complications

- Most studies have not indicated any pregnancy complications related to beta-thalassemia minor.
- The possible fetal complication is the inheritance of homozygous beta-thalassemia (Cooley's anemia).

## Patient Teaching

- The patient with beta-thalassemia minor should be given information about the cause of the condition and reassurance about her own well-being. Arrangements should be made for evaluation of the woman's partner, and the importance of such evaluation should be stressed.
- If the partner evaluation is negative for beta-thalassemia minor, the couple can be reassured that, while the baby may inherit beta-thalassemia minor, there is no risk of bearing a child affected with Cooley's anemia.
- If the partner is also heterozygous for beta-thalassemia, the couple must be informed that the fetus has a 25% chance of having a normal complement of globin genes (no hemoglobinopathy), a 50% chance of having beta-thalassemia minor, and a 25% chance of inheriting beta-thalassemia major (Cooley's anemia). The problems and probable life span usually associated with Cooley's anemia should be explained to the woman and partner. Prenatal diagnosis is offered if the woman is less than 20 weeks pregnant and desires therapeutic abortion in case such diagnosis reveals an affected fetus. The couple should also be informed that a fetal loss rate of about 10% is associated with prenatal diagnosis.

- If the woman chooses to undergo prenatal diagnosis, the amniocentesis procedure and the technique for aspiration and evaluation of fetal blood should be fully explained.
- The woman who is past the twentieth week of pregnancy and whose partner is heterozygous for beta-thalassemia needs encouragement and help in dealing with her fears of bearing an affected child.
- Aid in the grief and grieving process is needed when therapeutic abortion is necessary or when an affected baby is born.
- The couple in which both partners are heterozygous for beta-thalassemia requires genetic counseling about future pregnancies. The risk factors (as described above) are the same for *each* succeeding pregnancy.

## REFERENCES

Alger LS, Golbus MS, Laros RK: Thalassemia and pregnancy: Results of an antenatal screening program. *Am J Obstet Gynecol* 134:662, 1979.

Horowitz JJ, Laros RK: Anemia and pregnancy: A review of the pathophysiology, diagnosis, and treatment. *JCE Ob/Gyn,* Feb 1979, pp. 9–30.

Laros RK: Lecture notes. University of California, San Francisco, 1979.

Lee GR, Wintrobe MM, Bumn HF: Iron deficiency anemia and the sideroblastic anemias, in Thorn GW, Adams RD, Braunwald E, et al (ed): *Harrison's Principles of Internal Medicine,* ed 8. New York, McGraw-Hill Book Company, 1977, p 1652.

McFee JC: Iron metabolism and iron deficiency during pregnancy. *Clin Obstet Gynecol* 22:799, 1979.

Morrison JC: Hemoglobinopathies and pregnancy. *Clin Obstet Gynecol* 22:819, 1979.

Peck TM, Arias F: Hematologic changes associated with pregnancy. *Clin Obstet Gynecol* 22:785, 1979.

Pritchard JA, MacDonald PC: *Williams Obstetrics,* ed 15. New York, Appleton-Century-Crofts, 1976, pp 595, 606.

# 5
# Urinary Tract Infection

For a complete discussion of urinary tract infections the practitioner should refer to Chapter 13. This chapter will cover certain aspects of predisposing factors and treatment in urinary tract infection as they apply to pregnancy as well as asymptomatic bacteriuria.

### General Considerations in Pregnancy

During pregnancy several anatomic and physiologic changes impede the complete and unhindered emptying of the urinary tract, which is the main defense of this system against infection. These changes include:

- Diminished ureteral peristalsis due to hormonal influences on smooth muscle
- Compression of the ureters at the pelvic brim by the growing uterus
- Dextro-rotation of the pregnant uterus, which places mechanical pressure on the right kidney and ureter.

These changes encourage dilatation of the renal pelvises and ureters leading to stasis and increased susceptibility to urinary tract infection. Trauma to the bladder during delivery and routine catheterization before birth are factors predisposing to postpartum infections of the urinary system.

Pyelonephritis occurs in 2% of all pregnancies and is the major cause of prenatal hospitalization. Acute pyelonephritis may be related to increased risks of premature birth and low birthweight with an attendant increase in fetal perinatal morbidity and mortality. Thus, prevention of acute pyelonephritis during pregnancy is of utmost importance. Prompt recognition and adequate treatment of cystitis can help to prevent the ascension of the infection. Most importantly, the incidence of acute pyelonephritis can be reduced by approximately 80% by the appropriate treatment of asymptomatic bacteriuria.

Asymptomatic bacteriuria is the presence of significant bacteriuria without symptoms of a urinary tract infection. In about 50% of the cases the bacteriuria is limited to the bladder, but the remaining half have kidney involvement with the potential for serious renal disease. The incidence of asymptomatic bacteriuria in pregnancy is 2–10%. The incidence is higher in black women (pregnant or nonpregnant) and in women with low hematocrits. Less than 2% of the women with negative urine cultures at the first prenatal visit subsequently develop asymptomatic bacteriuria. However, these women probably account for a large percentage of cases of acute pyelonephritis since their bacteriuria goes untreated. Approximately 25–40% of the women with untreated asymptomatic bacteriuria develop acute pyelonephritis during the course of pregnancy or the puerperium.

## Clinical Features

Signs and symptoms of cystitis and pyelonephritis are outlined in Chapter 13. There are no signs or symptoms associated with asymptomatic bacteriuria.

## Differential Diagnosis

(See also Chap. 13.)

- Pyelonephritis
    Labor
    Appendicitis
    Abruptio placenta
    Postpartum uterine infection
    Cholecystitis
- Cystitis
    Normal frequency and dysuria of pregnancy
    Vaginitis, cervicitis

## Diagnostic Studies as Clinically Indicated

Diagnostic studies for pyelonephritis and cystitis are discussed in Chapter 13. Diagnosis of asymptomatic bacteriuria is based on the culture of more than

$10^5$ colonies of the same bacterial species per milliliter of clean-voided urine on two consecutive occasions.

## Management and Treatment Clinically Indicated

- Infections confined to the lower urinary tract are treated on an outpatient basis during pregnancy. Treatment is initiated in cystitis before return of the culture results since the organisms usually causing both cystitis and asymptomatic bacteriuria are sensitive to treatment with a short (10- to 14-day) course of any of the following:

    Sulfisoxazole (Gantrisin): 1 g four times a day (except in last weeks of pregnancy when sulfonamides may cause or increase jaundice in the newborn)

    Ampicillin: 250 mg four times a day

    Nitrofurantoin (Furadantin): 100 mg three times a day (except in women who have a G6PD deficiency and may develop drug-induced hemolytic anemia)

- After return of the culture results, a change of therapy is instituted if the pathogen is insensitive to the chosen medication.
- Because approximately 20% of cases of asymptomatic bacteriuria recur or are resistant to treatment, follow-up cultures should be obtained after treatment of any lower urinary tract infection. If follow-up culture results are positive, physician consultation is indicated. Sensitivity studies are done and retreatment with the appropriate drug initiated. Resistant or recurring infections may indicate renal involvement and may require suppressive therapy for the duration of the pregnancy.
- Physician referral is indicated for all patients with symptoms suggestive of acute pyelneophritis since hospitalization is necessary until clinical improvement is observed.

    Intravenous ampicillin (1–2 g qid) is given for 48–72 hours or until the temperature is normal. Oral medication is contraindicated since bacteremia may cause partial paralytic ileus with associated drug malabsorption. (A change in medication may be indicated after the sensitivity report is known). Oral ampicillin (500 mg qid for one week, then 250 mg qid for two weeks) is prescribed after the acute phase has passed.

    During hospitalization, the patient is observed for signs of bacterial shock. Intake and output are recorded along with frequent blood pressure readings.

    Since recurrence of pyelonephritis has been reported to be as high as 60–75% in women not maintained on suppressive therapy, antimicrobial treatment is often continued. Nitrofurantoin (50 mg tid) is often the drug of choice. Other practitioners follow the patient's urine culture reports and initiate further treatment only in the presence of bacteriuria.

- Postpartum renal evaluation by intravenous pyelography 6-12 weeks postpartum is indicated in patients who have pyelonephritis or resistant/recurrent lower urinary tract infections. Many of these women have underlying urinary tract abnormalities or evidence of chronic disease.

## Complications

- Bacterial shock may occur in acute pyelonephritis.
- Chronic pyelonephritis may result from repeated acute infections or chronic cystitis.
- Asymptomatic bacteriuria may progress to acute pyelonephritis.
- Premature labor and delivery may be related to acute pyelonephritis.

## Patient Teaching

(See also Chap. 13.)

- Asymptomatic patients with positive urine cultures should be contacted immediately, told of the results, and urged to return for a repeat culture within 48 hours to prevent progression to acute infection.
- Patients with cultures repeatedly contaminated by several organisms even after careful collection explanations may require practitioner supervision to obtain a clean-voided, midstream specimen.
- Patients with asymptomatic bacteriuria or cystitis should be counseled about the importance of treatment to prevent acute pyelonephritis. Many women without this knowledge fail to complete the course of treatment after any bladder symptoms cease. Patients with asymptomatic bacteriuria often do not understand why they should take antibiotics when they do not feel ill.
- Patients with pyelonephritis should be urged to rest in bed on the unaffected side if the condition is unilateral.
- Patients with acute infection need a complete explanation of the treatment and procedures as well as emotional support. Hospitalization during pregnancy is doubly frightening since the woman is very concerned about the condition of her baby as well as her own illness.
- Patients with acute pyelonephritis should be told about the possibility of premature labor after febrile illness and should be urged to report promptly any signs of beginning labor.

- Symptoms of urinary tract infection should be discussed with all pregnant women, especially those with histories of prior infection.

## REFERENCES

Davidson JM, Lindheimer MD: Renal disease in pregnant women. *Clin Obstet Gynecol* 21:411, 1978.

Harding GK, Marrie TJ, Ronald AR, et al: Urinary tract infection localized in women. *JAMA* 240:1174, 1978.

Harris RE: Urinary tract infections during pregnancy. Part 1: asymptomatic bacteriuria. *The Female Patient* 3(11):47-61, 1977.

Harris RE: Urinary tract infections during pregnancy. Part 11: acute infections. *The Female Patient* 3(12):11-15, 1977.

Harris RE, Thomas VL, Underwood JM, et al: A comparison of two indirect methods for localizing the site of a urinary tract infection. *Am J Obstet Gynecol* 131:647, 1978.

Marchant DJ: Alterations in anatomy and function of the urinary tract during pregnancy. *Clin Obstet Gynecol* 21:855, 1978.

Marchant DJ: Urinary tract infections in pregnancy. *Clin Obstet Gynecol* 21:921, 1978.

Naeye RL: Causes of the excessive rates of perinatal mortality and prematurity in pregnancies complicated by maternal urinary tract infections. *New Engl J Med* 300: 819, 1979.

Niswander KR: *Obstetrics—Essentials of Clinical Practice,* ed 1. Boston, Little, Brown and Company, 1976, pp 583-589.

Polk BF: Urinary tract infection during pregnancy. *Clin Obstet Gynecol* 22:285, 1979.

Pritchard JA, MacDonald PC: *Williams Obstetrics,* ed 15. New York, Appleton-Century-Crofts, 1976, pp 583-589.

Riff L: Evaluation and treatment of urinary infection. *Med Clin North Am* 62:1183, 1978.

# 6

# Variations in Uterine Growth Patterns

The practitioner confronted with a pregnancy in which uterine growth seems to be at variance with normal progression is faced with a problem in differential diagnosis that is common in clinical practice and is often crucial to the pregnancy outcome. In the past several years, much research time has been devoted to the classification and etiology of intrauterine growth retardation, the first section in this chapter. However, clinical diagnosis and management of this complication remain difficult and, to a large extent, empiric. The second section deviates somewhat from the format of the remainder of the book in that a clinical sign (uterine size larger than expected for dates) is presented with discussion of several possible causative complications. Although some of the complications leading to a large uterine size have been discussed elsewhere in this book and others may fall into the realm of physician management, reference to this section will be of use to the clinician in differential diagnosis.

## INTRAUTERINE GROWTH RETARDATION

### Definition

The infant who has experienced intrauterine growth retardation (IUGR) is classified as small-for-gestational age (SGA). The SGA fetus is one whose birth-weight is below the tenth percentile of mean weight for gestational age. Therefore, a fetus born at any gestational age (premature, term, postmature) may be classified as growth retarded or SGA if his/her birthweight falls into the lower 10% of birthweights for infants of that gestation.

The two main types of IUGR are:

- Symmetrical growth retardation: The head circumference, body circumference, and length of the fetus are usually all reduced. Symmetric growth retardation may be noted as early as the twentieth week of gestation and is usually associated with decreased potential for normal fetal development.
- Asymmetrical growth retardation: This type usually begins in the third trimester and results from the fetal potential for "brain sparing." In the absence of adequate nutrient transfer for continued normal growth, the fetal brain is provided with nourishment at the expense of the rest of the body, resulting in near normal head circumference and small body circumference. Asymmetric growth retardation is usually associated with a normal potential for fetal growth that is stunted by a condition causing uteroplacental insufficiency.

Intrauterine growth retardation occurs in approximately 5–7% of all pregnancies. The long-term prognosis for the baby depends on the cause of the growth retardation. In general, the growth-retarded fetus is at greater risk in the perinatal period for:

- Intrauterine death
- Anoxia in labor and delivery
- Meconium aspiration
- Hypothermia
- Hypoglycemia
- Hypocalcemia
- Polycythemia and hyperbilirubinemia
- Hemorrhage due to reduced blood coagulation factors

## Etiology

Four major mechanisms that may lead to IUGR are:

- Reduced placental or umbilical blood flow
- Abnormally low levels of nutrients in maternal circulation
- Decreased placental surface area
- Reduced transport of nutrients across the placental membrane

In many cases, the etiology of IUGR is unknown. Fetal, maternal, and environmental conditions known to be associated with IUGR are:

- Maternal hypertension: Severe pre-eclampsia–eclampsia or chronic hyper-

tension are suspected to cause about 40% of cases of asymmetric growth retardation.
- Chronic maternal renal disease
- Long-standing severe maternal diabetes associated with vascular changes
- Postdates pregnancy with placental senescence
- Multiple pregnancies
- Chronic maternal antepartum hemorrhage: Rarely, cases of placenta previa or abruptio placenta may cause IUGR.
- Maternal drug ingestion (aminopterin, heroin, Coumadin, Dilantin, methadone)
- Maternal smoking
- Maternal alcohol ingestion: There is a 10% risk of fetal abnormalities with ingestion of 1-2 ounces of absolute alcohol per day and a 44% risk of fetal abnormalities, including IUGR, in cases of chronic alcoholism.
- Fetal chromosomal abnormalities
- Intrauterine fetal disease (rubella, cytomegalic inclusion disease, syphilis, toxoplasmosis)
- Fetal anomalies: About 10% of the cases of IUGR are associated with an anomalous fetus.
- Severe maternal malnutrition
- Heavy radiation exposure
- High altitude
- Maternal cyanotic heart disease
- Maternal hemoglobinopathy
- Placental anomalies (abnormal cord insertions, hemangiomatous tumors)

## Clinical Features

### Symptoms

- No symptoms
- Symptoms related to various maternal conditions associated with IUGR

### Signs

- History of maternal smoking, alcoholism, drug addiction, hypertension, chronic renal disease, diabetes, cyanotic heart disease, rubella or other viral diseases during pregnancy, or previous pregnancy with IUGR may be noted.

- Signs related to the above conditions may occur.
- In some cases, signs of pre-eclampsia are present (see section on pregnancy-induced hypertension in Chap. 3).
- Inadequate maternal weight gain (less than 10 pounds in the third trimester) or low prepregnancy weight may be a sign associated with IUGR.
- Fundal height measurements are inappropriate for gestational age (except in cases involving multiple pregnancies). Inappropriate fundal measurements may begin in the second trimester in cases of symmetric growth retardation or after the thirty-second week of gestation in asymmetric IUGR. Usual increase in fundal height in pregnancies without IUGR is almost 1 cm/week, resulting in an average fundal height at term of about 36 cm. Anytime the fundal measurement fails to increase by 2 cm in four weeks (especially when measured by the same caregiver), the possibility of IUGR should be considered, even if fetal growth has been adequate to that point. (Only one-third to one-half of all cases of IUGR are recognized in the prenatal period.)
- Clinical estimates of fetal weight may be smaller than expected for gestational age. However, accuracy in estimation of fetal weight varies greatly depending on the size of the baby, weight of the mother, fetal position, and skill of the practitioner. In general, clinical fetal weight estimates are accurate to within a pound only in 40-45% of the cases when the baby weighs less than 2,300 grams.

## Differential Diagnosis

- Inaccurate fundal measurements and/or inaccurate estimates of fetal weight
- Inaccurate pregnancy dating (see section on postdates pregnancy for methods of pregnancy dating).
- Oligohydramnios
- Transverse fetal lie
- Small but normal fetus

## Diagnostic Studies as Clinically Indicated

- Sonography may be used for several purposes (besides pregnancy dating, detection of multiple pregnancy, or abnormal fetal position):
    Total intrauterine volume (TIUV) determination may help to document both oligohydramnios (often seen in IUGR) and low fetal weight.

Head circumference/abdominal circumference ratio is helpful in discovering the presence of the "brain-sparing" syndrome. In the second trimester, the fetal head area is larger than the fetal abdominal area. In the third trimester (about 32–34 weeks), the fetal abdominal circumference catches up to and gradually surpasses the fetal head circumference. When this change in ratio fails to occur, brain growth at the expense of body growth is indicated. The head circumference/abdominal circumference ratio may also be used in conjunction with the TIUV determination to diagnose the symmetrically growth-retarded fetus whose head/abdomen ratio may be normal but who is small for gestational age.

Serial biparietal diameters may be used to determine normal or abnormal rates of head growth (especially in pregnancies that are not securely dated). The biparietal diameters are often used in conjunction with the above parameters to evaluate fetal growth.

Real-time sonography is used to look for gross fetal anomalies (craniospinal abnormalities, limb defects, renal agenesis, etc.) and placental abnormalities. Observation of fetal breathing movements may also be used as an aid in determining fetal well-being. Absence of fetal breathing movements in a 30-minute observation period in conjunction with a nonreactive nonstress test has been associated with poor fetal toleration of labor stress.

- Serial serum estriol or 24-hour urine collections for estriol level determinations may be useful in predicting fetal size before the thirty-eighth week of pregnancy. The levels are most often used to monitor fetal well-being in cases of IUGR. A drop of 30–50% from the average of the two previous levels is considered to indicate compromise of fetal well-being.
- Human placental lactogen (HPL) levels determinations are not useful alone in predicting IUGR, but they may be used in conjunction with other tests to monitor the fetal condition in IUGR.
- Nonstress test (NST) or oxytocin challenge test (OCT) are not used in diagnosis of IUGR. However, the NST (followed by an OCT if results are suspicious or nonreactive) is used in many institutions to evaluate fetal condition.

## Management and Treatment as Clinically Indicated

- Physician consultation is indicated in all cases of IUGR.
- Treatment of the woman with an IUGR pregnancy varies with the cause (if known) of the growth retardation and may include:
  Cessation of maternal smoking

Intake of protein-rich, well-balanced diet (necessitates nutritional counseling and, frequently, financial assistance)

Bed rest on the left side to increase placental perfusion

Treatment and/or control of underlying illness

- Management, in most cases of IUGR, may include:

Monitoring of fetal well-being by weekly NST, twice weekly determinations of serum or urinary estriol levels and/or HPL levels, and serial sonography for estimation of fetal growth and observation of fetal breathing movements

Careful timing and management of delivery as discussed below:

1. A positive OCT (after a nonreactive NST), possibly in conjunction with falling estriol levels or lack of fetal breathing movements during sonography, is considered to be an indication for prompt delivery.
2. Slowing of fetal head growth in cases of asymmetric growth retardation indicates worsening fetal condition and also indicates the need for delivery.
3. In certain cases, maternal illness may be aggravated by pregnancy to such an extent that delivery is mandated on the basis of maternal condition.
4. In cases of maternal (insulin-dependent) diabetes, early delivery is routine to prevent intrauterine demise.
5. Amniocentesis is done to determine fetal lung maturity if any question exists as to the dating of pregnancy. However, even if the shake test or L/S ratio indicates that the fetal lungs are not mature, delivery may still be effected if the physician judges that the continuation of pregnancy would further compromise the fetal or maternal condition. Steroids may be administered to the mother to attempt to hasten fetal lung maturity.
6. In spontaneous or induced labor, the fetus is monitored by attachment of a scalp electrode and insertion of an intrauterine catheter.
7. Drugs that may cause a decrease in beat-to-beat variability of the fetal heart (Valium, Demerol) and anesthesia methods that may induce maternal hypotension (epidural, spinal) are not used in labor and delivery of the growth-retarded fetus.
8. Resort to cesarean-section delivery is prompt if fetal distress is present, induction fails, or cephalopelvic disproportion is suspected. (Resort to cesarean-section delivery is not indicated on the basis of fetal condition if previous testing has revealed a fetal diagnosis that is incompatible with extrauterine life, such as renal agenesis or anencephaly.)
9. If vaginal delivery is permitted, a wide episiotomy and delivery by low forceps is often done to reduce the chance of cerebral hemorrhage.

10. The infant's mouth and nares are suctioned before delivery of the thorax to prevent possible meconium aspiration.
11. Well-trained personnel are present to visualize fetal vocal cords and to direct tracheal suction when meconium is present.
12. The baby is dried thoroughly and wrapped well to prevent hypothermia and is transferred promptly to the nursery for observation and treatment of possible complications.

## Complications

- Maternal

    Complications related to possible underlying disease process

    Higher incidence of cesarean-section delivery

- Fetal

    Complications related to possible anomalies or intrauterine infection. IUGR babies are more prone to intrauterine demise, labor hypoxia, hypothermia, hypoglycemia, polycythemia and hyperbilirubinemia, meconium aspiration, hypocalcemia, and cerebral or pulmonary hemorrhage. Long-term prognosis of SGA babies varies, but, in general the prognosis is poor for symmetrically growth-retarded infants and good for nonasphyxiated babies with asymmetric growth retardation.

## Patient Teaching

- Because of the myriad of conditions associated with IUGR, education and support for the pregnant woman with this complication must be individualized. Many of these women need referral for social, medical, psychologic, and financial evaluation and assistance.
- The patient with a growth-retarded fetus is faced with a multitude of evaluative tests and incomprehensible laboratory values as well as feelings of guilt and/or concern about the condition of her baby. Careful and repeated explanation of the test purposes, the interpretation of results, and the plan of care is necessary. Additionally, demonstrated concern about the woman's fears and concerns is needed to help the woman (and family) to cope in this situation.
- Testing procedures (NST, OCT, estriol determinations, serial sonography, labor monitoring) must be fully explained, and instructions must be given about any patient preparation or responsibility for these procedures.

- The woman with a growth-retarded fetus may be advised to monitor fetal movements. This opportunity to participate in her cure is reassuring to many women and aids in clinical evaluation of fetal well-being. The woman begins by becoming aware of the baby's activity and sleep cycles. She may then count the number of times the fetus moves during a specified period each day (corresponding to a usually active fetal period) or screen total activity over a period of hours. She should be reassured that, as the pregnancy progresses, wide, sweeping fetal movements become less frequent due to constraints of intrauterine space. The woman should notify the practitioner if the baby's activity suddenly decreases or if she fails to feel movement in a specified length of time (usually 10-12 hours). However, the woman who is extremely anxious about fetal well-being may become obsessed with this monitoring and may not benefit from this activity.
- The woman should have dietary evaluation and should be given instructions for a well-balanced, high-protein diet.
- The patient is advised to rest as much as possible in the left lateral recumbent posture to maximize placental perfusion. Arrangements for childcare and/or work disability payments may be necessary to permit such rest.
- The period of labor and delivery is a time of extreme stress for patients with a growth-retarded fetus. The patient and her support person need detailed information about the possible testing, monitoring, and treatment required during labor. If the woman has no available support person, arrangements should be made to provide a constant, empathetic attendant for labor and delivery.
- After delivery, the woman (and family) should be kept fully informed about the baby's condition and prognosis. If intensive neonatal medical treatment is necessary, provision should be made for nursery visitation by the mother and family.
- Assistance in working through the grieving process is necessary if the fetus dies or is premature, ill, anomalous, or neurologically damaged.

## UTERINE SIZE LARGER THAN EXPECTED FOR DATES

### Definition

This section deals not with a well-defined condition, but with a sign—a uterus which is large for dates. The causes for this sign are numerous, and the treatment varies with the cause. However, for the sake of brevity and to aid the practitioner in clinical practice, all the possible conditions associated with large uterine size will be dealt with in this section, with appropriate cross references to other sections.

## Etiology and Differential Diagnosis

- Error in pregnancy dating (see section on postdates pregnancy for points on accurate pregnancy dating)
- Maternal obesity: Thick abdominal walls may lead to inaccurate estimations of fetal weight and large uterine measurements. In cases of maternal obesity (overweight 20% or more for body height and build), screening for possible maternal diabetes is indicated.
- Large fetus without associated disease process: Diagnosis is usually made on the basis of exclusion of other possible causes of fetal macrosomia.
- Hydramnios (or polyhydramnios)—an excessive amount of amniotic fluid (over 2,000 or 3,000 ml), usually accumulating gradually (chronic hydramnios)—is often associated with fetal anomalies (especially CNS malformations and esophogeal atresia), multiple pregnancies, maternal diabetes, and erythroblastosis fetalis, but often occurs without known cause.
- Maternal diabetes is often associated with a large uterine size because of the increased incidence of hydramnios and fetal macrosomia, especially in classes A-C (see section on class A diabetes in Chap. 7).
- Multiple gestation can cause increased uterine size not only because of the bulk of more than one fetus but also because of possible associated hydramnios.
- Hydatidiform mole often causes uterine size to be larger than expected for dates (in about 50% of the cases; see the section on hydatidiform mole in Chap. 2 for more information).
- Uterine myomas usually increase in size with advancing gestation, at times becoming quite large.
- Fetal hydrocephalus: An excessive amount of cerebrospinal fluid causes enlargement of the cranium. The large, unengageable head displaces the fetal body upward in vertex presentations, causing large uterine measurements. Breech presentations are common in cases of fetal hydrocephalus.

## Clinical Features

### Symptoms

- In cases of multiple gestation, the pregnant woman may report a great deal of fetal activity felt over the entire abdomen.

## VARIATIONS IN UTERINE GROWTH PATTERNS

- The patient with overt diabetes may have symptoms associated with the disease—weight loss, extreme thirst, excessive urination, abnormally large appetite.
- The woman with a molar pregnancy often experiences severe nausea and vomiting. Failure of occurrence of quickening and possible vaginal spotting or passage of grapelike vesicles are other symptoms of this condition.
- Occasionally, a woman may develop acute (rapidly developing) hydramnios, which can cause abdominal pain and dyspnea.
- Most often, the woman reports no symptoms (except for a possible feeling that she is "too big".)

### Signs

- Uterine measurements that are larger than expected for gestational stage may be the only sign readily apparent.
- A large fetus can be palpated in some cases involving maternal diabetes. Persistent glycosuria may also be noted. Maternal obesity is often present.
- In cases of multiple gestation, more than one fetal head and many fetal small parts are often felt on abdominal palpation in the third trimester. More than one fetal heart tone (auscultated simultaneously and varying by more than 10 beats per minute) is almost diagnostic of multiple gestation.
- If hydramnios is present, fetal parts may be difficult to palpate, fetal heart tones may sound muffled or faint, and abnormal fetal position may occur.
- In molar pregnancies, fetal parts cannot be felt and no fetal heart tones are heard. Maternal weight loss may occur due to nausea and vomiting. Signs of pre-eclampsia may occur, often before the twentieth to twenty-fourth week of pregnancy.
- When uterine myomas are present, irregularity of uterine outline and abnormal fetal position are often noted.
- In cases involving a hydrocephalic fetus, breech presentations are common. In vertex presentations, the enlarged fetal head usually does not engage near term or in labor. Diagnosis of fetal position on abdominal palpation may be difficult since it is not possible to feel the firm, hard, globular mass usually associated with the fetal cranium.
- Family or clinical history may alert the clinician to the possibility of diabetes, multiple pregnancy, myomas, or Rh-sensitized pregnancy.

## Diagnostic Studies as Clinically Indicated

- Sonography is a very useful diagnostic tool in cases presenting with large uterine size. Multiple pregnancy, fetal macrosomia, gross fetal anomalies (in-

cluding hydrocephalus), hydramnios, hydatidiform mole, and some uterine myomas can be diagnosed by real-time or static sonography. Sonography also aids in pregnancy dating and in the calculation of normalcy of fetal growth (see information on sonography in section on intrauterine fetal growth retardation).
- Other diagnostic studies may include:
    Maternal antibody titers and/or bilirubin level determinations in amniotic fluid (in cases of Rh-sensitized women)
    Oral or intravenous glucose tolerance testing for detection of maternal diabetes (in cases of fetal macrosomia)
    Radioimmunossay for hCG levels (in cases of hydatidiform mole)

## Management and Treatment as Clinically Indicated

- Management of large uterine size depends on the diagnosed cause.
- Physician consultation and management is indicated in many of the causative conditions.
- Diabetes (see section on class A diabetes in Chap. 7 for more information)
- Multiple gestation is managed by:
    Adjustment of normal pregnancy diet to provide for the increased nutrient demands of more than one fetus
    Maternal iron supplementation to prevent anemia from iron demands, which are increased over those for a singleton pregnancy
    Frequent bed rest in the left lateral recumbent position to increase uterine perfusion
    Observation for and treatment of signs of premature labor (occurs more frequently in multiple gestation)
    Observation for signs of pre-eclampsia (incidence increased in multiple gestation)
    Monitoring of fetal well-being and growth by serial sonography and non-stress testing if indicated
    Careful monitoring of labor (combination of external and internal methods) with prompt resort to cesarean-section delivery should maternal or fetal condition warrant. (Uterine dysfunction due to overdistension may also necessitate surgical delivery. If either twin is a breech, cesarean-section delivery is often routine, especially in primiparous women. Delivery of more than two fetuses is usually by cesarean section).
    Typing and crossmatching for two units of whole blood for treatment of possible postpartum uterine atony and hemorrhage

Avoiding the use of labor analgesia/anesthesia methods that may cause maternal hypotension or fetal depression

Attendance of an anesthesiologist at the birth for initiation of anesthesia should fetal extraction or cesarean-section delivery become necessary

Delivery and resuscitation of the newborns by a knowledgeable, skilled team
- Uterine myomas are managed by:

    Observation of location and size of myomas

    Treatment of possible hemorrhagic infarction of myoma by bed rest and administration of pain relievers.

    Delivery by cesarean section if myomas cause labor obstruction or if the patient has previously undergone myomectomy
- Hydatidiform mole management is discussed in Chapter 2.
- Fetal hydrocephalus is managed by:

    Drainage of fetal cerebrospinal fluid (to permit delivery) by tapping the ventricles with a trocar or spinal needle when the cervix is dilated 3-4 cm and the presentation is vertex

    Delivery of the body in breech presentations and drainage of fluid (vaginally or transabdominally) from the fetal head to permit completion of delivery

    Vaginal delivery without drainage of cerebrospinal fluid (possible in some cases of very mild degrees of hydrocephalus)
- Erythroblastosis fetalis (fetal hemolytic disease caused by maternal Rh sensitization) is diagnosed and managed by:

    Frequent determination of maternal antibody titers

    Spectrophotometric analyses of amniotic fluid for optical density to determine the amount of bilirubin present in the fluid (in cases of high maternal antibody titers—1:16 or over)

    Intrauterine transfusions between 24 and 30 weeks' gestation if monitoring of fetal condition indicates that the fetus will die before the point at which his/her chances for extrauterine survival are fairly good

    Preterm delivery for the affected fetus to prevent further hemolysis, followed by intensive nursery care and exchange transfusions as necessary
- Hydramnios of undiagnosed origin is managed by:

    Careful observation for signs of premature labor

    Use of sonography for detection of possible fetal anomalies and for evaluation of fetal well-being and growth (if necessary)

    Observation and examination for possible placental abruption or cord prolapse at the time of rupture of the membranes

    Evaluation of the newborn for possible anomalies

## Complications

- Hydramnios is associated with an increased incidence of:
    Fetal anomalies
    Premature labor
    Abnormal fetal position
    Umbilical cord prolapse
    Placental abruption
    Labor inertia
    Postpartum uterine atony and hemorrhage
- Maternal diabetes is associated with an increased incidence of:
    Pre-eclampsia
    Birth trauma
    Cesarean-section births
    Fetal anomalies
    Stillbirth and neonatal death
    Neonatal respiratory distress syndrome, hyperbilirubinemia, hypoglycemia, hypocalcemia
    Postpartum uterine atony and hemorrhage
- Erythroblastosis fetalis is associated with an increased incidence of:
    Stillbirth
    Neonatal death
    Hydramnios
    Iatrogenic prematurity
    Fetal anemia
    Fetal hyperbilirubinemia and neonatal kernicterus
- Multiple gestation is associated with an increased incidence of:
    Abnormal fetal position
    Cesarean-section birth
    Prematurity
    Uterine labor inertia
    Intrauterine growth retardation
    Maternal anemia
    Hydramnios
    Pre-eclampsia
    Postpartum uterine atony and hemorrhage

- Hydrocephalus is associated with an increased incidence of:
    Labor dystocia and possible uterine rupture (if condition is undiagnosed and untreated in labor)
    Neonatal death and stillbirth (prognosis is very poor if the condition is severe enough to require drainage of cerebrospinal fluid)
    Permanent neurologic impairment in surviving infants

## Patient Teaching

- Patient teaching and counseling must be individualized according to the underlying cause of the large uterine size.
- See sections on class A diabetes (Chap. 7) and hydatidiform mole (Chap. 2) for guides to counseling in these diagnoses.
- The patient should be informed of:
    The possible causes and diagnostic procedures used when the uterus is larger than expected for gestational age
    The results of the diagnostic tests
    The future plan of care, including methods of maternal/fetal assessment and available treatment methods
    The possible maternal/fetal effects of the condition
- If multiple gestation and/or hydramnios is diagnosed, the woman should be told about:
    The possibility of premature labor
    The signs and symptoms of labor
    The necessity for more frequent cervical checks to monitor for the onset of preterm labor
    The importance of reporting promptly any signs of labor
    The necessity of coming to the hospital immediately should her membranes rupture before the onset of labor
- When assessment of fetal condition is important, the woman may be taught to monitor fetal movement patterns (see the patient teaching section for intrauterine growth retardation).
- Feelings of guilt, fear, and grief occur in patients with pathologic fetal conditions. Support and the opportunity for ventilation of feelings is important in the care of these patients (and families). Referral for professional counseling is often advisable.

- In the postpartum period, the woman and family should be kept informed about the condition of the baby and the results of any infant testing/treatment.
- Assistance in working through the grieving process is necessary if the fetus dies or is premature, ill, anomalous, or neurologically damaged.

## REFERENCES

Baggish M: Gestational trophoblastic neoplasia. *Clin Obstet Gynecol* 17:259, 1974.

Cefalo RC: The hazards of labor and delivery for the intrauterine-growth-retarded fetus. *J Reprod Med* 21:300, 1978.

Gabbe SG: Diabetes in pregnancy: Clinical controversies. *Clin Obstet Gynecol* 21:443, 1978.

Galbraith RS, Karchmar EJ, Peircy WN, et al: The clinical prediction of intrauterine growth retardation. *Am J Obstet Gynecol* 133:281, 1979.

Hill DE: Physical growth and development after intrauterine growth retardation. *J Reprod Med* 21:335, 1978.

Hobbins JC, Berkowitz RL, Grannum PA: Diagnosis and antepartum management of intrauterine growth retardation. *J Reprod Med* 21:319, 1978.

Jones KL, Chernoff GF: Drugs and chemicals associated with intrauterine growth deficiency. *J Reprod Med* 21:365, 1978.

Jones OW: Genetic factors in the determination of fetal size. *Am J Reprod Med* 21:305, 1978.

Kohorn EI: Gestational trophoblastic disease: Diagnosis and management. *Contemp Obstet Gynecol* 13:165, 1979.

Koops BL: Neurological sequelae in infants with intrauterine growth retardation. *J Reprod Med* 21:343, 1978.

Niswander K: *Obstetrics: Essentials of Clinical Practice,* ed 1. Boston, Little, Brown and Company, 1976, pp 121, 306, 314, 443, 459.

Pritchard JA, MacDonald PC: *Williams Obstetrics,* ed 15. New York, Appleton-Century-Crofts, 1976, pp 453, 476, 529, 690 801.

Resnik R: Maternal diseases associated with abnormal fetal growth. *J Reprod Med* 21:315, 1978.

Tejani N, Mann LI: Diagnosis and management of the small-for-gestational-age fetus. *Clin Obstet Gynecol* 20: 943, 1977.

Waldimiroff JW, Bloemsma CA, Wallenburg HC: Ultrasonic assessment of fetal growth. *Acta Obstet Gynecol Scand* 56:37, 1977.

Wittman BK, Robinson HP, Aitchison T, et al: The value of diagnostic ultrasound as a screening text for intrauterine growth retardation: Comparison of nine parameters. *Am J Obstet Gynecol* 134:30, 1979.

# 7

# Other Complications of Pregnancy

Class A diabetes mellitus and the postdates pregnancy are two complications of pregnancy discussed in this chapter. Cases of class A diabetes in pregnancy comprise 80-90% of all diabetic gestations and, as long as overt diabetes is absent, are candidates for joint practitioner/physician management in the ambulatory setting. Diagnosis of postdates pregnancy and screening for the development of the fetal postmaturity syndrome are common occurrences in clinical prenatal practice. Early detection and appropriate management of both these complications can contribute significantly to an improved pregnancy outcome for mother and baby.

## POSTDATES PREGNANCY

### Definition

The average length of human gestation is 278-281 days (40 weeks) from the first day of the last normal menstrual period (LNMP). The prolonged or postdates pregnancy is one which lasts more than 295 days (42 weeks) after the first day of the LNMP. Estimates of occurrence for postdates pregnancies range from 6-12% of all pregnancies.

## General Considerations

Clinical concern about postdates pregnancy is based on the fact that fetal perinatal mortality and morbidity are two to three times higher in prolonged pregnancies than in gestations of normal length (38-42 weeks). Most of the increased risk to the fetus of a postdates pregnancy is attributed to the development of the fetal postmaturity (dysmaturity) syndrome. This syndrome (which occurs in only 20-30% of postdates pregnancies) is theoretically due to the aging of the placenta which, in some cases of prolonged pregnancy, may result in placental senescence with markedly impaired oxygen diffusion and transfer of nutrients to the fetus.

The fetus with postmaturity syndrome is typically long and thin, with long nails, abundant hair, and thin, dry, peeling skin. Fetal mortality may be as high as 35% if evidence of intrauterine fetal hypoxia is also present (meconium staining of umbilical cord, membranes, skin, and nails). However, 70-80% of the fetuses from postdates pregnancies do not demonstrate signs of dysmaturity but continue to grow well in utero, many to the point of macrosomia (birthweight over 4,000 grams). This macrosomia may result in labor dystocia, birth trauma, and increased incidence of cesarean-section delivery.

## Etiology

The initiation and continuation of human labor is probably triggered by a complex interplay of both fetal and maternal factors. The reason for the failure of labor initiation at the usual time is unknown in most cases of postdates pregnancy. Prolonged pregnancy is common in cases of fetal anencephaly. This is probably related to the lack of a fetal labor initiation factor from the fetal adrenals, which are hypoplastic in anencephaly. Prolonged pregnancy is also observed more frequently in women over 35 years of age. The reason for this correlation is unknown.

## Clinical Features

### *Symptoms*

- None

### *Signs*

- Usually none
- Decrease in fundal height may be noted in cases of fetal postmaturity. (How-

ever, a decrease in fundal height is often noted in normal pregnancy as the fetal head enters the pelvis.)

## Differential Diagnosis

The diagnosis of postdates pregnancy is often difficult since many women are unsure of the date of their last normal menstrual period. It is estimated that uncertain dating occurs in 20-30% of all pregnancies. The following factors should be taken into consideration when attempting to distinguish a postdates pregnancy from a misdated pregnancy:

- The date of the last menstrual period

    How certain is the patient about her dates?

    Was the period shorter and earlier than expected? (possible implantation bleeding)

- The length of menstrual cycles

    Are her periods regular?

    Are her cycles generally more or less than 28 days?

    Was she using oral contraceptives before or at the time of conception? (makes probable time of conception more difficult to determine)

- Sexual history

    Was the patient sexually active on a regular basis before conception?

    Does the patient know the approximate time of conception due to infrequent sexual intercourse?

- Early examinations

    Was a urine or serum pregnancy test done?

    When was the test positive?

    Was a pelvic exam done at the time of pregnancy testing, and if so, what did the examiner say about the size of the uterus?

    How early was the first prenatal visit and was the size of the uterus consistent with dates at that time?

    *Note:* The most accurate pregnancy dating is possible when the first examination is done before 12 weeks' gestation.

- Growth pattern

    Has the uterus consistently seemed small, large, or appropriate for dates at the prenatal visits?

- Fetal heart tones (FHT)

    When was the FHT first heard by ultrasonic device? (usually 12-14 weeks' gestation)

When was the FHT first noted with the fetoscope (usually 18-20 weeks' gestation)

*Note:* It should be remembered that these FHT guidelines may be of questionable value since the monthly patient visits may not coincide with the timing discussed above.

- Quickening

  When did quickening occur? (usually felt by primigravidas at 18-20 weeks' gestation and by multigravidas at 16-18 weeks' gestation)

  *Note:* When the first prenatal visit occurs before the time of quickening, the practitioner should always ask the woman to note the date of quickening for future reference.

- Sonographic evaluation

  Was a sonogram ordered earlier in pregnancy and, if so, what was the gestation reported?

  When was the sonogram done? (The sonogram is most accurate for pregnancy dating at 22-28 weeks' gestation.)

  *Note:* In many institutions, a woman with uncertain dates is sent for sonography at least once to avoid confusion about her estimated date of confinement (EDC).

- Pelvic examinations near EDC

  Is the cervix soft, anterior, effaced, dilated?

  If the patient is a primigravida, is the fetal head engaged or dipping well into the pelvis?

## Diagnostic Studies as Clinically Indicated

The studies discussed below are used for diagnosis of fetal postmaturity syndrome since it is this syndrome, not prolonged pregnancy in itself, that causes most of the increased perinatal mortality and morbidity. Controversy exists as to the most sensitive predictors of fetal well-being, and the tests are often used in combination.

- Nonstress test (NST) is used as an indicator of fetal well-being and placental function.
- Oxytocin challenge test (OCT) most commonly is used as a follow-up study to a nonreactive or suspicious NST.
- Serum estriol or 24-hour urine collection for estriol determinations are usually done in conjunction with weekly NST or OCT as an indication of placental function. To be a helpful diagnostic tool estriol level determinations must be done

two or three times a week (with facilities for prompt test reporting). The efficacy of estriol levels alone in determining fetal well-being in prolonged pregnancy is questionable.
- Amnioscopy or amniocentesis is used in some institutions to detect the presence of meconium in amniotic fluid. Oligohydramnios often accompanies postdates pregnancies, adding to the usual potential complications of amniocentesis. Amnioscopy can only be performed in cases of an anterior, partially dilated cervix and may lead to rupture of the membranes. For these reasons, and because of lack of agreement about the significance of the results, amniocentesis and amnioscopy are not commonly used.
- Sonography is sometimes used to detect oligohydramnios, gross fetal anomalies (especially anencephaly), and/or signs of placental senescence. Measurement of fetal head circumference/abdominal circumference ratio can help to identify the fetus who is undergoing wastage of subcutaneous fat deposits.
- Human placental lactogen (HPL) level determinations may sometimes be used. A low HPL level in association with other test results can help to confirm placental compromise.

## Management and Treatment as Clinically Indicated

- Physician consultation is necessary in cases of postdates pregnancy.
- The management of prolonged pregnancy varies greatly. Some physicians are aggressive in management, inducing labor at 41 weeks' gestation if the patient's cervix is ripe.
- The potential complications of routine oxytocin induction (fetal distress, iatrogenic prematurity, higher incidence of cesarean-section delivery in failed inductions) lead other practitioners to manage prolonged pregnancy more conservatively with:

    Weekly nonstress testing (beginning at 41–42 weeks' gestation)

    Oxytocin challenge testing within 24 hours of a nonreactive or suspicious NST

    Possible twice weekly estriol level determinations in conjunction with the above. If the estriol level falls by 25–30% from the average of the two preceding values, an OCT is scheduled within 24 hours.

    Possible use of real-time sonography to detect oligohydramnios, evidence of fetal dysmaturity, or excessive placental lobulation or calcification, followed by OCT if any of these conditions are found

    Regard of positive OCT as an indication of the need to deliver the baby because of possible compromise of placental function

Oxytocin induction of labor (when indicated) with continuous FHT monitoring

Vaginal delivery permitted if no evidence of fetal distress or labor dystocia

Presence of pediatric personnel in the delivery or operating room for infant resuscitation and/or thorough suctioning for meconium

Suctioning of baby's nares and pharynx before delivery of shoulders if meconium is present

## Complications

- Maternal

    Higher incidence of birth trauma and delivery by cesarean section (indicated by fetal condition or macrosomia)

- Fetal

    Higher incidence of birth trauma, respiratory distress syndrome (usually due to meconium aspiration)

    Evidence of cerebral anoxia, fetal mortality

    In the first year, postdates infants may also have increased incidence of minor illnesses, hospitalizations, feeding and sleep disturbances, impaired motor skills, and disturbed psychosocial interactions.

## Patient Teaching

- The woman whose pregnancy reaches 41 or 42 weeks' gestation should be told about the possibility of increased fetal risk in postdates pregnancies and about the tests that will be used to assure that her baby is continuing to thrive in the uterus. Reassurance should be given that the majority of babies experience no ill effects from prolonged pregnancy.
- The NST or OCT should be described in detail—where it is done, when to come in for the test, how long it takes, what equipment is involved, how the test is evaluated, what will be considered if the test is suspicious or indicates fetal compromise. If an OCT is to be done, the patient should also be told about the IV insertion, what oxytocin is and the reason for its use, and that the contractions produced are perhaps a bit uncomfortable but not really painful.
- If urine is to be collected for estriol level determination, the patient needs verbal and written instructions on how to properly collect and store the urine as well as where to bring the specimen when completed.

- The patient should be informed of the results of all tests and of the continued plan of care.
- The patient needs emotional support since she is not only concerned about the baby's well-being but is also frequently upset and tired of being pregnant. Often she is bombarded by phone calls and visits from well-meaning friends and relatives who want to know "why you haven't had this baby yet."
- It has often been observed that some cases of prolonged pregnancy occur in women who are emotionally unready for the baby to be born. Some of these women are very fearful of the birth itself, some feel unprepared for parenthood, some may have financial problems or interpersonal difficulties which are distracting. In counseling the woman with a postdates pregnancy, the practitioner may discuss the possibility of "maternal unreadiness" and advise the patient to think about whether or not any of these factors are operant in her situation. Discussion of the situation or help in financial matters may be indicated.

## CLASS A DIABETES MELLITUS

### Definition

Diabetes mellitus is a relative or absolute lack of endogenous insulin, which causes an inappropriate elevation of blood glucose levels and alterations in fat and protein metabolism. Long-standing diabetes is also associated with vascular changes including accelerated nonspecific atherosclerosis and specific disease of the small blood vessels, particularly in the eye and kidney.

### General Considerations in Pregnancy

Pregnancy is considered to be a diabetogenic state. The pregnancy hormones (particularly human placental lactogen and estrogen) interfere with the action of maternal insulin. These hormones are secreted in ever-increasing amounts throughout pregnancy, thereby increasing the diabetogenicity of pregnancy during the last 20 weeks of gestation.

The White classification system, commonly used for diabetes during pregnancy is:

- Class A: Chemical diabetes, asymptomatic

- Class B: Overt diabetes, maturity onset (over 20), duration less than 10 years, no vascular disease
- Class C: Overt diabetes, onset before age 20, duration 10-20 years, no vascular disease
- Class D: Overt diabetes, onset under age 10 or duration more than 20 years, benign retinopathy
- Class F: Nephropathy present (proteinuria, azotemia)
- Class R: Proliferative retinopathy present

This classification is helpful in predicting fetal outcome, with the incidence of stillbirths and neonatal deaths increasing from normal in class A diabetes to well over 50% in class F. The pathophysiology responsible for much of the perinatal mortality seen in infants of overt diabetics is poorly understood. Fetal macrosomia, more commonly seen in classes A-C, may be due to fetal hyperglycemia and hyperinsulinemia, which result in increased deposition of subcutaneous fat.

Class A diabetes probably accounts for 80-90% of all diabetes seen in pregnancy. However, much of the information on the effects of diabetes on pregnancy has not separated the class A diabetic woman from women with more severe classifications of diabetes. The class A diabetic:

- Has normal fasting blood glucose levels
- Has an abnormal glucose tolerance test (elevation of two of the three post-glucose-ingestion levels)
- Does not require insulin
- Requires minimal dietary regulation

Diabetes of pregnancy onset (gestational diabetes) can be either class A or class B. Since classes B-F and R require insulin therapy and management by a skilled medical team, this section will deal with class A diabetes in pregnancy.

## Etiology

It is generally accepted that diabetes (or susceptibility to diabetes) is transmitted genetically. However, the specific mode of inheritance is unknown and probably is multifactoral. Historical and clinical factors known to be associated with diabetes in pregnancy are:

- History of stillborn or malformed infants
- History of macrosomic infants (over 4,000 g)
- Family history of diabetes
- History of recurrent pre-eclampsia–eclampsia

- Marked obesity (20% or more over normal weight for height and body build)
- Polyhydramnios
- Glycosuria in pregnancy (usually defined as glycosuria occurring on two or more occasions)

## Clinical Features

### Symptoms

- No symptoms present in class A diabetes

### Signs

- Patient may have no signs.
- Obesity may be present.
- Large fetus may be noted.
- Polyhydramnios may occur.

## Differential Diagnosis

- Renal glycosuria
- Polyhydramnios
- Multiple pregnancy

## Diagnostic Studies as Clinically Indicated

Most institutions have developed criteria for screening pregnant women for diabetes. These criteria vary but are usually drawn from the historical and clinical factors known to be associated with pregnancy diabetes, which are listed above. Some authorities believe that screening should be done for all pregnant women since only 50% of women diagnosed as diabetic fulfill any of the criteria for screening. Screening is usually done at about the twenty-eighth to thirty-second week of pregnancy. Much controversy exists about the most effective manner to screen for diabetes. Some of the currently used tests are:

- Fasting blood sugar (FBS) and two-hour postprandial glucose level (2-hr PP): If the FBS (normal 90 mg/dl) or the 2-hr PP level (normal 120 mg/dl)

is elevated, a glucose tolerance test is ordered for final diagnosis. However, the lack of control over dietary carbohydrate intake preceding the postprandial specimen makes this test of questionable value as a screening tool.
- Blood glucose level one hour after ingestion of 50 ml of concentrated glucose liquid: Elevated blood glucose levels (upper limit of normal 160 gm/dl) require further screening by glucose tolerance testing.
- Glucose tolerance test: Controversy exists as to whether the IV injection of glucose solution (IV GTT) or oral glucose ingestion (OGTT) provides the most accurate picture of glucose metabolism in pregnancy. In both methods, the patient is placed on a high-carbohydrate diet for three days before testing. Blood is drawn to determine the fasting glucose level. Then blood and urinary glucose levels are measured one, two, and three hours after glucose loading. The normal values for glucose tolerance tests vary depending on the institution. The following levels provide a general guide to normal levels:

| *Period* | *Values (mg/dl of Whole Blood)* |
|---|---|
| Fasting | 90 |
| 1 hour | 165 |
| 2 hours | 145 |
| 3 hours | 125 |

(*Note:* If the test is performed on serum, values will be approximately 15% higher. A normal FBS level and an elevation of two of the other three values is considered diagnostic of class A diabetes.

## Management and Treatment as Clinically Indicated

- Physician consultation and comanagement is indicated in cases of class A diabetes.
- The general principles of management are:

    The patient is seen every two weeks from the time of diagnosis until the thirty-sixth week when weekly visits are begun.

    The patient is placed on an 1,800–2,200 calorie diet (based on age and weight) with no concentrated sweets. If acetonuria occurs, the caloric intake is increased.

    The patient tests her urine (second-voided morning specimen) every day for acetone and glucose and records the results.

    Urine is checked for acetone and sugar at each clinic visit. An FBS level is also determined each time. (Ten–fifteen percent of class A diabetics may develop overt diabetes later in pregnancy. The urine and FBS tests aid in detecting this change in classification.)

If the FBS level is over 110 mg/dl on two separate occasions, the patient is considered to be an overt diabetic with an attendant greater risk of perinatal mortality and morbidity. Physician management is then mandated.

The patient should be monitored carefully for signs and symptoms of pre-eclampsia and urinary tract infection, which are more common in diabetic women.

The class A diabetic woman whose FBS levels remain normal may be allowed to go to term, unlike patients with overt diabetes in whom early delivery is often considered necessary to attempt to prevent intrauterine death. Some physicians, however, prefer to induce labor at 40 weeks' gestation.

The woman with class A diabetes who has a history of previous stillbirth will probably be managed with delivery at the time of fetal lung maturity.

After 40 weeks' gestation, the class A diabetic woman is followed with urinary estriol level measurements and/or weekly nonstress tests for determination of fetal well-being.

Vaginal delivery is permitted if all remains normal. The macrosomia common in babies of class A diabetics may result in labor dystocia, birth trauma, shoulder dystocia, and postpartum hemorrhage. The incidence of indicated cesarean-section delivery is much higher in women with diabetes than in the general pregnant population.

The woman with class A diabetes should be evaluated post partum by a glucose tolerance test to determine if the diabetic condition persists, requiring physician management.

(*Note:* Some physicians place the class A diabetic patient on small daily amounts of insulin in an attempt to prevent fetal macrosomia. In some institutions, the class A diabetic woman may be given insulin during labor to decrease the incidence of hypoglycemia in the neonate.)

## Complications

- Maternal

    Higher incidence of birth trauma and cesarean-section delivery (due to fetal macrosomia), pre-eclampsia, urinary tract infections, hydramnios

    Increased incidence of overt diabetes later in life

- Fetal

    Higher incidence of birth trauma, neonatal hypoglycemia, hyperbilirubinemia, and congenital anomalies

## Patient Teaching

- The woman with class A diabetes should be informed about:
  How the diagnosis was reached
  What diabetes is (including discussion of basic glucose metabolism and the effects of insulin deficiency)
  The planned treatment of her condition
  How her disease will affect her pregnancy (including reassurance about probability of good fetal outcome)
  The importance of compliance with the plan of care
  The possibility of progression of the disease to overt diabetes, either during pregnancy or at a later period in life
- Dietary counseling (preferably with a nutritionist) should emphasize not only the actual components of the planned diet but also the patient's responsibility for control of her condition through diet.
- Prompt attention is required for possible severe nausea and vomiting in pregnancy since it may lead to acidosis. See section on common complaints of pregnancy (Chap. 1) for medical, nutritional, and behavioral treatment measures for control of nausea.
- The patient should be instructed in urine testing and charting of results. She should be given materials for such testing.
- Since the woman has no symptoms of diabetes, she may need repeated explanation of her condition and the importance of close medical supervision and evaluation.
- The woman (and family) requires emotional support and reassurance since the diagnosis of diabetes can be very frightening, carrying with it a highly charged negative emotional component.
- The patient should be kept informed at each visit about the results of laboratory testing and the progress of the pregnancy.
- The woman should be told about the necessity of observing the baby in the postpartum period for evidence of hypoglycemia or hyperbilirubinemia and about the usual treatment for these conditions.
- The patient needs explanation of the importance of postpartum evaluation of her condition and follow-up yearly testing for glucose metabolism.
- The woman should be informed about the mild diabetogenic properties of birth control pills and that they may be contraindicated in her situation.

## REFERENCES

Adashi EY, Humberto P, Tyson JE: Impact of euglycemia on fetal outcome in diabetic pregnancy. *Am J Obstet Gynecol* 133:269, 1979.

Field TM, Dabiri C, Hallock N, et al: Developmental effects of prolonged pregnancy and the postmaturity syndrome. *J Pediatr* 90:836, 1977.

Gabbe SG: Diabetes in pregnancy: Clinical controversies. *Clin Obstet Gynecol* 21:443, 1978.

Granat M, Sharf J, Cooper A: Glucose intolerance during pregnancy: A reappraisal of alleged screening criteria. *Obstet Gynecol* 53:157, 1979.

Green JN, Paul RH: The value of amniocentesis in prolonged pregnancy. *Obstet Gynecol* 51:293, 1978.

Hertz RH, Sokol RJ, Knoke JD, et al: Clinical estimation of gestational age: Rules for avoiding preterm delivery. *Am J Obstet Gynecol* 131:395, 1978.

Ismach JM: Diabetes in pregnancy: New group discusses management problems. *Contemp Obstet Gynecol* 11(2):31, 1978.

Klapholz H, Friedman EA: The incidence of intrapartum fetal distress with advancing gestational age. *Am J Obstet Gynecol* 127:405, 1977.

Knox GE, Huddleston JF, Flowers CE: Management of prolonged gestations. *Am J Obstet Gynecol* 134:376, 1979.

Naeye RL: Causes of perinatal mortality excess in prolonged gestations. *Am J Epidemiol* 108:429, 1978.

Pritchard JA, MacDonald PC: *Williams Obstetrics,* ed 15. New York, Appleton-Century-Crofts, 1976, pp 618-625.

Schneider JM, Olson RW, Curet LB: Screening of fetal and neonatal risk in the postdate pregnancy. *Am J Obstet Gynecol* 131:473, 1978.

Steinke J, Soeldner JS: Diabetes mellitus, in Thron GW, Adams RD, Braunwald E, et al (ed): *Harrison's Principles of Internal Medicine,* ed 8. New York, McGraw-Hill Book Company, 1977, pp 564-582.

Weiner S, Librizzi RJ, Bolognese RJ: Postdates pregnancy: Its risks and management. *Contemp Obstet Gynecol* 14:133, 1979.

White P: Pregnancy complicating diabetes. *Am J Med* 7:609, 1949.

# 8

## Common Postpartum Complications

Two of the most common medical complications of the puerperium seen in the ambulatory setting are considered in this chapter—subinvolution of the uterus and postpartum mastitis. Although it is not within the scope of this book to consider all the marked and rapid physiologic, emotional, and social readjustments considered normal for the puerperium, the practitioner plays a vital role in easing these transitions, as well as in diagnosing and managing possible medical problems. Sensitive, supportive attention and referral to available sources of childbirth education, relevant literature, and parenting and lactation support groups play an important part in ensuring the emotional and physical health of the families in the practitioner's care.

### SUBINVOLUTION OF THE UTERUS

#### Definition

Uterine involution is the process by which the postpartum uterus returns to normal nonpregnant size and proportions. In general, the uterus is no longer palpable as an abdominal organ after 9-12 days postpartum, and total involution occurs over a four- to six-week period after term delivery. Involution after abortion and preterm delivery is usually accomplished in a shorter period of time. Subinvolution is an arrest or prolongation of the normal involution process.

## Etiology

- Retained placental fragments
- Endometritis (see Chap. 9 for full discussion)
- Cesarean section
- Uterine myomas

## Clinical Features

### Symptoms

- Excessive or prolonged flow of lochia and/or uterine bleeding
- Possible delayed postpartum hemorrhage (occurs more than one week after delivery)
- Possible chills and fever
- Possible pelvic and/or back pain
- Possible leukorrhea

### Signs

- Uterus is larger than expected for the period of the puerperium when examination is performed.
- Uterus feels boggy, soft.
- Uterine tenderness may be present.
- Uterine bleeding, excessive lochia, or leukorrhea may be observed.
- Fever may be present.

## Differential Diagnosis

- Ovarian cyst
- Pelvic adhesions
- Malignant uterine tumors
- Cystitis
- Gestational trophoblastic disease

## Diagnostic Studies as Clinically Indicated

- A CBC and sedimentation rate is indicated in cases suggestive of endometritis.
- Culture of cervical discharge may be performed when endometritis is suspected.
- Histologic examination of endometrial tissue may be done if dilatation and curretage is necessary.

## Management and Treatment as Clinically Indicated

- If the uterus is nontender, there is no fever or chills, the uterine discharge is not foul-smelling, and bleeding is minimal to moderate, the patient is usually given an ergot preparation (Ergotrate, 0.2 mg every four to six hours) for two to three days. Uterine size is rechecked in one or two weeks.
- If uterine tenderness, foul-smelling lochia or leukorrhea, and fever or chills suggest endometritis, culture of the discharge is done to identify the endometrial pathogen. Treatment with a broad-spectrum antibiotic is begun pending results of the culture (ampicillin, 500 mg qid for 7–10 days). Concomitant treatment with Ergotrate may be indicated. Hospitalization is necessary in cases in which the endometrial infection is severe or has spread to other pelvic structures. Adnexal tenderness, abdominal rigidity and rebound pain, high fever, and extreme malaise are all suggestive of extension of the endometritis.
- If uterine hemorrhage is brisk, hospitalization for dilatation and curettage (D&C) may be necessary to remove retained placental fragments. Blood and fluid replacement may be needed if hemorrhage is severe. If the patient's condition permits delay, administration of antibiotics is started before the D&C. The patient is given an ergot preparation and antibiotic therapy for several days after surgery.
- In certain cases (especially after cesarean-section delivery or when uterine myomas are present) the uterus may feel larger than normal, but symptoms of infection and excessive bleeding are absent. The clinician may elect simply to inform the patient of symptoms of possible complications and to schedule her for a visit to recheck uterine size in one to two weeks.

## Complications

- Hemorrhage
- Pelvic peritonitis, salpingitis, abscess formation in cases of endometritis

### Patient Teaching

- The patient should be informed of the diagnosis, suspected etiology, and plan for treatment.
- The woman should be told that Ergotrate commonly causes uncomfortable or painful uterine contractions.
- The patient should be advised to avoid overexertion and to rest in bed as much as possible in cases of subinvolution caused by endometritis.
- If hospitalization is necessary, the woman (and family) need emotional support and explanation of probable procedures and treatment. If the woman is to be separated from an infant, she may need help in arranging for child care. Provisions should be made for maintenance of lactation via manual or mechanical expression of milk. If possible, arrangements should be made for visitation by the infant and other children on a daily basis to moderate the trauma of mother-child separation.
- In ambulatory treatment, the woman should be told of the importance of completing the course of medication and of informing the practitioner promptly if symptoms of complications occur or if her condition seems to be worsening.

## POSTPARTUM MASTITIS

### Definition

Postpartum mastitis is inflammation of the breast, usually unilateral, which occurs almost exclusively in breastfeeding women. This condition occurs in about 2.5% of all nursing mothers.

The two main types of postpartum mastitis are:

- Epidemic mastitis: Inflammation affects the lactiferous apparatus of the breast, often with infection present in several nonadjacent lobes, progressing quickly to abscess formation in untreated cases. This type of infection is usually not seen after the first 3-5 days after delivery.
- Sporadic mastitis: Inflammation occurs most frequently three to four weeks after delivery, although it may occur earlier or later (especially at the time of weaning). The cellulitis is at first confined to the interlobular connective tissue with infection progressing to abscess formation in the majority of untreated cases.

This section will deal mainly with the sporadic type of postpartum mastitis since this is the classification most often seen on an ambulatory basis.

## Etiology

The causative organism in both types of postpartum mastitis is usually a strain of *Staphlycoccus aureus*. In epidemic mastitis, a highly virulent strain of *S. aureus* is carried by nursery personnel and spread by cross-contamination to babies born in the hospital. The organism is harbored in the baby's nasopharynx and is introduced into the breast ducts during nursing. The baby may become clinically infected, usually beginning at the umbilical stump.

In sporadic mastitis, the nursing woman is usually predisposed to infection by less virulent strains of *S. aureus* normally present in the infant's nasopharynx by:

- Engorgement and stasis of milk associated with missed feedings or weaning
- Cracked or irritated nipples

## Clinical Features (Sporadic Mastitis)

### Symptoms

- Initial "flulike" aching and malaise
- Fever and chills
- Later, breast redness and soreness

### Signs

- Fever, often 39–40° C
- Redness and warmth of breast skin, usually in a V-shaped area at the demarcation between breast lobes
- Breast tenderness to palpation
- Inability to express pus from the nipple
- Possible fissured or irritated nipple
- Possible pitting edema and fluctuation on palpation of affected area (in cases of abscess formation)

## Differential Diagnosis

- Epidemic mastitis usually develops in the first few days following delivery; nonadjacent lobes may be affected; pus can be expressed from the nipple.
- Focal breast engorgement develops due to blocked duct; breast lobe is swollen, firm, and tender; no fever or breast erythema. This engorgement can progress to mastitis unless relief measures are instituted.

## Diagnostic Studies as Clinically Indicated

- Culture of milk from affected breast may grow causative organism. However, since the initial inflammation is limited to the connective tissue, the milk culture may be negative.

## Management and Treatment as Clinically Indicated

- Treatment of sporadic mastitis consists of:
    Emptying of the breasts to relieve stasis
    Antibiotic treatment of the causative organism
- In the past, women with sporadic mastitis were advised to discontinue breastfeeding and to suppress lactation. This is no longer considered necessary and is thought to lead to increased incidence of abscess formation due to congestion and stasis of blood and milk in the breast. Currently, the woman with sporadic mastitis is advised to:
    Empty the breast frequently, by nursing her baby or by breast pump or manual expression
    Rest as much as possible
    Relieve discomfort with non-aspirin pain relievers as directed
- Antibiotic treatment may be based on the sensitivity of the cultured organism. However, initiation of antibiotic therapy after diagnosis with cephalosporin (250-500 mg q6h for 7-10 days) or dicloxacillin (125-250 mg q6h for 7-10 days) is most often indicated, with a change in agent, if necessary, when the culture report is received.
- Signs and symptoms usually disappear within 24-48 hours of initiation of antibiotic treatment.
- Abscess formation, which occurs in about 5-10% of mastitis cases, is treated by wide incision and drainage with loose gauze packing of the abscess cavity.

Nursing from the affected breast is contraindicated, but lactation may be maintained in the contralateral breast if desired.
- In the epidemic type of mastitis, nursing is usually contraindicated due to the chance of reinfection. The breasts are emptied by breast pump or manual expression until the inflammation is resolved. If the baby is being treated for clinical infection at the same time as the mother, nursing may be resumed after both have completed therapy.

## Complications

- Abscess formation
- Possible recurrence at a later time

## Patient Teaching

- Prevention of mastitis should be the aim of the practitioner. Every woman who plans to breastfeed should be taught:

    The technique of manual expression to relieve breast engorgement and to reduce tension in the engorged areola before putting the baby to breast.

    To decrease nipple soreness and cracking by:
    1. Making sure that the baby has in his/her mouth as much of the areola as possible during feeding
    2. Changing nursing positions often to alternate points of maximum sucking pressure
    3. Avoiding the use of soap or other drying agents on the nipples
    4. Applying ointment, such as anhydrous lanolin, to the nipple and areola after nursing
    5. Washing the nipples with clear water frequently to avoid the thickening and drying of milk on the nipples
    6. Exposing the nipples to air as much as possible
    7. Using correct technique for removing the baby from the breast (inserting finger at the side of the baby's mouth to release suction)
    8. Nursing at the least sore breast first
    9. Avoiding engorgement

    To deal with engorgement by:
    1. More frequent nursing

2. Expression of milk to soften areola before nursing
3. Gentle massage of the firm breast areas when nursing
4. Use of a correctly fitted nursing bra, which supports the breasts separately, does not bind, and encloses all of the breast tissue within the cups.
5. Frequent warm showers, baths, or wet packs to the breasts to relieve discomfort and to promote milk flow
6. Possible use of oxytocin nasal spray to initiate "letdown" until this reflex is well established
7. Very gradual weaning (giving up one feeding every week, beginning with the one when breasts are least full)
8. Prompt reporting of any symptoms of mastitis

- All the above points should be stressed in cases of postpartum mastitis.
- The woman with mastitis who wishes to continue breastfeeding should be reassured that, even in cases of staphylococcal pyolactia, infant illness from the infection is very rare.

## REFERENCES

Barden TP: Perinatal care, in Romney SL, Gray MJ, Little AB, et al (eds): *Gynecology and Obstetrics: The Health Care of Women*. New York, McGraw-Hill Book Company, 1975, p 708.

Jensen M, Benson R, Bobak I: *Maternity Care—The Nurse and the Family*. St Louis, The CV Mosby Company, 1977, p 427.

Ledger W: Infectious disease, in Romney SL, Gray MJ, Little AB, et al (eds): *Gynecology and Obstetrics: The Health Care of Women*. New York, McGraw-Hill Book Company, 1975, p 463.

Marshall BR, Hepper JK, Zirbel CC: Sporadic puerperal mastitis: an infection that need not interrupt lactation. *JAMA* 233: 1377, 1975.

Niebyl JR, Spence MR, Parmley TH: Sporadic (nonepidemic) puerperal mastitis. *J Reprod Med* 20:97, 1978.

Pritchard J, MacDonald P: *Williams Obstetrics*, ed 15. New York, Appleton-Century-Crofts, 1976, pp 759–781.

Puerperal mastitis, editorial. *Br Med J* 1:920, 1976.

Romney S, Ober W, Moyer D: Uterus, in Romney SL, Gray MJ, Little AB, et al (eds): *Gynecology and Obstetrics: The Health Care of Women*. New York, McGraw-Hil Book Company, 1975, p 1037.

# Section II

# Problems in Ambulatory Gynecology

# 9
# Gynecologic Infections

Gynecologic infections are among the most common problems encountered in the practice of women's health care and may range from the simple to the complex to diagnose and to manage. Symptoms produced by some gynecologic infections can be extremely troublesome but have no long-term serious consequences, while other infections may not only be troublesome but also may produce long-lasting effects on the woman's general health and fertility.

The anatomic arrangement of the female pelvic organs provides easy passage for infection. Infection, which may begin in the lower structures of the vagina and cervix, may readily ascend through the uterus and fallopian tubes into the peritoneal cavity. Bacterial pelvic infection becomes a serious problem when it is not treated early with the proper antibiotic. Delay in diagnosis or treatment may result in chronic pelvic disease, the need for surgical intervention, and permanent infertility. Thus, the importance of early diagnosis and effective treatment of genital tract infections cannot be overstressed.

## VAGINAL INFECTIONS

The normal vaginal ecology depends on a delicate physiologic balance of hormonal and bacterial interaction. Four factors that work in harmonious action to accomplish this are (1) normal estrogen secretion, which maintains (2) a thick, protective squamous epithelium containing glycogen contributing to the growth of (3) Döderlein's bacilli (lactobacilli), which metabolize glycogen to form (4) lactic acid, which maintains the normal vaginal acidity at a pH of 4.0-

5.0. Disruption of any of these factors causes changes in the normal vaginal environment and predisposes to infection.

Other influences that affect the occurrence of vaginal infections are:

- Age of the patient: Premenarchal and postmenopausal women do not produce sufficient estrogen to maintain the glycogen-rich vaginal epithelium. The epithelium is thin and the vaginal pH is alkaline, leaving the vagina vulnerable to infection.
- Pregnancy: Due to increased hormone production during pregnancy there is an overabundance of vaginal glycogen, increased physiologic vaginal discharge, and local tissue edema from increased vascularity. These normal changes make vaginal infections more common during pregnancy.
- Menstruation: The nutrient value of the menstrual flow, in conjunction with the alkaline environment caused by the presence of blood, makes a favorable growth medium for pathologic bacteria.

Vaginal infections continue to be one of the most common complaints of women seeking health care. Factors that may be responsible for the increasing incidence are:

- Increased use of oral contraceptives causing change in the normal physiology of the vagina
- Increased sexual activity of the younger population
- Decreased use of condoms for contraception and prevention of venereal transmission of infection
- Increased use of antibiotics causing change in vaginal flora

Although trichomoniasis and *Hemophilus vaginalis* vaginitis are sexually transmitted diseases they are included in this section because of their common occurrence and their method of diagnosis is the same as discussed for other infections included in this section.

## CANDIDIASIS (MONILIASIS)

### Definition

Candidiasis is inflammation of the vagina caused by a fungus of the genus *Candida*.

## Etiology

*Candida albicans* is a yeastlike fungus formerly called *Monilia albicans*. It is a common ingredient of soil, vegetation, and many dairy products. Vaginal cultures reveal its occurrence in 4-6% of nonpregnant women and in 10-30% of pregnant women. It is considered a common vaginal and rectal inhabitant, and infection is attributed to a change in host resistance rather than to a contagious factor.

Infection is caused by alteration of the vaginal environment by increasing its glycogen content or by changing its normal acid pH to an alkaline pH. Predisposing factors include:

- Pregnancy
- Diabetes
- Oral contraceptive use
- Frequent douching
- Allergic reactions
- Antibiotic therapy
- Metronidazole (Flagyl) therapy
- Excessive carbohydrate intake
- Psychogenic problems
- Obesity
- Poor hygiene practices
- Debilitation
- Hypoparathyroidism

## Clinical Features

### Symptoms

- Leukorrhea
- Moderate to severe pruritus
- Burning and frequency of urination
- Dyspareunia (painful intercourse)
- Onset before the menses with aggravation during menses

*Signs*

- Vulvar erythema, edema, and excoriation from scratching
- White curdlike, odorless discharge found in the labial folds
- Reddened, irritated vaginal mucosa
- Thrush patches adherent to vaginal mucosa that bleed when scraped (12% of patients only)
- Vaginal pH of 4.0-4.7

## Differential Diagnosis

- Vaginal infection from bacteria or viruses
- Venereal disease
- Cervicitis
- Uterine infection
- Allergic reaction
- Foreign body in the vagina
- Sexual or social problems
- Tumors of the vagina or uterus
- Pinworms

## Diagnostic Studies as Clinically Indicated

Before collecting specimens be sure the patient has used no intravaginal medication, contraceptive foam, or diaphragm jelly, and has not douched in the past 48 hours.

- A 10-20% KOH (dissolves cellular debris) wet mount shows branching pseudomycelia, yeast buds of *Candida,* and an increased number of leukocytes.
- An isotonic saline or Ringer's wet mount shows no trichomonads or "clue cells" (epithelial cells with a stippled or granulated surface).
- A Gram stained smear shows gram-positive pseudohyphae and yeast buds.
- Sabouraud's or Nickerson's culture medium grows colonies within 48 hours at room temperature.
- A culture for *Neisseria gonorrhoeae* on Thayer-Martin medium is indicated.

- Urine is tested with a dipstick for glucose. If it is positive for glucose, check the patient's family history of diabetes and follow-up with a fasting blood sugar, two-hour postprandial blood sugar test, or a glucose tolerance test.

## Management and Treatment as Clinically Indicated

- Consult or refer to a physician as necessary.
- Clotrimazole vaginal tablets (Gyne-Lotrimin): One tablet is inserted at bedtime for seven days.
- Miconazole nitrate cream (Monistat): One applicatorful is inserted at bedtime for seven days.
- Nystatin vaginal tablets (Mycostatin or Nilstat): One tablet (100,000 units) is inserted twice a day for two weeks.
- Nystatin cream or Mycolog Cream (nystatin, neomycin, gramicidin, and triamcinolone acetonide) is applied twice a day for three to five days for relief of vulvar irritation. *Use Mycolog Cream with caution in pregnant patients, since it contains a corticosteroid.*
- Candicidin vaginal ointment (Candeptin or Vanobid): One applicatorful is inserted at bedtime for two weeks.
- Gentipax tampons: One tampon is inserted in the vagina twice a day for seven days; or for severe discomfort, a 1-2% solution of gentian violet painted on the vagina during clinic visits daily or every other day will offer quick relief from itching. Caution the patient about staining of clothing and about the need to wear a perineal pad. *This treatment may cause chemical irritation.*
- Vinegar douche: Two tablespoonfuls to 1 quart of lukewarm water is used once daily for one week.
- Povidone-iodine douche (Betadine): Two tablespoonfuls to 1 quart of lukewarm water is used once daily for one week.
- Cultured plain yogurt: One applicatorful or 2 tablespoonfuls are inserted twice daily (*Lactobacillus acidophilus* contained in the yogurt restores lactobacilli to the vagina.)
- Acidophilus tablets: One tablet is inserted at bedtime for one to two weeks (may be obtained in a health food store).
- Aci-Jel Therapeutic Vaginal Jelly: One applicatorful is inserted twice a day for three weeks to restore acidity to the vagina.
- Premarin Vaginal Cream: One applicatorful is inserted at bedtime for 10 days for atrophic changes in the postmenopausal patient.

## Complications

- A superimposed bacterial or viral vaginal infection may occur.
- Chronic dermatitis of the skin on the vulva and thighs may occur from irritation by the vaginal discharge.
- Infection of the mother at parturition may predispose the neonate to develop skin and/or mucous membrane infection and, rarely, serious systemic candidiasis
- Balantitis (infection of the glans penis) in the male sexual partner may occur.

## Patient Teaching

(for care of current infection and prevention of a recurrence)

- Discuss with the patient the nature, predisposing factors, and treatment of the infection.
- Advise warm sitz baths for patients with vulvar irritation.
- Advise the patient to practice good personal hygiene with frequent bathing and hand washing. Cleansing from front to back after a bowel movement prevents vaginal contamination.
- Advise against wearing pantyhose and clothes that fit tightly in the crotch. Loose-fitting cotton underwear is porous and retains less moisture and heat than polyester underwear.
- Advise against using feminine hygiene sprays, bath oils, or strong soaps on the vulva or in the vagina; they may cause allergy or irritation.
- Stress the importance of continuing the ordered medication throughout the menstrual cycle and of not stopping treatment when symptoms disappear.
- Suggest to patients with chronic or recurrent infections to use the medication at bedtime 7-10 days before the menses.
- Advise the patient to refrain from intercourse during treatment or to use a condom.
- Caution against reinfection from contact with fomites such as bath towels, soiled clothing, and used douche tips.
- Discuss with the patient the correct method of douching and caution her against its daily use except when infection is present. Once-a-week douching using a vinegar solution when no infection is present is adequate; overuse can cause drying and changes in the normal vaginal environment.
- Advise oral contraceptive users with recurrent or chronic infection that they may need to consider an alternative birth control method.

GYNECOLOGIC INFECTIONS

## TRICHOMONIASIS

### Definition

Trichomoniasis is inflammation of the vagina caused by a parasitic protozoa and is considered the most common of all vaginal infections.

### Etiology

*Trichomonas vaginalis,* the causative organism, may affect the vagina, Skene's glands, Bartholin's glands, and lower genitourinary tract of women and the prostate gland in men. The protozoa feeds on the vaginal mucosa and ingests bacteria and leukocytes. During menstruation the blood in the vagina causes a rise in pH to 6.0-6.5, producing a favorable environment in which the organism will grow. Emotional stress may also predispose to infection by causing physiologic change in the vaginal environment. Many patients are asymptomatic and are possible carriers of the infection, which is transmitted sexually. The role of fomites such as toilet seats, washcloths, and douche tips in transmission of infection is questionable.

### Clinical Features

#### Symptoms

- Profuse leukorrhea is common.
- Pruritus of the vulva and vagina occurs when acute infection is present.
- Urinary symptoms of frequency, urgency, and dysuria are common in the patient and in her sexual partner.
- Dyspareunia occurs from sensitivity of the infected vaginal mucosa to friction.
- A feeling of fullness in the genitals results from increased vascularity of the tissue and vulvar edema.

#### Signs

(usually follow the menses)

- Copious greenish-gray vaginal discharge, which is usually malodorous and may be frothy ($CO_2$ from carbohydrate metabolism of the trichomonad), is present.

- Diffuse vaginal and vulvar inflammation and edema is common.
- "Strawberry patches" may be evident in the vagina or on the cervical portio.
- Inflammation of the Skene's, Bartholin's glands, and the urethral meatus may occur.
- Pain, which is dull and poorly localized and may be felt in the lower abdomen, is a rare finding.
- A thin, gray pseudomembrane that cannot be wiped away is sometimes found in the vagina.
- Swollen inguinal nodes (inguinal adenopathy) may be palpable.
- Alkalinity of the vagina occurs with a pH of 5.0-5.5.

## Differential Diagnosis

- Vaginal infection from bacteria, yeast, viruses, or allergens
- Sexually transmitted disease from other organisms
- Uterine infection
- Cervicitis
- Urinary tract infection

## Diagnostic Studies as Clinically Indicated

- A warm isotonic saline wet mount specimen should be collected from the vagina rather than from the cervix for increased reliability. It should be examined as soon after preparation as possible for positive identification of the motile, flagellated, undulating trichomonad. When cold, the organism stops moving and is difficult to differentiate from a white blood cell since it assumes a rounded shape.
- A KOH wet mount is done to exclude *Candida albicans.*
- Urine is tested with a dipstick for pH and glucose.
- A culture for *Neisseria gonorrhoeae* is collected on Thayer-Martin (TM) or Transgrow transport medium.
- A Pap smear is indicated if one has not been done in the past year. (Cytologic reporting of trichomonads is only 60-80% reliable.)
- A sedimented urine specimen may reveal the trichomonad when examined microscopically.
- A WBC is indicated after treatment with Flagyl. It is especially important before retreatment with the drug is considered.

## Management and Treatment as Clinically Indicated

- Consult with a physician when necessary.
- Metronidazole (Flagyl), 2 g, is given orally at one time (eight 250-mg tablets) to the patient and her partner. *This treatment is contraindicated in pregnant and lactating women since the drug passes the placental barrier and is excreted in mother's milk.* Teratogenic effects are unknown.
- When Flagyl is contraindicated, a "shotgun" approach to treatment may achieve a 50% cure. It involves treating the male partner with Flagyl and using a topical method of treatment in the patient for two weeks. Some spontaneous eradication may also occur during this time.
- Povidone-iodine douche (Betadine): Two tablespoonfuls to a quart of lukewarm water is used once daily until the infection clears. OR
- Povidone-iodine vaginal gel (Betadine): One applicatorful is inserted at bedtime for two weeks. OR
- Aci-Jel Therapeutic Vaginal Jelly: One applicatorful is inserted twice daily for three weeks to restore vaginal acidity.
- Floraquin Vaginal Suppositories: Two suppositories are inserted at bedtime for two weeks.
- Topical steroid cream (Mycolog) may be used sparingly three times a day for relief of severe vulvar irritation. *Use with caution in pregnant patients since it contains a corticosteroid.*

## Complications

- Vaginal candidiasis resulting from treatment with Flagyl may occur. Also, Flagyl therapy adversely affects the response to nystatin treatment for infection due to *Candida*. *This infection should be ruled out before oral treatment is begun.*
- A decrease in the WBC to below 5,000 cells/cu mm. (leukopenia) may occur after treatment with Flagyl, but the count usually returns to normal when the drug is discontinued.
- Trichomonal urethritis, cystitis, or bartholinitis may occur.
- Chronic cervicitis with repeated trichomonal infection may predispose to malignant transformation. Cytologic reports of a Class II Pap smear with inflammatory atypical cells is common.
- Acute trichomoniasis is often associated with vaginal flora harboring pathogenic bacteria such as enterocci, staphylococci, *vaginalis*, coliform organisms, gonococci, and *Bacteroides*.

- Prostatitis or nonspecific urethritis may result from infection of the male partner.
- Reversible sterility may occur from toxicity of the parasite inhibiting sperm motility (probably a rare phenomenon).

### Patient Teaching

- Advise that Flagyl should be taken simultaneously by both partners for optimum effectiveness.
    Alcohol consumption is contraindicated when taking this medication due to its Antabuse effect.
    The drug may cause anorexia, unpleasant taste in the mouth, nausea, diarrhea, abdominal cramping, headache, vomiting, or dizziness.
- Advise the patient with multiple sexual partners that systemic treatment is of little value since reinfection might occur. Local treatment with vaginal medications and use of a condom by the partner is recommended.
- Advise the patient to refrain from intercourse during treatment or to use a condom.
- Advise the patient against using vaginal tampons since they block the passage of air into the vagina, which helps destroy the organism; they also absorb any vaginal medication.
- Inform the patient that a strongly acidic douche (2 tablespoonfuls of vinegar to 1 quart of warm water) immediately after intercourse with an infected male may be helpful in preventing infection.
- Inform the patient that reinfection may occur after local treatment since the organism remains in 96% of the extravaginal sites such as the paraurethral glands, urethra, and endocervix.
- Explain that eating one container of cultured plain yogurt every day during antibiotic therapy may prevent gastric upset.

## *HEMOPHILUS* VAGINITIS OR *CORYNEBACTERIUM* VAGINITIS (NONSPECIFIC VAGINITIS)

### Definition

*Hemophilus* vaginitis is inflammation of the vagina caused by the bacterium *Hemophilus vaginalis*.

## Etiology

The organism, *H. vaginalis,* is a pleomorphic (many-shaped), gram-negative, non-motile bacillus that grows best in a low-oxygen atmosphere. This bacillus does not fit into either the genus *Hemophilus* or the genus *Corynebacterium;* its proper classification has yet to be determined. When a vaginal infection cannot be identified as candidiasis or trichomoniasis, it is diagnosed as "nonspecific" or "*Hemophilus* vaginitis."

Transmission of the infection is probably through sexual contact, with its incidence high in populations identified with other sexually transmitted diseases. Both partners are frequently infected, and the *Hemophilus* organism has been isolated from 79% of the male partners of infected women. Ten to forty percent of the women are asymptomatic.

## Clinical Features

### Symptoms

- Malodorous leukorrhea (the most common symptom)
- Pruritus from irritation of the vaginal discharge
- Erythema of the vulva and vagina (may be slight or absent)

### Signs

- A grayish-green, thin, pasty discharge (which may be blood-streaked and malodorous) adhering to the vaginal wall
- Inflammation and irritation of the vaginal tissue and introitus
- A rare gross infection of the vagina
- A vaginal pH of 5.0–5.5
- No relationship of infection to the menses

## Differential Diagnosis

- Vaginal infection from a nonsexually related cause
- Sexually transmitted infection
- Cervicitis
- Uterine infection or tumor
- Foreign body in the posterior fornix (tampon, diaphragm)

## Diagnostic Studies as Clinically Indicated

- A Pap smear should be done to rule out inflammatory changes.
- A KOH wet mount shows no branching pseudomycelia (characteristic of *Candida*).
- An isotonic saline wet mount shows no trichomonads.
- An isotonic saline wet mount shows "clue cells," which are epithelial cells with a stippled or granulated effect caused by bacilli adhering to the cell surface. Many leukocytes may be present, but lactobacilli are conspicuously absent after the first week of infection.
- A Gram stain, the diagnostic method of choice by many, reveals fine gram-negative bacilli with rounded ends in short chains, "school of fish," or granular cornified cells.
- Proteose Peptone #3 (Difco) or modified Stuart's medium (Amies) transport medium may be used for laboratory culture.
- A culture for *Neisseria gonorrhoeae* should be done because more than one sexually transmitted disease may be present at the same time.
- A blood sample for a VDRL test should be collected when indicated.

## Management and Treatment as Clinically Indicated

- Consult with a physician as indicated.
- Treatment of the sexual partner is important.
- Systemic treatment

    Metronidazole (Flagyl), 500 mg, is given orally twice a day for seven days to the patient and her partner. *This treatment is contraindicated in pregnancy* (see the patient teaching section for trichomoniasis). OR

    Ampicillin, 500 mg, is given orally every six hours for seven days to the patient and her partner. *Check for penicillin allergy.* This treatment may mask the presence of gonorrhea or syphilis; rule out these infections before treatment. OR

    Tetracycline, 250 mg, is given orally every six hours for seven days to the patient and her partner. *This treatment is contraindicated in pregnant and lactating women because of possible retardation of fetal skeletal development and permanent discoloration of the teeth.* OR

    Cephalexin (Keflex), 50 mg, is given orally every six hours for six days
- Local treatment

    Triple sulfa cream (Sultrin): One applicatorful is inserted into the vagina twice a day for two weeks. Check for sulfa allergy. OR

Sulfanilamide and aminacrine hydrochloride cream (AVC): One applicatorful is inserted into the vagina twice a day for two weeks. Check for sulfa allergy. *Note:* The February 1980 FDA Drug Bulletin (p 6) states: "there is no adequate evidence that sulfanilamide and sulfisoxazole vaginal creams are effective in treating vaginitis caused by *Candida albicans, Trichomonas vaginalis,* and *Hemophilus vaginalis.*" However, the FDA is requesting manufacturers to review the studies that have shown these findings "so that a determination can be made on whether *H. vaginalis* vaginitis can be included as an indication in the labeling or whether additional studies are needed."

Vagitrol suppositories: One suppository is inserted twice a day for two weeks.

Nitrofurazone vaginal suppositories (Furacin): One suppository is inserted twice a day for two weeks.

Povidone-iodine vaginal gel (Betadine): One applicatorful is inserted twice a day for two weeks.

Terramycin vaginal tablets: One tablet is inserted at bedtime for one week.

Povidone-iodine douche (Betadine): Two tablespoons to 1 quart of lukewarm water is used once daily for one week.

Vinegar douche: Two tablespoons to 1 quart of lukewarm water is used once daily for one week.

Nystatin vaginal suppositories (Mycostatin, 1,000,000 units) may be used twice a day for two weeks prophylactically to prevent infection due to *Candida* when systemic treatment is given.

## Complications

- Superimposed viral or bacterial infection
- Vaginal candidiasis from oral antibiotic therapy or long-term use of terramycin vaginal tablets

## Patient Teaching

- Tell the patient what her infection is and how it is to be treated.
- Discuss the use of Flagyl. (Its use and side effects are discussed in the section on trichomoniasis.)
- Advise the patient for whom tetracycline has been prescribed to take the medication one hour before or two hours after meals. Food and some dairy products interfere with its absorption.

- Advise the patient to continue treatment through the menstrual period.
- Stress good personal hygiene and the need to cleanse from front to back after a bowel movement.
- Advise the patient to avoid sexual intercourse during the treatment or to use a condom until treatment is complete.
- Suggest the use of a perineal (mini) pad when vaginal creams or suppositories have been ordered.
- Advise the patient that her male partner will need treatment if urethral organisms are isolated, or she may be reinfected.
- Explain that eating one container of cultured plain yogurt every day during antibiotic therapy may prevent gastric upset and secondary yeast infection of the vagina.

## ATROPHIC VAGINITIS

### Definition

Atrophic vaginitis is a nonspecific inflammation of the vagina resulting from decreased estrogen stimulation to the vaginal mucosa.

### Etiology

Atrophic changes of the vagina and vulva occur postmenopausally. The amount of atrophy depends on the degree of estrogen deficiency and differs from woman to woman. Little atrophy occurs when estrogen production is adequate to maintain the acid pH of the vagina. In women not producing sufficient estrogen, the pH of the vagina becomes alkaline and results in thining of the vaginal mucosa, rendering it susceptible to trauma and infection.

### Clinical Features

#### Symptoms
- Bloody vaginal staining is the most common symptom.
- Pruritus, burning, and tenderness may occur from irritation or bacterial effect on atrophic tissue.

- A thin, scant vaginal discharge is common.
- Dysuria may occur from a bladder infection or atrophic change of the urethra.
- Contraction and dryness of the vagina may cause painful intercourse.

*Signs*

(Many of the signs listed are changes that occur normally in the postmenopausal state.)

- Sparce and brittle pubic hair
- Shrinking or disappearance of the labia minus
- Atrophy of the glans clitoris
- Pale vagina with few, or decreased, rugae
- Shrinking and dryness of the vaginal mucous membrane
- Vaginal pH of 5.5-7.0
- Thinning, excoriation, or fissuring of the vulvar tissue
- Narrowing and rigidity of introitus
- Development of localized areas of vaginitis in the posterior fornix and around the urethral orifice

## Differential Diagnosis

- Vaginal infections from bacteria, yeast, or viruses
- Venereal disease
- Irritation, trauma, or allergic reactions
- White lesions (leukoplakia, lichen sclerosis)
- Malignancy
- Atropic cervicitis
- Postmenopausal bleeding from other causes

## Diagnostic Studies as Clinically Indicated

- The history taking is to include questions about symptoms of menopause, hormone therapy, and history of vaginal bleeding.
- A Pap smear is done to rule out cervical changes.
- A saline wet mount is done to rule out trichomoniasis.
- KOH wet mount is done to rule out candidiasis.

- A specimen for culture of *Neisseria gonorrhoeae* should be collected on Thayer-Martin (TM) or Transgrow transport medium.
- A urinalysis is done to check for WBCs, bacteria, pH, and glucose.
- A maturation index (MI) shows a predominance of parabasal cells with few superficial squamous cells. (This test is not of great diagnostic value since it does not correlate with menopausal symptoms.)
- Any suspicious looking areas of the vagina, vulva, or cervix should be stained with Shiller's solution or toluidine blue, and a biopsy should be taken of negative staining areas.

## Management and Treatment as Clinically Indicated

- Physician consultation is necessary.
- Local treatment: Estrogen creams will cause thickening of the vaginal epithelium and decrease pruritus. However, these creams must be used carefully since systemic absorption may stimulate uterine bleeding or may produce other side effects

    Premarin Cream: One applicatorful is inserted into the vagina at bedtime for one or two weeks for symptom relief, then 1 applicatorful is inserted two to three times a week to maintain the vaginal mucosa. OR

    Dienestrol Cream: One or two applicatorfuls are inserted into the vagina at bedtime for 7-10 days, then one-half applicatorful is inserted once or twice a week. OR

    AVC/Dienestrol Cream or Suppositories: One applicatorful or 1 suppository is inserted intravaginally once or twice daily.

    *Note:* The use of topical estrogen creams in patients for whom estrogen is contraindicated is now under scrutiny. A recent study by Martin et al. (1979, p 2699) confirms previous studies which show that ". . . estrogens applied locally in the vagina are absorbed systemically with rapidity and efficiency. Within 12 hours of the first vaginal cream application, serum estrogen reached levels that are normal for the follicular phase in ovulating women." It would appear that contraindications to estrogen be considered before using topical estrogen creams.

- Systemic estrogen treatment may be given depending on the patient's history, physical examination, severity of symptoms, and consideration of contraindications. With fully informed consent the patient should be able to make a decision about use of the drug. Two commonly used estrogens are:

    Premarin, 1.25 mg/day, is given orally for three weeks, then one week off in a cyclic fashion. Reassessment of the dose level downward should be done at least yearly. OR

Diethylstilbestrol, 0.5-2.0 mg/day, is given orally in a cyclic fashion as above.

For contraindications of systemic estrogen use see Chapter 16.

## Complications

- Vulvovaginitis from bacterial, fungal, allergic, traumatic or psychogenic cause
- Bacterial urethritis or cystitis
- Vulvar fissuring
- Labial or vaginal adhesions

## Patient Teaching

- Discuss the etiology, symptoms, and treatment of atrophic vaginitis.
- Stress good personal hygiene to prevent future vaginal infections by keeping the vulva clean and dry and by wiping from front to back after bowel movements.
- Explain that scratching can create superimposed infection.
- Discuss the need for lubrication (K-Y gel, saliva, or vegetable oil) during intercourse to prevent friction and trauma to the vaginal mucosa.
- Instruct the patient on the method of vaginal cream insertion.
- Encourage the patient to return for regular medical check-ups, with a Pap smear every six months. Be sure the patient understands that any vaginal bleeding is indication for immediate evaluation by a physician.

# VULVAR INFECTIONS
# (PRURITUS VULVAE)

## Definition

Pruritus vulvae is itching of the female external genitalia for which relief is instinctively attempted by scratching. Rather than a disease, it is a symptom common to many health problems and is caused by a variety of conditions.

## Etiology

Single or multiple conditions causing itching may include:

- Underlying systemic illness such as diabetes, psoriasis, thyroid dysfunction, leukemia, cancer
- Bacterial, fungal, viral, or allergic vaginitis
- Parasitic infestation
- Contact dermatitis from polyester underwear, female deodorants, douche powders, perfumed soap and toilet tissue, contraceptive creams, rubber, exposure to industrial chemicals
- Urinary incontinence or infection
- Poor hygiene
- Postmenopause or surgical menopausal sensitivity
- Hemorrhoids
- Psychogenic causes
- Reaction to systemically administered drugs
- Radiation therapy
- Drug withdrawal (heroin, methadone)
- Malnutrition (causes decreased bactericidal activity of leukocytes)
    Vitamin A, B, or C deficiencies
    Iron-deficiency anemia, which causes
    1. Dry vulvar tissue
    2. Fissuring at the angles of the mouth
- Fox-Fordyce disease
    Rare, chronic intensely pruritic skin disease, cause unknown
    Found in women during reproductive years
    Precipitated by emotional upset, clears spontaneously

## Clinical Features

*Symptoms*

- Vulvar itching and/or burning
- Sensitivity of the skin
- Pain from lesions or excoriations

## GYNECOLOGIC INFECTIONS

*Signs*

- Erythema of tissue
- Excoriated papules
- Fissures, crusts, wheals, scaling
- Lesions on other body surfaces (may indicate systemic problems)
- Secondary infection of lesions

### Management and Treatment as Clinically Indicated

- Treat the underlying cause of itching.
- Discontinue previous medication used in treatment of the pruritus.
- Rule out reaction to a systemically administered drug or local irritant.
- Take a diet history and refer the patient for counseling if necessary.
- Take a sexual and social history
- Biopsy should be performed on suspicious lesions.

### Patient Teaching

- To help the patient decrease itching and to avoid exacerbation advise her to
    Keep the skin clean and dry
    Avoid tight clothing and polyester underwear
    Avoid scratching and frequent and vigorous washing
    Avoid using feminine hygiene sprays, bath oils, or strong soaps on the vulva or in the vagina
    Take warm sitz baths for vulvar irritation

## FOLLICULITIS, FURUNCULOSIS

### Definition

Folliculitis is a local papular or pustular inflammation of the hair follicle. Furunculosis (boil) is a local pyogenic infection involving the perifollicular tissue.

## Etiology

Hair follicles in the genital region are prone to infection because the area is moist and easily traumatized. Pathogenic bacteria enter the skin when it is irritated by friction or scratching. The majority of infections are caused by *Staphylococcus aureus* organisms entering the hair follicle when the following conditions exist:

- Pediculosis pubis
- An ingrown hair
- Diabetes
- A prior lesion or trauma

## Clinical Features

### Symptoms

- Pain and irritation
- Itching

### Signs

- Lesions occur in hairy areas of outer labia majora and mons veneris.
- Lesions may be multiple and vary in size.
- Infected follicles are initally firm but progress to become fluctuant.
- Inguinal adenopathy may be present.
- Lesions are tender and inflamed.

## Differential Diagnosis

- Venereal lesions
- Impetigo
- Insect bites
- Foreign object with secondary infection
- Molluscum contagiosum

## Diagnostic Studies as Clinically Indicated

- Culture of the lesion is done when identification of the organism is necessary.

## Management and Treatment as Clinically Indicated

- Consult or refer to a physician as necessary.
- Wash the area with soap and water.
- Remove ingrown hairs when present.
- Treatment of folliculitis.
    Apply hot compresses four times a day for 20 minutes.
    Apply antibiotic ointment such as gentamicin (Garamycin). 0.1% topically.
- Treatment of furunculosis:
    Apply hot compresses six times a day until the furuncle is fluctuant. It is then ready for incision and drainage. System antibiotic therapy may be necessary depending on the extent of infection.

## Complications

- Carbuncle
- Recurrence of the infection
- Bacteremia
- Cellulitis

## Patient Teaching

- Explain the cause of the infection.
- Stress the importance of keeping the area clean and dry.
- Teach the patient the method of applying hot compresses.
- Encourage the patient not to scratch the lesions, a superimposed infection might occur.
- Tell the patient not to squeeze the lesions. Further tissue injury or superimposed infection may result.
- Encourage the patient to inspect the vulvar hair frequently to be sure no hairs are growing inward into the tissue.

## BARTHOLINITIS
## (BARTHOLIN ADENITIS)

### Definition

Bartholinitis is an acute or chronic inflammation of the vulvovaginal Bartholin's glands. The Bartholin's glands are two pea- to bean-sized glands located beneath the vestibule, one on either side of the opening at the base of the labia majus. They secrete a clear, odorless mucus for lubrication of the vaginal orifice and canal.

### Etiology

The most common infecting organism is *Neisseria gonorrhoeae,* but other organisms such as *Staphylococcus, Streptococcus, Escherichia coli, trichomonads,* and *Bacteroides* may be involved. Unilateral acute infection arises from the duct of the gland, not from the gland itself. The lumen of the ducts are narrow and allow pyogenic organisms to become trapped in the passages causing infection.

In chronic inflammation of a gland, cysts may form. These postinflammatory pseudocysts cause permanent partial or complete closure of the duct. Accumulation and retention of mucus produced by the gland causes it to enlarge and become painful.

### Clinical Features

*Symptoms*

- Acute infection
    Unilateral swelling of the labia over the infection site
    Extreme tenderness and throbbing
    Dyspareunia
    Pain when walking or sitting
- Chronic infection
    Symptoms may persist for years, or no symptoms may exist.

Recurrent episodes of abscess formation may occur.
History of a prior acute infection may be lacking.

*Signs*

- Acute infection
  Inflammation and swelling of the labia
  Purplish discoloration and stretching of the skin
  Purulent discharge from the duct (expressed or spontaneous)
  Palpable, tender inguinal nodes
- Chronic infection
  A small, nontender nodule palpable deep in the posterior labia majora (can be rolled between the examining fingers)

## Differential Diagnosis

- Inclusion cyst
- Sebaceous cyst
- Primary cancer of Bartholin's gland or duct
- Secondary metastatic malignancy in vulvovaginal area

## Diagnostic Studies as Clinically Indicated

- History taking to establish a history of prior infection
- Inspection and palpation of vulvar swelling
- Culture of the discharge to identify infecting organism

## Management and Treatment as Clinically Indicated

- Physician consultation is necessary.
- An acute infection usually heals within a week. If the infection is not eradicated, it may remain as a source of chronic inflammation. Treatment is as follows:
  Bed rest is prescribed for patient comfort and prevention of irritation to the swollen gland from walking or sitting.

Symptom relief may be obtained by the application of heat by compresses or sitz baths. The application of heat will also increase the circulation to the infection and speed its consolidation.

Analgesics are given for pain relief.

Appropriate antibiotics should be given when inflammation is present.

Incision and drainage of the abscess offers temporary relief from pain, but obstruction tends to recur. Use of a Wurm catheter in the abscess cavity keeps it open and draining while healing, but it does not guarantee against recurrence.
- Chronic cysts may be small and asymptomatic and require no treatment. When acute repeated episodes of infection occur surgical intervention is indicated. This may include:

    Surgical excision of the cyst to remove the infection site

    Marsupialization of the cyst: When quiescent, an incision is made into the cyst and the edges of the cyst wall are sutured to the skin. This forms a pouch, which heals gradually by granulation, and prevents further episodes of infection.

## Complications

- Chronic bartholinitis
- Abscess formation with edema of entire labium
- Cellulitis of surrounding tissue
- Emotional and physical stress to the patient

## Patient Teaching

- Describe the process of the infection to the patient and discuss its acute and chronic aspects.
- Refer to the patient teaching section for gonorrhea if this disease is diagnosed.
- Explain the treatment to be used and its probable outcome. If the patient's infection is acute she will have to wait for healing before more permanent treatment. If a chronic cyst remains but does not cause further problems, future treatment may be unnecessary.
- Allow time for the patient to ask questions and to express her concerns.

## MOLLUSCUM CONTAGIOSUM

### Definition

Molluscum contagiosum is a benign viral infection that causes proliferation of the vulvar skin resembling a localized neoplasm.

### Etiology

The lesions are probably caused by a large virus of the pox group, but laboratory confirmation has not been established. Molluscum bodies containing viral inclusion bodies are seen within the epithelial cells of the lesion. This infection was formerly found primarily in children, with the lesions distributed widely over the body. Presently, infections caused by molluscum contagiosum are being found in the warm, moist genital areas of sexually active people. Its incubation period is from three to eight weeks. Infection is believed to be transmitted by direct or indirect contact, with sexual contact a possible factor; its incidence is believed to be more common than heretofore realized.

### Clinical Features

#### Symptoms
- Pruritus may be the only symptom.

#### Signs
- Individual painless lesions begin as seedlings 1-2 mm in diameter and grow over months from pinhead size to 1 cm in diameter. Lesions are usually multiple, varying in number from 1 to 20 in a haphazard distribution. They appear as dome-shaped, wavy papules with a central depression containing keratonized cells infected with the virus. The material within the lesion is semifluid caseous matter that can be expressed with pressure.
- Lesions are commonly found on the face, eyelids, breasts, vulva, and inner surface of the thigh.

## Differential Diagnosis

- Syphilitic chancre
- Vulvar folliculitis
- Bacterial skin infection
- Herpesvirus hominis type 2 infection

## Diagnostic Studies as Clinically Indicated

- Collect a Pap smear specifically for molluscum bodies from the central depression of the lesion.
- Collect specimens for culture of *Neisseria gonorrhoeae* and for the VDRL test to rule out other sexually transmitted disease.

## Management and Treatment as Clinically Indicated

- Consult with a physician as necessary.
- A thin coat of cantharidin (Cantharone) is used to coat each lesion. The patient returns in one week, and new lesions are treated. Resistant lesions are coated with the medication and are covered with a piece of tape that is to be removed in six to eight hours. *This medication may produce blisters if spilled on skin or mucous membranes* and should be wiped off immediately with acetone or alcohol, then washed with soap and water. OR
- The lesions are opened, their contents expressed, and the base scraped. Nevitol (trichloroacetic acid) is applied to the lesion cavity. OR
- The individual papule is removed with a dermal curette, and the cavity is painted with Monsel's solution (a liquid astringent of ferric subsulfate, sold over the counter).

## Complications

- Secondary infection with suppuration and breakdown that may cause ulcerations

## Patient Teaching

- Explain what the papules are and the possible mode of transmission.
- Suggest that the patient examine her sexual partner for similar lesions, which may need examination and treatment.
- Explain the method of treatment to be used, and that further treatment may be needed as new lesions occur.
- Stress the need for good personal hygiene to prevent further infection. Bathing the genitals before and after sexual intercourse is helpful in preventing infections.
- Tell the patient to return if the infection continues or if secondary infection occurs.

# TINEA CRURIS

## Definition

Tinea cruris is a well-delineated pink or red, scaly, superficial fungal skin infection. Synonyms include: trichophytosis vulvae, Eczema marginatum, tinea vulvae, and ringworm of the vulva.

## Etiology

Tinea cruris is caused by a variety of ringworms, especially *Epidermophyton floccosum,* and spreads by direct contact or contaminated clothing. Tight clothing and obesity, which produce a warm moist medium, favor growth of the organisms. It is known as "jock itch" in men.

## Clinical Features

### Symptom

- Mild to intense pruritus

### Signs

- Lesions are well-circumscribed erythematous patches with vesication, crusting, and scale formation.
- Lesions spread, coalesce, and tend to heal in the center as they enlarge.
- Lesions are located on the skin of the vulva, pubis, lower abdomen, groin, or inner thighs.
- Eruption of the lesions is usually asymmetric.
- Tissues are easily traumatized, excoriated, and fissured.
- Infection may recur, especially during the summer months.

## Differential Diagnosis

- Contact or seborrheic dermatitis
- Psoriasis
- Candidiasis
- Arythrasma (bacterial infection)
- Allergic reaction
- Psychogenic origin

## Diagnostic Studies as Clinically Indicated

- KOH (20%) wet mount of superficial scales from the skin shows branching mycelia; no conidia are seen.
- Culture of the scales on Sabouraud's medium grows the yeast.

## Management and Treatment as Clinically Indicated

- Tolnaftate 1% powder or powder aerosol (Tinactin) is applied twice a day for two to three weeks, but may be used for four to six weeks if necessary. (Tinactin also comes in solution and cream, but the powder is more effective for the moist vulvar area.) If this treatment does not cure, the diagnosis needs reevaluation. Tinactin is not an effective treatment for bacterial infections or candidiasis. OR
- Clotrimazole 1% (Gyne-Lotrimin cream or Lotrimin solution) is applied twice a day in the morning and evening. If infection is not cleared in four weeks, the

diagnosis should be re-evaluated. *This medication should not be used during the first trimester of pregnancy.* OR
- Pragmatar ointment (alcohol-coal tar distillate, sulfur and salicylic acid) is applied sparingly but thoroughly, to the affected area using caution around genitals. Wash with soap and water (rinse carefully) in 12 hours. *Apply ointment no more than once a day.* OR
- Whitfield's ointment (benzoic and salicylic acid) is applied to the affected area twice a day.
- Griseofulvin (Fulvicin U/F, Grifulvin V, Grisactin), 500 mg/per day, is given for two to four weeks, but longer treatment may be necessary. This drug is *used for chronic or resistant cases only.* An oral antibiotic, it reaches the skin keratin through the bloodstream. *Its safe use in pregnancy has not been established.* It may cause mild heartburn, nausea, headache, or diarrhea.

## Complications

- Scratch dermatitis
- Lichenification (hardening and thickening of the skin from constant irritation)
- Secondary bacterial infection
- Allergy to systemic or topical antifungal agent

## Patient Teaching

- Discuss the contagious nature of the infection with the patient. She needs to find out where it was contracted and to refer all contacts for treatment. All exposed clothing and bed linen should be thoroughly washed or dry cleaned.
- Discuss the importance of using the prescribed medication as directed for a more rapid cure. If redness or swelling of the skin occurs from use of the cream or lotion, discontinue its use. Carefully wash off all medication left on the skin, and call for advice.
- Stress the importance of keeping the infected area *dry.* Second to medical treatment this is the most important factor in discouraging growth of the fungus.
- Advise the patient to wear loose cotton underwear; it is cooler than polyester underwear and absorbs more moisture. Tight slacks prevents ventilation of the area and may cause irritation to the infected skin.

## CERVICAL INFECTION—CERVICITIS (TRACHELITIS)

### Definition

Cervicitis is an acute or chronic inflammation of the cervix. It is one of the most common gynecologic lesions, with a high percentage of parous women showing some evidence of infection.

### Etiology

The infection is usually bacterial with the gonococcus being the most common offender. Other organisms normally present in the vagina, or introduced from the outside, can also cause acute cervicitis when host resistance is low. Non-gonoccal infection is usually related to (1) recent trauma such as childbirth or abortion, (2) anal-vaginal contamination, and (3) diminished resistance to infection as in hypoestrogenism, hypovitaminosis, or irritation from the presence of a foreign body.

### Clinical Features

#### Symptoms

- Acute cervicitis
    - Profuse leukorrhea
    - Backache (lympangitis of uterosacral structures with referred pain to sacrum)
    - Bearing-down sensation in pelvic structures
    - Dull lower abdominal pain, dyspareunia, dysmenorrhea
    - Dysuria, urinary frequency, trigonitis (lymphatic spread)
    - Slight temperature elevation
- Chronic cervicitis
    - May be absent
    - Thick, tenacious, persistent leukorrhea
    - Spotting or bleeding after intercourse or douching
    - Vulvovaginitis resulting from irritating discharge
    - Metrorrhagia (hyperemia of cervix with increased bleeding surfaces)

*Signs*

- Acute cervicitis
  Cervical motion tenderness
  Profuse, white-to-yellowish, purulent, malodorous discharge from the endocervix
  Inflamed cervix, boggy, edematous
  A normal appearing portio and upper vagina (particularly with gonorrheal infection)
  Thick mucus packed with leukocytes in the cervical canal during preovulatory phase (normally thin and clear at this time)
  Vulvovaginal irritation
- Chronic cervicitis
  Ulcerated or normal-appearing cervix (there is no characteristic picture)
  Mucopurulent discharge from endocervix
  Ectropion (usually present)
  Nabothian cysts (retention cysts)

## Differential Diagnosis

- Cervical carcinoma
- Chronic vaginitis
- Salpingitis, parametritis
- Herpesvirus hominis infection, gonorrhea, syphilis, chancroid, granuloma venereum, chlamydial infection

## Diagnostic Studies as Clinically Indicated

- KOH and saline wet mount to rule out candidiasis or trichomoniasis
- Culture for *Neisseria gonorrhoeae* on Thayer-Martin (TM) or Transgrow transport medium
- Pap smear (may also be done for suspected herpetic infection)
- Bacteria smear for staphylococci, streptococci, *E coli, Chlamydia, Aerobacter aerogenes, Bacteroides*
- WBC (slightly elevated with a shift to the left)
- Hemoglobin and hematocrit

- Sedimentation rate to rule out chronic infection
- Schiller test if indicated
- Colposcopic examination
- Biopsy of suspicious lesions

## Management and Treatment as Clinically Indicated

- Physician consultation or referral as necessary
- Antibiotic therapy (see the section on treatment of gonorrhea)
- Antibiotic therapy for specific other bacteria
- Pelvic rest for acute infection (no instrumentation or topical treatment during acute phase before menses when spread of infection upward may occur)
- Specific therapy for associated vaginitis
- Prevention of recurrent vaginal infections to control chronic infection
- Aci-Jel Therapeutic Vaginal Jelly: 1 applicatorful inserted at bedtime for three weeks (will help to restore vaginal acidity)
- Cryosurgery, electrocauterization, or surgery

## Complications

- Salpingitis (especially in gonococcal infections and post-abortion patients)
- Pelvic cellulitis
- Pelvic congestion and parametritis
- Abortion of a pregnancy (ascending infection of the uterine decidua and placenta)
- Cervical dystocia (fibrosis and stenosis from chronic infection)
- Infertility (thick, viscid, acid, pus-ladened mucus kills sperm)
- Chronic urinary tract infections
- Dyspareunia (chronic undiagnosed endocervicitis)
- Polyp formation
- Causal relationship between chronic cervicitis and cervical carcinoma

### Patient Teaching

- Review with the patient the location of the infection using pictures or diagrams of the female pelvic organs for clarity.
- Refer to the patient teaching section for gonorrhea when counseling a patient with this diagnosis.
- Explain to the patient who does not have a gonococcal infection the type of bacteria causing her symptoms, when it is known, and its etiology.
- Impress upon the patient with an acute infection who is not to be hospitalized, the need for bed rest to prevent spread of infection to her uterus, fallopian tubes, or abdominal cavity.
- Tell the patient to avoid sexual intercourse until the infection has cleared, or advise the use of condom if abstinence is unlikely.
- Stress the necessity of using the prescribed oral antibiotic or local treatment as ordered to ensure optimum recovery.
- Explain the use of electrocautery or cryosurgery if one of these is to be used (see Chap. 17).
- Explain that with good treatment and follow-up cervical infections are usually cleared. If mild, the infection should clear in four to eight weeks; severe infections may take two to three months of treatment to clear fully.
- Stress the importance of Pap smears at least once a year.

## UTERINE INFECTION (ENDOMETRITIS)

### Definition

Endometritis is an acute or chronic inflammation of the endometrial lining of the uterus.

### Etiology

Infection is caused by invasion of the uterine endometrium by staphylococci, *E coli,* gonococci, or *Mycobacterium tuberculosis.* Predisposing factors include:

- Trauma to the uterus

- Therapeutic abortion
- Use of an IUD
- Retained products of conception after an abortion
- Sexual exposure to *Neisseria gonorrhoeae*
- Intrauterine instrumentation
- General physical debilitation
- Submucous leiomyoma
- Endometrial polyps
- Postmenopausal endometrial atrophy
- Prolonged rupture of the membranes during labor, prolonged labor, or frequent vaginal examinations

## Clinical Features

### Symptoms

- Acute infection
    An elevated temperature
    Low back and/or lower abdominal pain
    Malaise
    Dysmenorrhea
    Menorrhagia
- Chronic infection
    Scant, serosanguineous leukorrhea
    Symptoms as in acute infection but to a lesser degree
    Infertility

### Signs

- Acute infection
    Uterine tenderness on bimanual examination
    Leukorrhea, which may have foul odor
- Chronic infection
    Attenuation of infection after each menses (desquamation of the endometrium)
    Sterility

## Differential Diagnosis

- Pelvic adhesions
- Benign or malignant tumors
- Pelvic congestion
- Cystitis

## Diagnostic Studies as Clinically Indicated

- CBC, sedimentation rate, VDRL test
- Pap smear
- Cuture for *Neisseria gonorrhoeae* on Thayer-Martin (TM) or Transgrow transport medium
- Histologic examination of endometrial curettings (not usually done due to possible spread of infection resulting from endometrial instrumentation)
- Culture of menstrual blood if *M. tuberculosis* is suspected

## Management and Treatment as Clinically Indicated

- Physician consultation is necessary.
- Hospitalization may be indicated for severe acute infection.
- In acute infection it is necessary to determine if the cervix is patent to allow drainage from the uterus.
- Broad-spectrum antibiotic therapy may be indicated until a specific organism is identified by culture results.
- Pelvic rest is necessary to prevent spread of infection.
- An acute infection with an IUD in place should be treated with antibiotics before removal of the device.
- Chronic infection may clear spontaneously with successive menses due to endometrial shedding.
- A D&C for removal of retained products of conception post partum or post abortion may be necessary.
- A diet history or referral to a nutritionist is necessary for debilitated patients or for those with iron-deficiency anemia. Oral iron supplementation with ferrous sulfate (325 mg bid) is indicated in anemic patients. *Inform the patient her stools will be black from the iron supplement.*

## Complications

- Pelvic peritonitis
- Paralytic ileus
- Pelvic cellulitis
- Subinvolution of the uterus post abortion or post pregnancy
- Thrombophlebitis with possible emboli from puerperal infection

## Patient Teaching

- Explain to the patient the location of the infection, its possible cause, and treatment.
- Refer to the patient teaching section for gonorrhea if this organism has been identified as the causative organism.
- Explain to the patient who is to be hospitalized for acute infection, the need for complete bed rest and parental medication. The patient's future fertility may depend on preventing progress of the infection to the fallopian tubes and peritoneum.
- Stress to the patient being treated on an ambulatory basis the importance of taking the prescribed medication on time and the necessity to complete the entire course of medicine. She should remain on bed rest (with possible bathroom privileges) until the symptoms have cleared. If increased abdominal pain or temperature elevation occurs she should contact the practitioner as soon as possible.
- Assess the desire for pregnancy in patients who return with repeated endometrial infections. These patients need to know that with each infection their chance of future fertility is diminished. A sexual history with counseling may be indicated.

# PARASITIC INFESTATIONS (PEDICULOSIS PUBIS)

## Definition

Pediculosis pubis is an infestation of the vulvar hair by a louse. Usually it confines itself to the genital hair but may involve hair of the axilla, eyebrows, eyelashes, beard, or body.

## Etiology

The parasite, the *Phthirus pubis* or crab louse, attaches firmly to the base of the hair. It buries its head in the hair follicle where it lives on the host's blood. The ova(nits) are attached to the hair shaft and should not be confused with dandruff. Other lice infecting the body are *Pediculus humanis* var. *corporis* (body louse) and *P humanis* var. *capitis* (head louse). Predisposing factors include:

- Crowded living conditions
- Infrequent bathing or poor hygiene
- Sexual intercourse with an infected person
- Contaminated bed clothes, toilet seats, clothing

## Clinical Features

### Symptom

- Intense itching of the vulva or other infected body surfaces

### Signs

- No visible lesions
- Bluish macules in pubic areas or other skin surfaces (produced by toxin secreted by the parasite)
- Maculopapular inflammation with crust formation
- Excoriation
- Nits may be seen on shaft of the hair

## Differential Diagnosis

- Body or head lice
- Glycosuria (causing vulvar itching)
- Allergic reaction
- Lichenification (thickening and hardening of skin due to chronic irritation)

## Diagnostic Studies as Clinically Indicated

- Visualization of the nits or crab lice. A magnifying glass or a microscope may be used if necessary.

### Management and Treatment as Clinically Indicated

- Consult or refer to a physician as necessary
- Physically remove all visible lice and nits with a fine comb.
- Apply gamma benzene hexachloride cream, lotion, or shampoo (Kwell). Use lotion for the treatment of *P pubis* applying it to the hairy areas and surrounding skin. Shampoo is used for head lice and cream or lotion for body lice. *Leave on for 12 hours, no less, but not more than 24 hours.* Wash thoroughly; wear freshly laundered or dry-cleaned clothing, and launder bed clothes. (If repeated application is necessary, wait four days). The *Use of Kwell in pregnancy is not recommended.* OR
- Apply A-200 Pyrinate (Norcliff Thayer Inc) liquid or gel. (It may be purchased without a prescription). Use sufficient gel to completely wet the pubic hair, rubbing vigorously for two to three minutes to ensure thorough distribution. Leave gel on no longer than ten minutes, then rise with warm water. *Do not use gel more than twice in 24 hours.* Reapply 7-10 days after initial application. This product may be used by the pregnant patient.

### Complications

- Secondary skin infection
- Skin eruption from sensitivity or too frequent use of the antiparasitic agent
- "Vagabond's disease," a bronzed pigmentation of the skin from prolonged infestations
- Louse acts as a vector for typhus, trench fever, and possibly other diseases.

### Patient Teaching

- Discuss the parasitic nature of the infection and its transmission.
- Advise the patient to use no more of the medication than is indicated on the package insert; the skin absorbs the drug. If skin sensitivity results, wash the skin thoroughly and call the practitioner immediately.
- Advise the patient to refrain from scratching to prevent secondary infection. Pinching the skin or applying firm pressure with a closed fist over the area of itching sometimes helps.
- Stress the need for other family members to be examined and treated if infected.

- Explain that all exposed clothing and bed linen must be laundered or dry cleaned. The louse lives 24 hours after removal from the body, and the ova survive six days.
- Stress the importance of preventing reinfection by personal cleanliness and frequent laundering of clothing, bed linen, and towels.

## SCABIES

### Definition

Scabies is a communicable skin disease caused by an arachnid.

### Etiology

This skin disease is caused by the impregnated itch mite (*Sarcoptes scabiei*), which burrows into the stratum corneum of the skin leaving erythematous tracts. These tracts may be several millimeters to several centimeters in length and serve as depositories for eggs of the female mite, which hatch in four to eight days. The mite is transferred by personal contact, especially in crowded living conditions, or by indirect contact with contaminated clothing, bed linen, or towels. In cool weather the mite can survive one week away from the body.

### Clinical Features

#### Symptoms

- Intense itching, especially at night (worsened by warmth and perspiration)
- Fever, malaise, headache with severe infection

#### Signs

- Excoriation of the skin from scratching
- Punctate lesions with eczematous changes at lesion sites
- Skin areas most commonly affected are the palms, finger spaces, nipples,

wrists, waistline, buttocks, axillae, external genitalia, and inner aspect of the thighs
- Skin burrows from one-half to three centimeters in length

## Differential Diagnosis

- Pediculosis corporis
- Mosquito, tick, chigger, flea, or bed bug bites
- Impetigo
- Eczema, urticaria, allergy
- Lichen planus

## Diagnostic Studies as Clinically Indicated

- Clinical diagnosis is made by visualization of the tunneling mite with a head lens. Lifting the upper layer of skin with a needle reveals a white, glistening body visible at the end of the burrow. The burrow or vesicle should be scraped and the specimen placed on a slide in mineral oil or saline and visualized microscopically.

## Management and Treatment as Clinically Indicated

- Consult or refer to a physician referral as necessary
- A thorough soap and water bath is recommended.
- Gamma benzene hexachloride cream or lotion (Kwell) is applied to affected skin sites. The medication is left on for no less than 12 hours but not more than 24 hours. It is necessary to wait four days if repeated application is necessary. OR
- Benzyl benzoate ointment (Eurax) is applied by massaging it into the skin of the whole body, being especially careful to cover folds and creases. A second application is applied 24 hours later. Forty-eight hours after the second application a cleansing bath should be taken. Lesions respond to treatment in one or two weeks.
- Triamcinolone ointment may be ordered for severe itching.

## Complications

- Secondary skin infection
- Allergic reaction to medication
- Eczema

## Patient Teaching

- Refer to the patient teaching section for Pediculosis pubis.

# SEXUALLY TRANSMITTED DISEASES
# HERPES GENITALIS
# (HOMINIS, PROGENITALIS)

## Definition

Herpes genitalis is an acute primary or recurrent herpesvirus infection of the cervix, vagina, or genitalia.

## Etiology

Genital herpes infections have become the second most prevalent sexually transmitted disease in this country. There are many types of herpesvirus causing a variety of symptoms. The offending organism in the etiology of genital infections is primarily herpesvirus hominis type 2 (HVH-2). Ninety-five percent of virus strains isolated from the female genital tract are of this type.

The infection may be primary or recurrent. A primary infection usually occurs when sexual activity begins, and the patient may be acutely ill with viremia and multiple genital lesions. However, some patients with primary infections are unaware of its presence and have minor "flulike" symptoms. Once the virus has entered the body it never leaves and remains dormant in the neurons of sensory ganglia nearest the primary infection site.

Recurrent HVH-2 infections occur when the virus becomes reactivated and are local rather than systemic. Lesions of recurrent infection usually occur in the area of the initial lesion and may be symptomatic or asymptomatic. Some women never experience recurrent infection, while others have frequent attacks that are physically and mentally debilitating.

When conditions exist that favor its reactivation, a recurrent infection occurs. The predisposing factors initiating a primary or recurrent infection include:

- Exposure to an infected person
- Exposure to heat or sunshine
- Premenstrual phase of the menstrual cycle
- Emotional stress
- Trauma or friction to the genital area
- Infections causing temperature elevation
- Gastrointestinal disturbances

## Clinical Features

### Symptoms

- Hyperesthesia of the area where the lesion will erupt
- Itching, burning of infection site
- Dyspareunia
- Leukorrhea
- Temperature elevation
- Painful lesions (as distinguished from other lesions of the vulva which are usually painless)
- Viremia with primary infection

### Signs

- Absence of symptoms in 50% of the patients
- Indurated papules, vesicles, and/or ulcerations
- Lesions occurring on the vulva, perianal skin, vagina, and cervix
    Vesicular vulvar lesions
    Vaginal and cervical lesions resembling mucous patches or having elevated circumferences with necrotic centers
    Recurrent lesions occurring at the site of the primary lesion

- Vulvovaginal edema
- Inquinal adenopathy
- Healing in 7-10 days

## Differential Diagnosis

- Other vaginal infections
- Venereal disease (often found in association with lymphogranuloma venereum)
- Allergic reaction
- Herpes zoster
- Cervicitis

## Diagnostic Studies as Clinically Indicated

- Pap smear: Vesicular fluid is obtained by swabbing or aspirating fluid from the vesicle and rolling it on a slide. Giant multinucleated cells with inclusion bodies characteristic of viral infection are identified.
- Tzank test: A scraping from the crater of the vesicle is placed on a slide and stained with Wright's or Giemsa stain. Cells are identified as found in the Pap smear.
- Serologic studies: These studies show a rise in neutralizing antibodies but are rarely done.
- Virus culture: Eagle's medium with 5% calf serum is a virologic culture medium. A specimen is obtained with a cotton-tipped applicator from the base of the ulcerated lesion or cervix to inoculate the culture.
- VDRL test: This serologic test is done to rule out syphilis.
- Culture: A culture for for *Neisseria gonorrhoeae* should be done to rule out gonorrhea.

## Management and Treatment as Clinically Indicated

There is no known cure for herpesvirus infections, and no treatment is completely effective in promoting more rapid healing or preventing recurrent infection. A variety of palliative measures are used to reduce discomfort.

**172** PROBLEMS IN AMBULATORY OBSTETRICS AND GYNECOLOGY

- Consult or refer to a physician as necessary.
- Burow's solution (Domeboro) compresses are applied to the lesions for 30 minutes four times a day. The solution is made by dissolving 1 to 2 Domeboro tablets or powder packets in 1 pint of water; let the medication dissolve and then shake.
- Aspirin (2 tablets qid) will relieve pain and lower the body temperature. For patients with recurrent infection related to menstrual periods, aspirin may be taken starting five days before the menses.
- Lysine (an amino acid that is normally found in the body) suppresses clinical symptoms, accelerates recovery, and suppresses recurrent infections in some patients. It comes in 500-mg tablets and may be purchased in health food stores. When prodromal symptoms or an acute infection occur, 1,000 mg. is taken immediately, than one-half tablet is taken every day for maintenance and prevention of further attacks. This treatment, still under study, is said to block arginine receptor sites necessary for herpesvirus replication. Foods such as seeds, grain, and chocolate are arginine-rich and should be avoided when lysine treatment is used.
- Cold milk compresses applied to the lesions may be cooling and soothing.
- Topical application of ether to the lesions until the skin blanches causes penetration of the lipid membrane of the virus and acts as a local anesthetic.
- Anesthetic ointments (Lidocaine, Amercaine) may help to relieve pain when applied to the lesion.
- Warm to cool sitz baths are cooling and soothing to inflamed tissue and help to prevent secondary infection. (Oilated Aveeno may be added to the water.)
- Listerine may be applied to lesions with a cotton-tipped applicator and allowed to dry. Aloe vera gel is then applied and will offer relief of symptoms.
- Systemic treatment with smallpox vaccine between episodes of recurrent infection has been effective in decreasing the number of recurrent attacks in some patients.
- Secondary or concurrent vaginal infection needs appropriate treatment.
- *Use of photodynamic inactivation of the virus may be carcinogenic, and its use is controversial.*

## Complications

- Superimposed bacterial infection
- Cervicitis

- Urinary retention
- Spread to other body sites or persons
- Possible susceptibility to cervical dysplasia and cancer in women with repeated genital herpesvirus infections
- Systemic infection
- Neonatal infection from vaginal delivery through an infected birth canal

## Patient Teaching

- Discuss the nature of the infection and its transmission and possible recurrence.
- Advise the patient to abstain from sexual intercourse (oral or genital) if either partner has signs of infection. If lesions are confined to the penis, vagina, or cervix, condoms should be used for six weeks or until all signs of infection have cleared.
- Discuss general hygiene measures with the patient to prevent secondary in-infection.
- Discuss factors that may prevent reactivation of the virus. Elevation of body temperature appears to be the most common predisposing factor of recurrent infection. Advise the patient to:
  Protect herself from the heat of the sun
  Avoid overheating of the vulva with hot baths or tight clothing
  Avoid friction from prolonged intercourse by using a lubricant (K-Y jelly, vegetable oil, saliva)
  Use aspirin to maintain lowered body temperature before the onset of the menses
- Advise the patient with burning during urination to pour warm water over the vulva or to sit in a tub of warm water while urinating.
- Recognize that patients with frequent recurrent attacks may need strong emotional support because of the psychologic and sociologic stresses resulting from repeated infections.
- Support for pregnant patients is crucial. When herpetic lesions are present on the vulva, in the vagina, or on the cervix in late pregnancy, cesarean-section delivery is indicated, and counseling of the patient is important.
- Refer interested patients to HELP, a national organization formed to help victims of HVH-2. Its newsletter provides information on the latest research and provides suggestions on how to cope with recurrent infections. Those wishing to join should write to HELP, Box 100, Palo Alto, CA 94302.

## CONDYLOMATA ACUMINATA (VENERAL WARTS)

### Definition

Condylomata acuminata, more commonly known as venereal or genital warts, are intradermal papillomas that are treelike in structure and are covered with hyperplastic epithelium.

### Etiology

The causative agent of these growths is verruca acuminata, the virus that causes the common wart. This is a sexually transmitted infection with warts appearing one to three months after initial contact with an infected partner. They are estrogen dependent and may appear on the vulva, vagina, anus, and less frequently the cervix.

### Clinical Features

#### Symptoms

- A profuse, irritating vaginal discharge
- Vulvitis with pruritus resulting from contact with the irritating discharge
- Accompanying vaginitis
- Dyspareunia from sensitive lesions or blockage of the vaginal canal

#### Signs

- Multiple warty growths of varying size on the vulva, perineum, buttocks, inner thighs, vagina, or cervix
- Lesions that first appear as small, discrete structures, then spread, enlarge, and coalesce to form narrow-based pedunculated cauliflowerlike growths
- A profuse vaginal discharge and secondary vulvitis
- Hypertropy of lesions during pregnancy, which regress after delivery
- Lesions that ulcerate, become infected, and have a foul odor

## Differential Diagnosis

- Melanoma
- Squamous papilloma
- Polyps

## Diagnostic Studies as Clinically Indicated

- Culture for *Neisseria gonorrhoeae* and a VDRL test are done to exclude the presence of other sexually transmitted disease.
- A saline and KOH wet mount is done to identify accompanying vaginitis.
- A Pap smear should be done, especially if lesions are located on the cervix.
- Biopsy of suspicious lesions or of lesions that are resistent to treatment is done as indicated.

## Management and Treatment as Clinically Indicated

- Consult or refer to a physician as necessary.
- Treat underlying vaginal infection as appropriate.
- Apply a 25% solution of podophyllin in tincture of benzoin on the individual growths of small lesions. Petrolatum applied on the surrounding skin will protect it from the strong treatment solution (contraindicated in pregnancy). OR
- Apply Nevitol (trichloroacetic acid) solution on small lesions as above, being cautious not to drip on the surrounding skin.
- Lesions larger than 1 cm are usually removed by cryocautery, with an electric cutting loop, or by surgical excision. One or two treatments with laser therapy is sometimes given.

## COMPLICATIONS

- Infection and necrosis of the lesions
- Vaginal outlet obstruction
- Difficult delivery in pregnant patients with large lesions
- Malignant change is rare

## Patient Teaching

- Explain what the lesions are and how they were contacted.
- Advise the patient that if she ever sees similar, or other lesions, on her sexual partner, to refrain from intercourse. Reinfection after cure is possible.
- Advise the patient to keep the vulva as clean and dry as possible. This is one of the most important ways of speeding recovery; a damp environment enhances growth of the wart.
- Stress the importance of using vaginal medication for treatment of vaginitis as directed. Treating this infection will many times cause spontaneous disappearance of small condylomata.
- Advise patients treated with podophyllin or Nevitol to wash it off carefully with soap and water in four to six hours or it will burn the skin.

    The lesions may also become painful several hours after this treatment, but the pain will not last long.

    The lesions will start sloughing two to four days after treatment.

    Treatment may have to continue every one to two weeks until all the lesions have cleared.
- Explain that the warts can be cured, especially if the patient completes treatment and her partner is treated at the same time. Reinfection can occur.

# CHLAMYDIOSIS

## Definition

Chlamydiosis is inflammation of the cervix caused by chlamydia, organisms not normally found in the genital tract.

## Etiology

The genus *Chlamydia* (TRIC agent; subgroup A chlamydia) was formerly called *Bedsonia*. The pathogenic organisms of this genus were previously thought to be large viruses but are presently considered gram-negative obligate intracellular bacteria. This group of organisms causes trachoma, psittacosis, lymphogranuloma venereum, and inclusion conjunctivitis. These intracellular parasites will not grow on artificial media. Tissue cultures are necessary for isolation and identification. Chlamydia have been identified in 40% of the men with nonspecific urethritis (NSU), and in over 35% of the women with cervicitis. The infection is sexually transmitted and is found more commonly in women with multiple sexual partners. Its role in pelvic infections is unknown.

## Clinical Features

### Symptoms

- May be absent
- Cervical congestion, edema, inflammation
- Mucopurulent discharge
- Rare urinary symptoms

### Signs

- The infection is commonly found in conjunction with other sexually transmitted disease.
- The cervix may appear normal.
- It is a persistant, asymptomatic, rather than an acute type infection, with organisms harbored in the cervix.
- A mucopurulent discharge may be draining from the cervical os.
- It is found more often in oral contraceptive users; the cause and effect is unknown.

## Differential Diagnosis

- Cervical carcinoma
- Herpesvirus hominis infection, gonorrhea, syphilis, chancroid, granuloma venereum
- Chronic vaginitis
- Salpingitis, parametritis

## Diagnostic Studies as Clinically Indicated

(Rule out patient use of intravaginal medications, contraceptive creams, or douching in the past 48 hours.)

- A Pap smear is collected (may also be done for suspected herpetic infection).
- A KOH and saline wet mount is done to rule out candidiasis or trichomoniasis.
- A specimen for culture of *Neisseria gonorrhoeae* should be collected on Thayer-Martin (TM) or Transgrow transport medium.
- A bacterial culture is taken by inoculating Sorbitol or other transport medium with a swab from the endocervix.
- Rule out nonspecific urethritis in the male sexual partner.

## Management and Treatment as Clinically Indicated

- Consult or refer to a physician as necessary.
- Tetracycline, 2 g/day, is given for 7-14 days to the patient and her partner. *This treatment is contraindicated in pregnant and lactating women because of possible retardation of fetal skeletal development and permanent discoloration of the teeth.* Side effects may include heartburn, abdominal discomfort, nausea, vomiting, diarrhea, and sensitivity to sunlight. These symptoms usually disappear after the first few pills are taken.
- There is currently no treatment for infection of the pregnant woman. The mother, and neonate if necessary, are treated after delivery.

## Complications

- Nonspecific urethritis may occur in the patient and her male sexual partner.
- Inflammatory changes of the cervix may occur.
- Salpingitis may occur from ascending infection.
- Inclusion conjunctivitis or pneumonia of the newborn may occur after delivery through an infected cervix.

## Patient Teaching

- Describe the nature of her infection and its treatment. Use pictures or diagrams of the female pelvic organs for clarity.
- Advise the patient to take the tetracycline one hour before or two hours after meals. Food and some dairy products interfere with its absorption.
- Advise the patient that she and her sexual partner should take the tetracycline

over the same period of time. Infection may reoccur after contact with untreated or multiple partners.
- Tell the patient to avoid sexual intercourse until the prescribed medication is completed, or advise the use of a condom if abstinence is unlikely.
- Advise the patient to return for a follow-up culture in six weeks. A Pap smear should also be repeated in six months if inflammatory changes were reported on the last smear.

# GONORRHEA

## Definition

Gonorrhea is a sexually transmitted infectious disease that may involve the mucous membrane of any structure of the body. It most commonly involves the cervix, rectum, urethra, and pharynx, but may invade the bloodstream and may spread to other columnar and transitional epithelium.

## Etiology

*Neisseria gonorrhoeae* is a gram-negative, intracellular diplococcus, an anaerobic organism that grows best under $CO_2$ stimulation at a pH of 7.2-7.6. The organism dies with cold or drying. Its incubation period is from two to five days, after which it may enter a prolonged incubation, an asymptomatic, or acute infectious state.

Gonorrhea ranks first among the reportable communicable diseases in the United States. It occurs most frequently in the 20- to 24-year-old age group, with teenagers 15-19 years of age constituting the second highest risk group. The incidence of gonorrhea infections has risen due to increased sexual activity among the young population and the decreased use of the condom as a contraceptive method.

Gonorrhea is the only sexually transmitted disease that involves both the upper tract (uterus, fallopian tubes, ovaries, and pelvic peritoneum) and the lower tract (cervix, vagina, urethra, Skene's and Bartholin's glands, and vulva) of the female reproductive system.

After a brief discussion of penicillinase-producing *N. gonorrhoeae* and (patient teaching information) acute lower tract infection, acute upper tract infection, (salpingitis PID), and chronic pelvic inflammatory disease, will be covered in separate sections.

## Penicillinase-Producing Neisseria Gonorrhoeae*

Penicillin has been the drug of choice against infections with *Neisseria gonorrhoeae* for the past 30 years. In March of 1976 an isolate of *N. gonorrhoeae* was cultured from a man in Maryland with urethritis who had failed treatment on an appropriate dose of penicillin. This isolate was resistant to penicillin. The isolate produced an enzyme called penicillinase, which destroyed penicillin. Although this enzyme has been identified in other bacteria (i.e., *Staphylococcus aureus*) that are resistant to penicillin, this was the first time it had been observed in *N. gonorrhoeae*.

During the period from March through November 1976, the Center for Disease Control confirmed 35 more cases of infection with penicillinase-producing *N. Gonorrhoeae* (PPNG) in 12 different states. This new strain has also been detected in England, Canada, Korea, Japan, Singapore, the Philippines, and Australia. Most cases in the United States are related to people who have sexual contact in the Far East; military personnel account for many of the cases.

The symptoms, signs, and complication rate of infection with penicillinase-producing *N. gonorrhoeae* so far appear to be no different from those observed with nonpenicillinase-producing strains. Most cases seen in the United States have been uncomplicated infection, although one case of disseminated infection and one case of localized abscess formation (Bartholin gland) have been observed. In England at least one case of PPNG infection associated with pelvic inflammatory disease has been reported.

Penicillin has been shown to be ineffective against this new strain. In 30 of the first 35 cases seen in the United States where penicillin therapy was used initially, it failed to eradicate the infection. In addition a small number of patients treated with tetracycline, a drug used as an alternative to penicillin in penicillin-allergic patients, also led to an unacceptable failure rate. Most cases in the United States have been cured with spectinomycin, a drug normally used for the few patients who fail initial therapy with penicillin or tetracycline. Although spectinomycin appears to be effective against this new strain, absolute resistance of *N. gonorrhoeae* to spectinomycin has been documented in the past and injudicious use of this drug could ultimately result in spectinomycin-resistant organisms.

Since the number of cases of this new strain in the United States is very low

*Source: HEW, PHS, Center for Disease Control, Atlanta, Georgia.

at the present time, the CDC still recommends 4.8 million units of aqueous procaine penicillin G intramuscularly, administered with 1 g of probenecid orally, as initial treatment of choice for uncomplicated gonorrhea. A follow-up test-of-cure culture should be obtained for all patients three to seven days after initial therapy. Patients who have a positive test-of-cure culture should be retreated with spectinomycin, 2 g IM, and a repeat culture should be done in three to seven days.

Surveillance for this new strain is being conducted through state health departments. Physicians requiring assistance in screening for PPNG or in case follow-up and contact referral should contact health department officials.

## Patient Teaching

- Tell the patient that she has gonorrhea, which is a highly infectious disease spread by sexual intercourse with an infected person. The contact person will need to be notified so that he/she may be examined and treated.
- Stress the importance of proper treatment. In lower tract disease medication will cure the disease, but if a prescription has been given for treatment at home, *all the medication must be taken as directed.* Have the patient return one week after completion of the medication for a repeat of the cervical culture to verify a cure.
- Discuss the importance of pelvic rest. The patient should not engage in intercourse or in any activity that jars the pelvis, which could cause spread of infection to the pelvic organs. Bed rest in a semi-Fowler's position is necessary to maintain downward pressure and prevent upward spread.
- Discuss the above information with patients who have salpingitis and who are to be treated on an ambulatory basis. However, stress the absolute need for bed rest in the semi-Fowler's position to maintain the infection as low in the pelvis as possible.
- Instruct all patients about the importance of maintaining adequate fluid intake and a diet high in protein and vitamins to help optimize recovery.
- Suggest that patients eat one container of cultured plain yogurt every day during antibiotic therapy to prevent gastric upset.
- Explain to the patient who is to be hospitalized why this is necessary. She needs parenteral antibiotic therapy to halt further spread of the infection and peritonitis and close surveillance of her infection to assure proper medication, bed rest, and control of painful symptoms. Swift and conservative action will also enhance her future fertility.

### Preventive Measures to Help Control Infection

- Suggest to the patient that if her sexual partner is not well known to her she should insist he wear a condom (she can carry some in her purse). If she notices any sores or discharge on the partner's genitals, refrain from intercourse.
- Suggest that washing with soap and water before intercourse will help prevent infection.
- Explain that drinking liquids before intercourse and voiding immediately afterward will help to flush organisms from the urethra.
- Advise the patient that contraceptive foams and jellies provide some protection against the gonococcus and, if used in conjunction with a condom, will offer added protection.
- Advise the patient to seek care immediately if there is possibility of reinfection.

## ACUTE LOWER TRACT GONORRHEAL INFECTION

Acute lower tract infection usually begins with infection of the urethra, cervix, Skene's and Bartholin's gland, or the rectum.

### Clinical Features

#### Symptoms

Eighty percent of women may be asymptomatic, but symptoms, if present, usually occur 1-14 days after sexual contact with an infected partner and may include:

- A profuse, purulent, irritating cervical discharge, which may be the only noticeable symptom
- Urethritis, urinary frequency, urgency, and dysuria, which may occur from urinary tract involvement. These symptoms may resolve spontaneously in a few days due to the acidity of the urine, which adversely effects the gonococcus.
- Vulvovaginitis, which occurs from contamination of the tissues by irritating vaginal discharge. This symptom is most severe in prepubertal and postmenopausal women who do not have the protective squamous vaginal

epithelium of the estrogen-producing woman. The organisms grow best on columnar epithelium and do not normally invade estrogen-rich vaginal squamous epithelium.
- Proctitis, which occurs from genitorectal intercourse with an infected partner
- Pharyngitis or tonsillitis, which occurs from oral-genital contact with an infected person
- Bartholin's and Skene's gland infections, which may accompany any of the above symptoms

### Signs

Signs of lower abdominal involvement are usually absent but may include:
- Redness and swelling at the contact site of infection 3-21 days after exposure
- A profuse, purulent vaginal discharge
- Purulent discharge oozing from the urethra when stripped during the pelvic examination
- Cervicitis, which may be difficult to differentiate from that due to other causes
- An edematous, inflamed posterior pharynx or tonsillitis with submaxillary lymphadenitis may occur from a gonococcal infection of the throat

## Differential Diagnosis

- Nongonococcal cervicitis
- Urinary tract infection
- Nongonococcal pharyngitis
- Cervical dysplasia

## Diagnostic Studies as Clinically Indicated

Definitive diagnosis is extremely important, not only because this is a reportable disease but also to prevent spreading of the infection upward to the pelvic organs.
- The patient history may reveal contact with an infected person.
- Blood studies include a CBC, a differential count, and a sedimentation rate.

- A blood specimen should be drawn for a VDRL test for syphilis because simultaneous infectious disease is not uncommon.
- A wet mount with saline and KOH should be done to rule out vaginal infection.
- Cervical and pharyngeal smears on Thayer-Martin (TM) or Transgrow transport medium should be done. The cervical smear is important and should be taken during any phase of the menstrual cycle. Two separate cotton-tipped applicators should be placed in the cervix (one after the other) and allowed to moisten, then smeared separately. This method of collection will increase the yield of positive results by 10%. The TM specimen should be incubated in a candle jar (to exclude oxygen) within 20 minutes or the gonococcus will chill and die. The transport medium should be incubated at 35°C before transport.
- In the female, Gram staining of the cervical discharge is not a reliable test since other gram-negative diplococci in the vaginal flora may confuse the diagnosis. In a male, however, the Gram stain is a valid test for gonorrhea.

## Management and Treatment as Clinically Indicated

- Warm sitz baths, with the vulva kept clean and dry should be recommended to the patient with vulvar irritation. For the prepubertal or postmenopausal woman, topical estrogen cream can be given for more rapid healing. However, this treatment should be temporary (especially in the young girl) and should be used only for extreme irritation because it may cause vaginal bleeding.
- Pelvic rest with no sexual intercourse or heavy exercise is advised to prevent the infection from ascending.
- The patient may be treated before positive culture results are obtained if (1) there has been an exposure to gonorrhea, (2) there is a strong history and clinical evidence of infection, and (3) there is strong suspicion the patient will not return. Consultation with the physician is necessary. The following treatment schedules for uncomplicated gonococcal infections in men and women are those recommended by the Center for Disease Control 1979.* *Note:* Physicians are cautioned to use no less than the recommended dosages of antibiotics.
- Drug regimens of choice

    Aqueous procaine penicillin G (APPG), 4.8 million units, is injected IM at two sites, and 1.0 g of probenecid is given orally. OR

---

*The source of the following section on drug regimens of choice is the Venereal Disease Control Division, Bureau of State Services, Center for Disease Control, Atlanta, Georgia.

Tetracycline hydrochloride, 0.5 g, is given orally four times a day for five days (total dose: 10.0 g). Other tetracyclines are not more effective than tetracycline hydrochloride. All tetracyclines are ineffective as a single-dose therapy. OR

Ampicillin, 3.5 g, or amoxicillin, 3.0 g, is given with 1 g of probenecid by mouth. Evidence shows that these regimens are slightly less effective than the other recommended regimens.

*Patients who are allergic to the penicillins or probenecid* should be treated with orally administered tetracycline as described above. Patients who cannot tolerate tetracycline may be treated with spectinomycin hydrochloride, 2.0 g, in one IM injection.

- Special considerations

    Single-dose treatment is preferred for patients who are unlikely to complete the multiple-dose tetracycline regimen.

    The APPG regimen is preferred for men with anorectal infection.

    Pharyngeal infection is difficult to treat. High failure rates have been reported with ampicillin and spectinomycin.

    Tetracycline treatment results in fewer cases of postgonococcal urethritis in men.

    Tetracycline may eliminate coexisting chlamydial infections in men and women.

    Patients with incubating syphilis (seronegative, without clinical signs of syphilis) are likely to be cured by all the above regimens except spectinomycin. A serologic test for syphilis should be done on all patients at the time of diagnosis.

    Patients with gonorrhea who also have syphilis should be given additional treatment appropriate to the stage of syphilis.

- Treatment of sexual partners: Men and women exposed to gonorrhea should be examined, have specimens cultured, and be treated at once with one of the regimens above.

- Follow-up cultures should be obtained from the infected site(s) three to seven days after completion of treatment. A specimen for culture should be obtained from the anal canal of every woman who has been treated for gonorrhea.

- Therapeutic failures

    When therapy with penicillin, ampicillin, amoxicillin, or tetracycline fails, the patient should be treated with spectinomycin, 2.0 g IM.

    Most recurrent infections after treatment with the recommended schedules are due to *reinfection* and indicate a need for improved contact tracing and patient education. Since infection by penicillinase ($\beta$-lactamase)-producing

*N. gonorrhoeae* is a cause of therapeutic failure, post-treatment isolates should be tested for penicillinase production.

*Although long-acting forms of penicillin (such as benzathine penicillin G) are effective in syphilotherapy, they have no place in the treatment of gonorrhea. Preparations of penicillin administered orally, such as penicillin V, are not recommended for the treatment of gonococcal infection.*

- Penicillinase-producing *N. gonorrhoeae* (PPNG): Patients with uncomplicated PPNG infections and their sexual contacts should receive spectinomycin, 2.0 g, in a single IM injection. Because gonococci are very rarely resistant to spectinomycin and reinfection is the most common cause of therapeutic failure, patients with positive cultures after spectinomycin therapy should be retreated with the same dose. A PPNG isolate that is resistant to spectinomycin may be treated with cefoxitin, 2.0 g, in a single IM injection, with probenecid, 1.0 g by mouth.
- Treatment in pregnancy

    Cultures of endocervical specimens for *N. gonorrhoeae* should be obtained for all pregnant women as an integral part of the prenatal care at the time of the first visit. Second cultures late in the third trimester should be obtained for women at high risk for gonococcal infection.

    Drug regimens of choice are APPG, ampicillin, or amoxicillin, each with probenecid as described above.

    Women who are allergic to penicillin or probenecid should be treated with spectinomycin.

    Refer to the sections on acute salpingitis and disseminated gonococcal infections for the treatment of these conditions during pregnancy. Tetracycline should not be administered to pregnant women because of potential toxic effects on mother and fetus.

## Complications

- "Ping-Pong" gonorrhea occurs with re-exposure to a gonorrheal infection after treatment and cure of a prior infection.
- Increased incidence of upper tract infection (especially in IUD wearers)
- A vaginal infection resulting from antibiotic therapy

## Patient Teaching

See p. 181.

# ACUTE PELVIC INFLAMMATORY DISEASE

## Definition

Acute pelvic inflammatory disease (PID) or salpingitis usually begins after the end of the menstrual period when a lower tract infection has not been treated or when treatment has been inadequate. The cervical mucous plug, which acts as a protective device, is lost during menstruation allowing infection to ascend to the upper organs.

## Clinical Features

### Symptoms

Symptoms may include those discussed in the section on acute lower tract gonorrheal infection in addition to those listed here.

- Bilateral lower pelvic tenderness and pain
- Temperature elevation to 102°-103°F
- Symptoms of acute illness may be absent

### Signs

Signs may include those discussed in the section on acute lower tract gonorrheal infection in addition to those listed here.

- A soft, boggy, enlarged uterus
- Cervical motion tenderness ("chandelier sign")
- Uterine fundus and adnexa are tender to palpation
- Adnexal thickening, abscess formation
- Tender inguinal adenopathy
- Involuntary guarding with abdominal palpation

## Differential Diagnosis

- Nongonococcal pelvic infection
- Diverticulitis, appendicitis

- Ectopic pregnancy
- Septic abortion
- Pelvic endometriosis
- Acute cholecystitis, pancreatitis
- Hemorrhagic ovarian cyst

## Diagnostic Studies as Clinically Indicated

- The patient history may reveal contact with an infected person.
- Blood studies include a CBC, a differential count, and a sedimentation rate. (The WBC may be 20–30,000/mm$^3$ with a shift to the left).
- A serum amylase level determination is done with upper tract infection to rule out perihepatic involvement.
- A blood culture may be indicated.
- A blood specimen should be drawn for a VDRL test for syphilis since simultaneous infection is not uncommon.
- Wet mounts with saline and KOH are done to rule out a vaginal infection.
- Cervical and pharyngeal smears on Thayer-Martin (TM) or Transgrow transport medium should be done. (For technique refer to the preceding section on acute lower tract gonorrheal infection.)
- Culdoscopy is done by the physician for definitive diagnosis.

## Management and Treatment as Clinically Indicated

- Pelvic rest is mandatory whether the patient is treated on an ambulatory basis or is hospitalized.
- The following treatment schedules for acute salpingitis are those recommended by the Center For Disease Control 1979.* There are no reliable clinical criteria by which to distinguish gonococcal from nongonococcal salpingitis. Endocervical cultures for *N. gonorrhoeae* are essential. Therapy should be initiated immediately.
- Hospitalization should be strongly considered in these situations:
    Uncertain diagnosis, in which surgical emergencies such as appendicitis and ectopic pregnancy must be excluded

*Source: Disease Control Division, Bureau of State Services, Center for Venereal Disease Control, Atlanta, Georgia.

Suspicion of pelvic abscess
Severely ill patients
Pregnancy
Inability of the patient to follow or to tolerate an outpatient regimen.
Failure to respond to outpatient therapy.
- Outpatient drug regimen

    Tetracycline, 0.5 g, is given orally four times a day for 10 days. This regimen should not be used for pregnant patients. OR

    APPG, 4.8 million units IM; ampicillin, 3.5 g; or amoxicillin, 3.0 g, each with probenecid, 1.0 g, is given. Either regimen is followed by ampicillin, 0.5 g, or amoxicillin, 0.5 g, orally four times a day for 10 days.
- Inpatient drug regimen

    Tetracycline, 0.25 g, is given IV four times a day until improvement occurs and is followed by 0.5 g orally four times a day to complete 10 days of therapy. This regimen should not be used for pregnant women. The dosage may have to be adjusted when renal function is depressed.

    Since optimal therapy for hospitalized patients has not been established, other antibiotics in addition to penicillin are frequently used.
- Special considerations

    Failure of the patient's condition to improve in response to the recommended regimens does not indicate the need for stepwise additional antibiotics, but necessitates clinical reassessment.

    The intrauterine device is a risk factor for the development of pelvic inflammatory disease. The effects of removing an intrauterine device on the response of acute salpingitis to antimicrobial therapy and on the risk of recurrent salpingitis are unknown.

    Adequate treatment of women with acute salpingitis must include examination and appropriate treatment of their sex partners because of the high prevalence of nonsymptomatic urethral infection in males. Failure to treat sex partners is a major cause of recurrent gonococcal salpingitis.

    Follow-up of patients with acute salpingitis is essential during and after treatment. All patients should have repeated cultures for *N. gonorrhoeae* after treatment.

## Complications

- "Ping-Pong" gonorrhea occurs with re-exposure to a gonorrheal infection after treatment and cure of a prior infection.

- Fitz-Hugh-Curtis syndrome, a gonococcal perihepatitis that mimics cholecystitis with referred pain to the right shoulder
- Pelvic abscess and hydrosalpinx, which may later require extensive pelvic surgery
- Periurethral abscess with possible urethral stenosis or urinary retention
- Infertility or ectopic pregnancy may result from scarring of the fallopian tubes after a pelvic infection.
- Gonococcal arthritis-dermatitis syndrome, which is manifested by painful, hot, swollen joints with purulent exudate or by painful joints with little swelling and inflammation but cultures that are positive for the gonococcus
- Chronic salpingitis, skenitis, or bartholinitis
- Nongonococcal salpingitis may occur two to four weeks after treatment for acute infection.
- Gonococcal septicemia, which may invade the joints or spinal fluid or cause skin lesions
- Abdominal and pelvic adhesions may result from healing of an upper tract infection.
- Gonorrhea in the parturient patient may cause:
    Premature rupture of the membranes and premature labor
    Infection of the neonate from ascending infection after prolonged rupture of the membranes or delivery through an infected birth canal
    Ophthalmia neonatorum, which is the most common gonococcal infection affecting the newborn. The stomach, oropharynx, the external ear, and the anal canal are other sites of possible infection of the neonate.

### Patient Teaching

See p.181.

## CHRONIC PELVIC INFLAMMATORY DISEASE

### Definition

Chronic pelvic inflammatory disease (PID) is the result of a locus of infection (gonococcal or other bacterial) that remains in the pelvis after an acute infection subsides. During the actue phase of PID, the uterus, fallopian tubes, ovaries, rectosigmoid, small bowel, and the omentum may become inflamed. In an attempt to localize the infection, the body's defense mechanism walls off its primary site; a process that causes fibrosis of the affected tissue. The fibrosis causes secondary complications of chronic pelvic disease. The patency of the tubes, which are always involved, become compromised by partial or total occlusion producing pockets that become the focus of low-grade symptomatic infection. These pockets are especially susceptible to secondary bacterial invaders ascending from the vagina and cervix.

## Clinical Features

### Symptoms

(result from a low-grade, long-term infection)

- Dysfunctional uterine bleeding results from endometritis or ovarian involvement.
- Chronic pelvic pain is due to the presence of pelvic scarring, adhesions, and localized areas of infection.
- Acute exacerbations of infection occur spontaneously or as a result of instrumentation of the uterus.
- Infertility occurs as a result of scarring and occlusion of the fallopian tubes.

### Signs

- Palpable masses in the pelvis
- Fixation of the uterus or adnexa
- Tenderness of the uterus and adnexa to palpation
- Inguinal adenopathy
- General physical debility from long-term infection

## Differential Diagnosis

- Nongonococcal pelvic infection
- "Ping-Pong" gonorrheal infection
- Pelvic malignancy

- Endometriosis
- Hemorrhagic ovarian cyst
- Ectopic pregnancy
- Diverticulitis, appendicitis

## Diagnostic Studies as Clinically Indicated

- Patient history may reveal past pelvic infection or a recent contact from an infected person. A symptom analysis of pelvic complaints is necessary.
- Abdominal and pelvic examination in conjunction with the history may strongly support a clinical diagnosis.
- A cervical smear on Thayer-Martin (TM) or Transgrow medium for *N. gonorrhoeae* should be done. (For technique refer to the section on acute lower gonorrheal infection.) A smear for bacteria may also be indicated.
- Blood studies should include a CBC, differential count, sedimentation rate, and a VDRL test, with other studies as indicated.
- A saline and KOH wet mount is done if vaginitis is suspected.
- A laparoscopy may be helpful in assessing the amount of infection or adhesions.

## Management and Treatment as Clinically Indicated

- Referral to a physician is necessary.
- Conservative management may involve the use of the appropriate antibiotic in conjunction with the administration of corticosteroid compounds. Ideally, the steroid therapy helps to inhibit the continued formation of fibrotic tissue, while the antibiotic therapy and the patient's defense mechanisms combat the chronic infection. This treatment may be effective in a first or second recurrent attack but its further use is questionable.
- Surgical treatment may be necessary to eradicate infection. Total abdominal hysterectomy and bilateral salpingectomy is usually done. The ovaries are not removed unless they are extensively involved, or if not removed, would remain as a source for future recurrent infection.
- The chronic inflammatory process may occasionally subside without further treatment. Infertility is usually a problem if this occurs.

## Complications

- Hydro- or pyosalpinx occurs when blockage of the tubes causes accumulation of mucus and inflammatory fluids.
- Tubo-ovarian abscess occurs when the fimbriated end of the tube fuses to an ovary creating a cavity that fills with fluids. It is a life-threatening event when it ruptures.
- Infertility from scarring and blockage of the tubes may occur.
- Ectopic pregnancy from trapping of the blastocyst in a partially blocked tube may occur.
- Chronic debilitation of the patient with malnutrition and iron-deficiency anemia may occur.

## Patient Teaching

See p.181.

# SYPHILIS

## Definition

Syphilis is both an acute and chronic sexually transmitted infectious disease that appears in three stages: primary, secondary latent, and tertiary.

## Etiology

The causative organism is *Treponema pallidum,* a spirochete that is spread primarily through sexual exposure (95%), through kissing and digital sex play, and prenatally through the placenta to the fetus. The organism must be identified microscopically since it will not grow in vitro, and is sensitive to heat, cold, drying, and antiseptics. It penetrates intact mucous membrane and abraded skin rapidly. It ranks third (after chickenpox and gonorrhea) among reportable communicable diseases in the United States. Since 1958 the number of reported cases among the young adult population has been steadily rising, especially in urban areas. This may be due in part to the increased sexual activity of the younger population and in part to the decreased use of the condom for contraception. Also, routine serologic testing for syphilis, formerly required on all hospital admissions, has been eliminated in many hospitals.

## Clinical Features

### Signs and Symptoms

- *Primary stage:* The incubation period is 9 to 90 days with a medium of 21 days. The serologic test results are not positive until the fourth week of infection.

    The chancre is the initial lesion, with single or multiple lesions occurring at the point of inoculation.

    1. The genitals are the most common site but lesions may also be found on the tongue, tonsils, face, breasts, fingers, and anus.
    2. The chancre begins as a papule, which erodes and becomes ulcerative. A painless, indurated ulcer with a raised border, it is smooth and discrete with a yellow serous discharge. The lesion may be easily overlooked if it is in an inconspicuous location.
    3. The chancre is extremely infectious at this stage and heals spontaneously in four to six weeks.

- *Secondary stage:* This stage occurs in an untreated person on an average of three weeks after the onset of the chancre, or six to eight weeks after exposure.

    Serologic test results are now positive.

    The chancre has healed or is in the process of healing.

    Early systemic complaints are flulike with headache, sore throat, runny nose, and generalized joint pain.

    Generalized nonpainful lymphadenopathy is a common finding; the nodes feel firm and rubbery.

    The temperature is slightly elevated.

    Weight loss is a common complaint.

    Leukocytosis occurs with an elevated sedimentation rate.

    The spleen is enlarged.

    A generalized skin rash occurs, which may be difficult to distinguish from other skin eruptions. The following signs are common:

1. The rash may recur in untreated persons one or more times during the first two years of infection.
2. The rash is nonpruritic and painless, discrete, and copper colored.
3. The rash occurs on the palms of the hand and soles of the feet. *This is a significant diagnostic sign.*
4. The rash occurs bilaterally, is symmetric and concentrated on the upper extremities, and may last a few weeks to twelve months.
5. Hair loss may occur from lesions on the scalp.

"Mucous patches" may appear in the mouth and on moist surfaces of the genitalia, with or without the generalized lesions. They are usually multiple, and appear as an oval, grayish-white ulcer with a raised dull red border. Condylomata lata appear as reddish brown, flat-topped, moist warty-appearing structures on the moist areas of the genitals. They may break down and present as a dull, red, oozing surface. These lesions are extremely contagious.

- *Latent stage:* This stage may last 10-20 years and is free from symptoms. Serologic test results are positive, but the results of spinal fluid and darkfield examination are negative for the organism.

    *Early latent stage*
    1. The patient has had a primary or secondary lesion in the past four years.
    2. The patient is less than 30 years old.
    3. The organism is invading the organ systems.
    4. The skin surface becomes noninfectious after one year, but blood and tissue products are contagious. A pregnant woman can infect the fetus.

    *Late latent stage*
    1. The patient has had a primary or secondary lesion four or more years previously.
    2. The patient is 30 years of age or older.

- *Late (tertiary) stage:* One or more body systems may be affected including the mucocutaneous, osseous, visceral, and cardiovascular systems. Lesions in these systems are progressive and destructive in about one-third of the infected population in this stage.

## Differential Diagnosis

- Skin rash from allergic reaction or other contagious disease
- Herpes simplex type 1 or 2

- Gonorrhea, chancroid, lymphogranuloma venereum
- Malignancy
- Infectious mononucleosis
- Painless lesions failing to heal within two weeks are suspect

## Diagnostic Studies as Clinically Indicated

Syphilis is known as the "great mimic" since it produces signs and symptoms similar to many other diseases, which makes its diagnosis difficult.

- A sexual history is an important diagnostic tool in assessing this disease.
- The VDRL (Venereal Disease Research Laboratory) test is a nontreponemal test and is 75% accurate. Treatment early in the course of the disease causes the VDRL titer to fall rapidly.

    This test should be done in all pregnant women at the first prenatal visit. In women suspected to be at high risk for infection, the VDRL test should be repeated in the third trimester.

    False-positive test results may be due to:

    1. Measles
    2. Chickenpox
    3. Viral hepatitis
    4. Lymphogranuloma venereum
    5. Heroin addiction
    6. Systemic lupus erythematosis (SLE)
    7. Infectious mononucleosis
    8. Rheumatoid arthritis

- The rapid plasma reagin card test (RPR) is a simplified nontreponemal test. Cards designed for hand mixing (teardrop card) or mechanical mixing (18-mm circle card) are available.
- The fluorescent treponemal antibody absorption test (FTA-ABS test) is used if results of the VDRL test are suspected to be false-positive or false-negative. It is:

    The most sensitive and reliable test for syphilis

    More expensive and difficult to perform than the VDRL test

    Not to be used for mass screening

    Used for patients with a suspicious history of lesions

- A darkfield microscopic examination of fluid from sores on sexual organs or

aspirate from buboes may be done. If the results are negative, this test should be repeated in three days.
- The treponemal immobilization (TPI) test is:
    The most specific blood test for syphilis
    Complex, difficult to perform, and expensive
    Used for difficult diagnostic problems only
- Spinal fluid examination is done with the VDRL and FTA-ABS tests for detection of latent disease.
- A culture for *Neisseria gonorrhoeae* should be done.
- A Pap smear should be done and may also be used for suspected herpes simplex type 2 infection.

## Management and Treatment as Clinically Indicated

Penicillin continues to be the drug of choice for all stages of syphilis. Every effort should be made to document penicillin allergy before choosing other antibiotics since these antibiotics have been studied less extensively in the treatment of syphilis than penicillin. Physicians are cautioned to use no less than the recommended dosages of antibiotics. The following minimum treatment standards have been recommended by the Center for Disease Control.

### Antibiotic Therapy for Syphilis

- Incubating syphilis: Patients exposed to infectious syphilis within the preceding three months or at high risk based on epidemiologic grounds should be treated as for early syphilis. Where possible a diagnosis should be established. Women who are culture-positive for gonorrhea with no lesion and nonreactive serologic tests must also be considered to be at high risk. The aqueous procaine penicillin G plus probenecid regimen for gonorrhea is also effective therapy for incubating syphilis. No other antibiotic regimen is known to be effective. A reagin test for syphilis should be repeated three months after the initial therapy.
- Treatment for syphilis of less than one year's duration
    Benzathine penicillin G, 2.4 million units total IM (1.2 million units in each buttock), has the advantage of a single visit treatment. Aqueous procaine penicillin G, 600,000 units/day for eight days for a total of 4.8 million units, is effective but requires multiple visits.
    For patients allergic to penicillin, two alternative regimens are recommended.

1. Oral erythromycin stearate, ethyl succinate, or base: 2 g/day for 15 days, a total of 30 g.
2. Oral tetracycline hydrochloride: 2 g/day for 15 days, a total of 30 g. These antibiotics have not been as extensively studied as penicillin.

If during the year following treatment clinical signs recur or persist, a spinal fluid examination should be done, and the patient should be retreated using the regimen for syphilis acquired more than one year previously. The same retreatment regimen is used if the initial nonspecific antibody titer is greater than 1:8 or fails to decrease to negative or by fourfold within a 12-month period.

- Treatment of syphilis of indeterminate length or more than one year's duration
  Benzathine penicillin G, 2.4 million units IM is given weekly (1.2 million units in each buttock) for three successive weeks for a total of 7.2 million units. This is a regimen with good patient compliance. Instead, the patient can be given aqueous procaine penicillin G, 600,000 units/day IM for 14 days, but the daily injections are a disadvantage. If the spinal fluid is positive, some investigators favor hospital admission and intravenous penicillin G therapy, 2.4 million units given every four hours for 10 days.

  For the patient allergic to penicillin, a spinal fluid examination must be performed before therapy. There are two alternative regimens: Tetracycline, 500 mg four times a day for 30 days, a total of 60 g, or the oral forms of erythromycin, except the estolate, 500 mg four times a day for 30 days, a total of 60 g.

  All patients with a positive spinal fluid should have spinal fluid testing at least every six months for three years.

- Treatment of syphilis in pregnancy: For pregnant patients not allergic to penicillin, treatment is the same as for the corresponding stage of syphilis in nonpregnant patients. For pregnant women who are allergic to penicillin, the only recommended therapy is erythromycin in the same form and dosage used for the same state of disease as in nonpregnant women. Women who have been treated for syphilis during pregnancy should have monthly quantitative nontreponemal serologic tests for the remainder of the pregnancy. Women who show a rise in titer of four dilutions or greater should be retreated.

### Congenital Syphilis

Every infant with suspected or proven congenital syphilis should have a cerebrospinal fluid examination before treatment and should be followed at monthly intervals until the results of nontreponemal serologic tests are negative. Symptomatic infants or infants with a positive spinal fluid should be treated with aqueous penicillin G, 500 units/kg/day IM or IV in two divided doses for a minimum of 10 days or aqueous procaine penicillin G, 50,000/kg/day IM for a minimum of 10 days.

Asymptomatic seropositive infants with a negative cerebrospinal fluid examination can be treated with penicillin G, 50,000 units/kg IM in a single dose.

Infants born of mothers treated with erythromycin for syphilis during pregnancy should be managed as though they have congenital syphilis.

### Drug Reactions Related to Syphilis Therapy

Penicillin reactions include skin rashes, urticaria, chills, fever, edema, arthralgia, prostration, and occasional fatal anaphylactoid reactions have occurred. Tetracyclines and erythromycin may cause skin rashes, or more commonly, gastrointestinal disturbances such as gastric intolerance, nausea, vomiting, cramps, and diarrhea. These may reduce patient compliance with the long dosage regimens. Because of maternal and fetal toxicity, tetracycline is not recommended for pregnant women. The estolate form of erythromycin is not recommended because of liver toxicity.

### Case Finding and Prevention

The best method for control of syphilis is by contact tracing through case interviewing. Syphilis is a reportable disease and help is available through local and state health agencies.

## Complications

- Secondary stage
    Syphilitic hepatitis
    Obliterative endarteritis
- Late state
    Cardiovascular complications
    1. Aortic valve insufficiency
    2. Saccular aortic aneurysm
    Central nervous system syphilis
    1. Paretic neurosyphilis resulting in loss of nerve cells
    2. Headaches, loss of memory, dysarthria, tremors of the lips, tongue, hands, progressing to personality changes and psychotic reactions

3. Tabes dorsalis, with weakening or loss of ankle and knee reflexes and various degrees of ataxia
4. General paresis

## Patient Teaching

- Explain to the patient what her infection is and how it was acquired. The patient may be embarrassed and uncommunicative, but giving her this information is important.
- Explain the necessity of completing medical treatment in order to halt progression of the disease, which although asymptomatic, will cause further dangerous health problems. When treated early, it is easily cured.
- Stress the need to notify her sexual partner(s) so they can be examined and treated as soon as possible. (The Department of Public Health tries to trace contacts to assure they receive treatment.)
- Explain that there is no immunity to the disease, and if contact is made with an infected partner, reinfection can occur. If possible reinfection has occurred, she should seek medical care immediately.
- Explain the need to refrain from sexual intercourse for one month, or until the results of follow-up tests are negative.
- Discuss with the patient the need to know her sexual partner. If there is any question of possible infection, examine the partner for genital lesions or discharge from the penis or vagina.
- Explain that use of a condom and contraceptive foams are helpful in preventing sexually transmitted disease. Again, their use is limited in prevention of syphilis.

# CHANCROID
# (SOFT CHANCRE, ULCUS MOLLE)

## Definition

Chancroid is an acute, self-limited, autoinoculable, sexually transmitted infection of the genitals.

## Etiology

The causative organism is *Hemophilus ducreyi,* a small gram-negative rod most commonly observed singly or in small clusters along strands of mucus. Chancroid is not commonly found in temperate zones but may be transported from tropical areas, usually by military personnel. The incubation period is five days or less. The disease is transmitted during sexual contact with open lesions and discharge from buboes. The organism does not penetrate intact, healthy epithelium. The infection is communicable as long as the organism is present in the ulcers or discharge, which is usually several weeks. When healing is complete the organism is no longer present. Infection offers no immunity. Fresh lesions occur by autoinoculation, and reinfection readily occurs immediately after cure.

## Clinical Features

### Symptoms

(Women are commonly asymptomatic.)

- Painful ulcers, usually confined to the genitalia, which are most commonly traumatized during sexual contact
- Tender inguinal nodes and swelling of the labia

### Signs

- Initial lesions are on or near the genitalia.
  Usually there are only one or two small, inflamed papules with erythematous borders.
  The lesion progresses to a pustule, which ruptures, leaving a painful shallow ulcer with a ragged, irregular edge. The ulcer base has grayish exudate, bleeds easily, and may be malodorous
  The lesion may be distinguished from chancre of primary syphilis by the presence of pain, softness, and lack of induration of the ulcer.
- Edema of the labia and bilateral adenopathy may occur.
- Spread of lesions to any area of the vulva, pubis, and abdomen or thighs occurs by autoinoculation.
- Bubo formation occurs in 25-60% of the cases. It is a large, erythematous, painful inguinal lesion that suppurates and drains.
- Lesions may heal spontaneously or become chronic.

## Differential Diagnosis

- Syphilis
- Granuloma inguinale
- Lymphogranuloma venereum
- Herpesvirus hominis type 2 infection
- Neoplasm

## Diagnostic Studies as Clinically Indicated

Diagnosis is usually made on the basis of history of exposure, typical signs and symptoms, and exclusion of other venereal disease.

- A smear of serous exudate from the bubo rolled on a glass slide and Gram stained shows gram-negative coccobacilli and polymorphonuclear leukocytes.
- A blood agar culture of pus from buboes incubated in a candle jar at 35°C for 48 hours will isolate the *H. ducreyi.*
- Biopsy of the lesion and culture of open lesions is difficult due to abundant secondary bacterial infection.
- A smear for gonococci and a VDRL test are indicated.

## Management and Treatment as Clinically Indicated

Treatment of the lesion before an inguinal mass becomes fluctuant and necrosis of the overlying skin occurs will avoid permanent scarring and deformity.

- Physician consultation or referral is always necessary.
- Oral sulfisoxazole, 1 g, is given every six hours for five to seven days. After a five-day interval the drug course should be repeated. *Check for sulfa allergy.*
- Tetracycline, 500 mg, is given orally four times a day for one to two weeks in resistant cases or in cases of infection with destructive lesions. This treatment:

    Masks the presence of syphilis. This disease should be ruled out before treatment begins.

    Is contraindicated in pregnancy because of possible retardation of fetal skeletal growth and permanent discoloration of the teeth.

    Should be taken one hour before or two hours after meals. Food and some dairy products interfere with its absorption.

- The bubo may be aspirated if large and fluctuant, but it should never be incised.
- Warm sitz baths are helpful in relieving local discomfort.
- Repeat the VDRL test in 6-10 weeks if it was initially nonreactive.

## Complications

- Extensive tissue destruction from persistent ulceration
- Secondary infection of the ulcers
- Strictures from scarring and keloid formation

## Patient Teaching

- Refer to the patient teaching section for syphilis.
- Discuss with the patient that sexual partner(s) of two weeks after the initial onset of symptoms should be contacted. They need to seek immediate medical examination and/or treatment.
- Stress the need to return for reexamination every three months for one year after completion of treatment.
- Tell the patient that correct use of a condom is helpful in prevention of chancroid because the initial lesion in the male is located on the penis.

# GRANULOMA INGUINALE
# (DONOVANOSIS, GRANULOMA VENEREUM, GRANULOMA PUDENDI, VENEREAL GRANULOMA, SCLEROSING GRANULOMA)

## Definition

Granuloma inguinale is a chronic, mildly contagious, sexually transmitted disease of the external genitalia and inguinal regions.

## Etiology

The causative organism, *Donovania granulomatis* (Donovan body), is a gram-negative, immobile, encapsulated body. A parasite of man, it has not been successfully grown in animals. The incubation period varies widely between eight days and 12 weeks. Transmission is questionable but presumed to be through contact with open lesions during sexual intercourse. Lack of clinical signs of disease in many exposed partners is unexplained. The disease is communicable as long as open lesions are present.

The disease has a low incidence and is usually found in tropical, subtropical, and temperate regions. It occurs most frequently in males and blacks between the ages of 20 and 40 years.

## Clinical Features

### Symptoms

- None
- A painless bump on the genitalia
- An open sore that bleeds easily
- A chronic ulcer on the genitalia that is getting larger

### Signs

If untreated, the clinical course of the disease is slowly progressive.

- The lesion begins as a macule and progresses to a papule, which breaks down to form a small, painless friable ulcer with a red granular base.
- The lesion is found on the vulva or vagina and spreads to the thighs, perineum, and anal regions.
- The lesion remains superficial in contrast to other forms of chronic ulcerative lesions.
- Lesions spread slowly becoming confluent, granulomatous, and destructive. They heal slowly and cause extensive fibrosis if untreated.
- Subcutaneous granuloma may form in the inguinal region.
- Extragenital lesions may be seen on the mouth, nose, and lips.
- Inguinal adenopathy is a rare finding.

## Differential Diagnosis

- Lymphogranuloma venereum
- Chancroid
- Syphilis
- Carcinoma
- Tuberculosis

## Diagnostic Studies as Clinically Indicated

- A tissue biopsy with cytologic examination shows Donovan bodies in mononuclear ("closed safety pin") cells.
- A Darkfield examination is done to exclude syphilis.
- A smear for gonococci should be done.
- A routine Pap smear should be done if indicated.

## Management and Treatment as Clinically Indicated

- Physician consultation or referral is necessary.
- Oxytetracycline, 500 mg, is given orally every six hours for 12 days. This treatment may be extended for two weeks if response is unsatisfactory. Patients should take the drug one hour before or two hours after meals. Food and some dairy products interfere with its absorption. *Oxytetracycline is contraindicated in pregnancy and masks the presence of syphilis, which must be ruled out before treatment.*
- Streptomycin, 1 g, is given IM every six hours for five days. Hospitalization is necessary for this treatment to observe for possible toxicity in the patient.
- Warm sitz baths with a 1:10,000 solution of potassium permanganate are taken three times a day for cleansing and prevention of secondary infection.
- Surgical excision and plastic repair are indicated in chronic cases.

## Complications

- Fibrosis and scarring of tissue
- Tissue depigmentation and keloid formation

- Lymphatic obstruction with elephantiasis
- Vaginal or anal stenosis
- Disseminated disease in the pregnant patient with cervical lesions (rare)
- Secondary infection
- Ophthalmologic, osseous, and dermatologic complications.

### Patient Teaching

- Refer to the patient teaching section for syphilis.
- Inform the patient that the lesions should be healed in six weeks (for those patients who seek early treatment and take the medicine as directed).
- Stress that if the lesions are not healing, the patient should return for reevaluation of the diagnosis.
- Stress the importance of three follow-up appointments for one year after treatment.

## LYMPHOGRANULOMA VENEREUM (LGV, LYMPHOGRANULOMA INGUINALE, LYMPHOPATHIA VENEREUM)

### Definition

Lymphogranuloma venereum is a sexually transmitted infectious disease characterized by a lesion of short duration followed by lymphadenitis. The disease primarily affects the lymph nodes and channels.

### Etiology

Members of the genus *Chlamydia (Bedsonia)* of the Psittacosis-LGV-Trachoma group are the infecting organisms. Chlamydia were previously thought to be large viruses but are presently considered gram-negative obligate intracellular bacteria. This group of organisms causes trachoma, psittacosis, inclusion conjunctivitis, as well as lymphogranuloma venereum. These intracellular parasites will not grow on artificial media, and tissue cultures are necessary for isolation and identification.

Primary inoculation may occur at any anatomic site involved in intimate contact, and its incubation period is 7-12 days. The disease is most commonly found in the more sexually active 20- to 40-year-old group and among the lower socioeconomic groups.

Transmission is by direct contact with a draining lesion, usually during sexual intercourse, or by indirect contact with contaminated clothing. Immunity develops after one clinical attack.

## Clinical Features

### Symptoms

- *Inguinal Syndrome* (The clinical course may be long and chronic.)
    Fever, chills
    Headache, abdominal pain
    Arthralgia, anorexia
    Splenomegaly
    Urticaria
    Generalized lymphadenopathy
- Genitoanorectal syndrome
    A bloody, mucopurulent anal discharge
    Fibrosis of ulcerative lesions with vaginal or urethral stenosis
    Proctitis with constipation or diarrhea

### Signs

- Inguinal syndrome

    A primary lesion appears at the inoculation site 10 days to three months after exposure.
    1. It is usually a single papule, small erosion, vesicular, painless lesion resembling that of herpes simplex type 2.
    2. It heals before the onset of lymphadenopathy.

    Regional lymphadenopathy occurs two weeks after the initial lesion.
    1. It may be unilateral or bilateral.
    2. A bubo appears 10 to 30 days after exposure.

Hyperglobulinemia may occur.

A groove ("groove sign") through the center of the mass, corresponding to the inguinal ligament, separates the mass into inguinal and femoral areas (pathogonomic finding of LGV).

The overlying skin breaks down draining seropurulent fluid from the multiple sinuses of the mass.

- Genitoanorectal syndrome

    Genitoanorectal problems occur primarily in women.

    Friable, edematous, hemorrhagic anorectal mucosa may be seen.

    Ulcerative lesions are evident on the vulva, vagina, and urethra.

## Differential Diagnosis

- Syphilis
- Chancroid
- Granuloma inguinale
- Tuberculosis
- Neoplasm
- Other chlamydial infection

## Diagnostic Studies as Clinically Indicated

- Frie test (0.1 ml of antigen is injected intradermally into the forearm.)

    The test is positive when an area of induration greater than 5 mm in diameter, surrounded by an erythematous zone, is seen after 48 hours. The test site should be checked for one week in case of delayed positive results.

    The test becomes positive 12–40 days after the primary lesion appears.

    The test remains positive for life and, without clinical signs, is not diagnostic. (The patient may have had an undiagnosed clinical case in the past.)

    If there is suspicion of the disease but the Frie test is negative, the test should be repeated in several weeks.

- The compliment fixation test is 97% accurate and becomes positive four weeks after an initial infection. A titer greater than 1:30 usually indicates active disease.
- The VDRL test may give false-positive results.

GYNECOLOGIC INFECTIONS 209

- Aspiration of inguinal bulboes with Giemsa staining of the fluid shows typical intracytoplasmic inclusions.
- The Lyngranum skin test antigen becomes positive in one to two weeks.
- A Pap smear and a smear for gonococci should be done.

## Management and Treatment as Clinically Indicated

(It is not certain if medications completely eradicate chlamydia from the body. The organisms may persist in a subclinical state.)
- Physician consultation or referral is necessary.
- Tetracycline, 2-4 g/day, is given orally for 10-15 days. Advise the patient to take this drug one hour before or two hours after meals. Food and some dairy products interfere with its absorption. *Tetracycline is contraindicated in pregnant and lactating women.*
- Sulfisoxazole, 1 g, is given orally four times a day for one to two weeks. Discontinue the medication for one week, then repeat the treatment. *Check for sulfa allergy.*
- The buboes may be drained by aspiration; they are not to be excised.
- Severe elephantiasis of the vulva requires surgical removal.

## Complications

- Genital elephantiasis
- Chronic buboes, perirectal abscess
- Rectal stricture (lymphatic drainage of infection to anorectal nodes)
- Possible increased risk for rectal or vulvar carcinoma
- Nonspecific urethritis
- Urethral or vaginal stricture
- Infection of newborn (contact with infected birth canal of mother)

## Patient Teaching

- Refer to the patient teaching section for syphilis (with the exception of the fourth point)

- Explain that the disease is characterized by remissions and exacerbations, and that follow-up every three months is necessary. Tell the patient that if recurrent signs appear, she should contact the physician immediately for resumption of medication.
- Explain that immunity results after one episode of the infection.

## REFERENCES

Aurelian L: Genital herpes update. *The Female Patient* 4:19, 1979.

Borrow G, Ferris T: *Medical Complications During Pregnancy.* Philadelphia, WB Saunders Company, 1975, pp 489-509.

Brown D, Daufman R: Pelvic infection and venereal disease, in Glass R (ed): *Office Gynecology.* Baltimore, Williams & Wilkins Company, 1976, pp 21-43.

Duncan W: Gonorrhea, chlamydia, and syphilis: New trends in diagnosis. *The Female Patient* 2:30, 1977.

Dykers J: Single-dose metronidazole for trichomonal vaginitis. *N Engl J Med* 293:23, 1975.

Edwards M: Venereal herpes: A nursing overview. *JOGN Nursing* 7:7, 1978.

*FDA Drug Bulletin* 10:6, 1980.

Fiumara N: Venereal diseases, in Charles D, Finland M (eds): *Obstetric and Perinatal Infections.* Philadelphia, Lea & Febiger, 1973, pp 447-477.

Garagusi V: Gonorrhea in genital and nongenital sites. *The Female Patient* 3:14, 1978.

Green T: *Gynecology: Essentials of Clinical Practice.* Boston, Little, Brown and Company, 1971, pp 181-188.

Greenhalf J: The problem of pelvic infection. *The Practitioner* 216:513, 1976.

Griffith R, Norins A, Kagan C: A multicentered study of lysine therapy in herpes simplex infection. *Dermatologica* 156:257, 1978.

Hill E: Disorders of the uterine cervix, in Benson R (ed): *Current Obstetrics and Gynecologic Diagnosis and Treatment.* Los Altos, Calif, Lange Medical Publications, 1978, pp 186-192.

Hilton A, et al: Chlamydia A in the female genital tract. *Br J Venereal Dis* 50:1, 1974.

Jaffee H: The laboratory diagnosis of syphilis: New concepts. *Ann Intern Med* 83:846, 1975.

Kern G: *Gynecology.* Chicago, Year Book Medical Publishers, 1976, pp 242-273.

Kibrick S: Herpes simplex, in Charles D, Finland M (eds): *Obstetric and Perinatal Infections.* Philadelphia, Lea & Febiger, 1973, pp 75-94.

Ledger W: Infections and infestations of the lower genital tract, in de Alvarez R (ed): *Textbook of Gynecology.* Philadelphia, Lea & Febiger, 1977, pp 399-429.

Lee L, Schmale J: Ampicillin therapy for *Corynebacterium vaginale (Haemophilus vaginalis)* vaginitis. *Am J Obstet Gynecol* 115:786, 1973.

Martin P, Yens S, Burnier A, et al: Systemic absorption and sustained effects of vaginal estrogen creams. *JAMA* 242:2699, 1979.

Mattingly R: *TeLinde's Operative Gynecology,* ed 5. Philadelphia, JB Lippincott Company, 1977, pp 259-266.

Neeson J: Herpesvirus genitalis: A nursing perspective. *Nursing Clin N Am* 10:599, 1975.

Palmer A: Vaginitis. *The Practitioner* 214:666, 1975.

Parsons L, Sommers D: *Gynecology,* ed 2. Philadelphia, WB Saunders Company, 1978, pp 828-877.

Pfeifer T, Forsyth P, Durfee M, et al: Nonspecific vaginitis, role of *Haemophilus vaginalis* and treatment with metronidazole. *N Engl J Med* 298:1429-1433, 1978.

Rein M, Chapel T: Trichomoniasis, candidiasis, and the minor venereal diseases. *Clin Obstet Gynec* 18:73, 1975.

Sabin A: Misery of recurrent herpes: what to do. *N Engl J Med* 297:986, 1975.

Schoode G: A vaginitis protocol that helps teach. *Nurse Practitioner* 1:64, 1975.

*STD Fact Sheet,* US Department of HEW, Public Health Service Center for Disease Control, Atlanta, Georgia, 1979, pp 6-8.

Tanowitz H: Parasitic gynecologic disease. *Medical Aspects of Human Sexuality* 8:1974.

# 10
# Menstrual Disorders

Disturbances of the menstrual cycle are common, and it is the rare woman who has never experienced abnormal vaginal bleeding or menstrual symptoms at some time in her life. Numerous physiologic and psychologic factors must function in perfect harmony to maintain normal menstrual cycles, and it is surprising that more women are not experiencing more problems.

Menstrual variation may result from dysfunction at any level of hormonal or physiologic function. Since symptoms of menstrual disorders may be similar regardless of the complexity of causes, differentiating and diagnosing these problems require sophisticated and supportive management skills.

This chapter covers only the most common menstrual disorders that are seen in the practice of women's health care and includes dysfunctional uterine bleeding, amenorrhea, dysmenorrhea, and premenstrual syndrome.

## AMENORRHEA*

### Definition

Amenorrhea is a symptom, not a disease. Traditionally it has been defined as primary and secondary, but more recent criteria have been developed to describe this disorder:

*The following section, up to "Management and Treatment as Clinically Indicated," is adapted from Speroff, L, et al: *Clinical Gynecologic Endocrinology and Infertility*, Baltimore, Williams & Wilkins Company, 1978. Used with permission of author and publisher.

- Absence or retardation of secondary sexual characteristics with failure to menstruate by age 14
- Presence of normal growth and development and secondary sexual characteristics, without menstruation by age 16
- Absence of menstruation for a time equivalent to a total of three previous cycle intervals, or six months of amenorrhea in a previously menstruating woman
- Physiologic amenorrhea:
    Delayed puberty
    Pregnancy
    Postpartum amenorrhea
    Menopause

## Etiology

Causes of amenorrhea are complex and involve four levels of functioning; dysfunction can occur at any of these four levels.

- Outflow tract and uterus resulting from:
    Congenital defects, trauma, or abnormality of the vagina, cervix, or uterus
    Absence or malfunction of the endometrium and/or dysfunctional estrogen or progesterone effect
- Ovary by alteration of:
    Secretion of estrogen and progesterone
    Follicular development, ovulation, or corpus luteum formation
- Anterior pituitary with alteration of:
    Follicle-stimulating hormone (FSH) secretion
    Luteinizing hormone (LH) secretion
- Central nervous system (hypothalamic factor) with alteration of gonadotropin-releasing hormone

### *Symptom*

- Initial or secondary absence of menstruation

### *Signs*

- Absence or malformation of pelvic organs
- Lack of ferning of cervical mucus

- Monophasic basal body temperature chart
- Galactorrhea

## Differential Diagnosis

- Pregnancy, pseudocyesis
- Premature menopause, hysterectomy
- Pituitary tumor
- Congenital absence or anomaly of pelvic organs
- Psychogenic or environmental factors
- Malnutrition, anorexia nervosa
- Oral contraceptive, psychotropic drug use
- Polycystic ovary syndrome
- Chromosomal abnormality
- Follicular cyst
- Cirrhosis, thyroid disease, tuberculosis
- Ovarian insufficiency
- Chiari-Frommel Syndrome

## Diagnostic Studies as Clinically Indicated

After a complete history taking and physical examination, diagnosis follows three logical steps (See Fig. 1).

### Step I

*Purpose*

- To assess endogenous estrogen level
- To assess competence of outflow tract/uterus
- To measure level of serum prolactin

*Method*

- Test the pituitary-ovarian system.

    Using a pure progestational agent (without estrogenic effects), a progesterone withdrawal test is done. Either of the following agents is administered:

    1. Progesterone in oil, 200 mg one dose IM OR
    2. Medroxyprogesterone acetate (Provera), 10 mg/day for five days

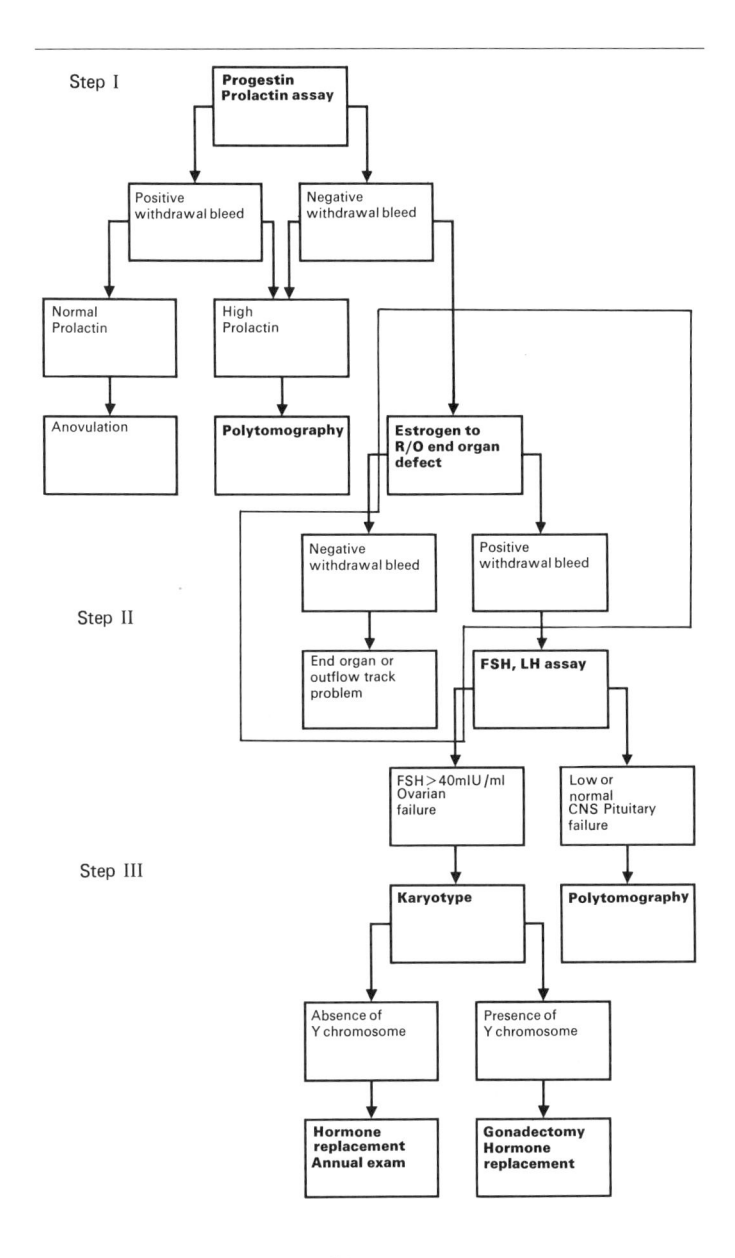

**Figure 1.**
Steps in the differential diagnosis of amenorrhea. (Adapted with permission from L. Speroff, R. Glass, and N. Kase: *Clinical Gynecologic Endocrinology and Infertility,* © 1978, The Williams & Wilkins Co., Baltimore.)

- Draw a specimen for a serum prolactin assay.

*Results:*

- If withdrawal bleeding occurs within two to seven days after completion of one of the above medications, it is diagnostic of:

  Anovulation

  A functional outflow tract with endometrial response to endogenous estrogen

  A functioning hypothalamic-pituitary-ovarian axis

- Bleeding may or may not occur, but a pituitary tumor may be ruled out if:

  There is absence of galatorrhea and

  Serum prolactin levels are normal ($< 20$ ng/ml)

- If withdrawal bleeding does not occur, it indicates either outflow tract dysfunction or lack of estrogen-primed endometrium

### *Step II*

Abnormalities in the outflow tract/uterus are uncommon, and Step II may be omitted if:

- The patient has normal external and internal genitalia.
- No history of trauma or infection of pelvic organs exists. If the above conditions do not exist, complete Step II.

*Purpose*

- To stimulate endometrial proliferation
- To assess the outflow tract

*Method*

- Give conjugated estrogen, 2.5 mg/day for 21 days (Conestron, Estrifol, Glyestrin, Premarin, Theogen). To achieve withdrawal, add medroxyprogesterone acetate (Provera), 10 mg/day for the last five days.
- If no withdrawal bleeding occurs, a second course of estrogen is recommended.

*Results*

- No withdrawal bleeding suggests:

  An outflow tract or uterine/endometrial dysfunction

  Inadequate estrogen stimulation

- Withdrawal bleeding indicates:

  An outflow tract with normal uterine/endometrium functioning when stimulated by estrogen

### Step III

*Purpose*

- To assess pituitary gonadotropin secretion and follicular activity to determine which is the source of decreased estrogen production and resulting dysfunction

*Method*

- Wait two weeks after Step II to proceed with Step III. This allows the patient's gonadotropins to return to baseline levels after the effects of the exogenous estrogens given in Step II have cleared.
- Collect a specimen for a serum gonadotropin radioimmunoassay. (Assay of urinary gonadotropins in a 24-hour specimen is not reliable.)

*Results*

- A normal FSH value (5-30 mIU/ml) indicates the presence of normal ovarian follicles.
- A FSH value of > 40 mIU/ml is abnormally high and occurs in:
    Gonadal failure with exhausted supply of ovarian follicles (Patient is considered sterile.)
    Ovarian failure in conjunction with elevated LH levels
    1. Repeat sampling is indicated in patients desiring fertility.
    2. In patients under 35 years of age karyotyping for the presence of a Y chromosome is indicated.
        a. If a Y chromosome is present, there is 25% chance that the patient has a malignant gonadal tumor, and gonadectomy is indicated.
        b. If a Y chromosome is not present, hormonal therapy and an annual pelvic examination is indicated.
    Women over 35 years of age who are undergoing premature menopause
- An LH value of < 5 mIU/ml indicates hypogonadism (normal: 5-25 mIU/ml).
- Low or normal gonadotropin levels with amenorrhea
    Polytomography is performed to rule out abnormalities of the sella turcica

## Possible Diagnoses

The possible diagnoses indicated by findings at each stage of the diagnostic process are given below. Addressing each of these problems separately is not within the scope of this book.

*Step I*

- Asherman's syndrome
- Mullerian anomalies
- Mullerian agenesis
- Testicular feminization

*Step II*

- Turner's syndrome
- Mosaicism
- Gonadal agenesis
- The resistant ovary syndrome

*Step III*

- Pituitary tumors
- The empty sella syndrome

## Management and Treatment as Clinically Indicated

The causes of amenorrhea are multiple and range in degree from those that are easily diagnosed and treated to those that are complex to diagnose and to treat. Often treatment for the various causative factors can only be palliative or cosmetic. The final diagnosis, reached with the aid of the sequential guide presented previously and in Figure 1, will determine the mode of therapy.

## Patient Teaching

- Discuss with the patient whose diagnosis has not been established what she can expect during future visits. She needs to know the different levels at which dysfunction can occur (uterus, vagina, ovaries, pituitary, and hypothalamus), and she needs to be made aware that diagnosis may take time.
- Review of the female anatomy and menstrual cycle may help some patients to better understand why diagnostic tests need to be done.
- Explain to patients who do not desire pregnancy the need to use contraception (ovulation may be occurring occasionally). Methods such as the condom

and foam and the diaphragm would be preferable to birth control pills, which would interfere with the diagnostic process.
- Explain to patients with postpill amenorrhea the need to wait six months for their period to return before seeking evaluation.
- Explore with the patient who has no physiologic basis for her lack of periods, possible causative psychologic or other stress factors. Appointments for counseling may be appropriate.
- Discuss with the obese amenorrheic patient that weight loss would be a positive factor in return of menses.

## DYSFUNCTIONAL UTERINE BLEEDING

### Definition

Dysfunctional uterine bleeding is abnormal, unpredictable bleeding of endometrial origin not resulting from an organic cause.

### Etiology

Dysfunctional uterine bleeding occurs primarily in women at the extremes of menstrual life; 20% of the cases occur in young women during puberty, 50% in women over 45 years of age, and 30% in women during the reproductive age. Seventy percent of the women with dysfunctional bleeding are anovulatory.

### Identified Causes

- Central, or neuroendocrine dysfunction, such as an immature hypothalamus in the adolescent resulting in alteration of estrogen and progesterone secretion by the ovaries
- Peripheral, or ovarian, dysfunction, as in the perimenopausal woman
- Anovulation, which may occur in any of the above age groups and may be due to:
    Follicular phase defect
    1. Immature follicle formation results in subnormal estrogen production and irregular, scanty cycles.

2. Persistent unruptured follicles result in prolonged, unopposed estrogen secretion with hyperplastic endometrium. The patient may experience two to three months of amenorrhea followed by prolonged and/or excessive bleeding.

Luteal phase defect
1. Premature corpus luteum degeneration causes shortening of the luteal phase, and polymenorrhea results.
2. Persistent corpus luteum causes prolonged progesterone stimulation of the endometrium resulting in polymenorrhea after a late menses.

Decreasing response to gonadotropin stimulation during the climacteric results in ovarian failure and less frequent ovulation.
- Temporary estrogen withdrawal at ovulation, causing endometrial breakdown and midcycle ovulatory bleeding
- Emotional lability, which may cause change in gonadotropin release at the hypothalamic level, resulting in an altered menstrual pattern
- Malnutrition, which may cause malfunction of gonadotropin release at the hypothalamic level

## Clinical Features

*Symptom*

- Irregular heavy or light bleeding with acute or chronic episodes

*Signs*

- Acyclic bleeding
- Absence of pelvic abnormalities
- Anovulatory bleeding (two to three months of amenorrhea followed by prolonged and/or excessive painless bleeding)
    Lack of premenstrual symptoms

## Differential Diagnosis

- Pregnancy complications
- IUD complications
- Psychogenic factors

# MENSTRUAL DISORDERS

- Benign or malignant lesions of the genital tract
- Obesity and weight fluctuations
- Thyroid dysfunction
- Polycystic ovary syndrome
- Premature menopause
- Exogenous steroids, psychotropic drugs, DES
- Chronic debilitative disease
- Blood dyscrasia, anticoagulant therapy
- Adrenal hypo/hyperfunction
- Gonadal dysgenesis
- Asherman's syndrome
- Rectal bleeding

## Diagnostic Studies as Clinically Indicated

- Consultation with a physician is necessary before diagnostic studies are ordered.
- Complete medical/menstrual/obstetric history. Sexual and social history may be indicated.
- Complete pelvic and rectal examinations. Observation of the estrogen effect on the pelvic organs, enlarged ovaries, or hirsutism, should be noted.
- A maturation index is done if indicated.
- A breast examination should be done with careful evaluation for galactorrhea.
- A Pap smear and a smear for gonococci are indicated.
- A pregnancy test is done to rule out bleeding from a problem pregnancy.
- A CBC, serum iron and total iron binding capacity determinations, quantitative electrophoresis, and platelet count are done to rule out iron-deficiency anemia or blood dyscrasias.
- T3, and T4 assays are done to assess thyroid function.
- The charting of a basal body temperature calendar will demonstrate hormone fluctuations and ovulation.
- Hormonal evaluation may include determination of levels of:
  Serum LH and FSH
  Serum estradiol (if no bleeding occurs after a progesterone withdrawal test)
  Serum progesterone, in selected cases
  Serum prolactin, in selected cases
- A progesterone withdrawal test may be indicated (see Chap. 17).

- An endometrial biopsy and/or D&C in the adult patient is done to assess endometrial function. This is not usually indicated in the adolescent patient.
- Laparoscopy may be indicated in selected cases.
- A hysterosalpingogram is ordered if genital tract abnormality is suspected.

## Management and Treatment as Clinically Indicated

The purpose of treatment is to control bleeding, to prevent recurrences, and to preserve fertility. Hormone therapy protocols are multiple and controversial, and some of the more common treatment schedules are included here. This does not mean that others are less effective or less appropriate. Physician consultation is necessary to determine individual treatment.

- Anovulatory cycles

    For heavy bleeding in women of reproductive age
    1. High-dose estrogen/progestin birth control pills (Norlestrin, 2.5 mg) are given as follows: one pill four times a day for five to seven days. Menstrual flow should cease within 12-14 hours, (if not, further diagnostic studies are indicated to rule out abnormalities). The patient will experience heavy, crampy flow two to seven days after this therapy.
    2. On the fifth day of the menses after this treatment, a low-dose combination birth control pill (Norinyl 1 + 50) is given for 21 days and is followed by a seven-day withdrawal bleeding period. This regimen is continued for three months.
    3. If no withdrawal bleeding occurs three months after stopping the above regimen, anovulation is to be suspected. Medroxyprogesterone acetate (Provera), 10 mg/day orally for five days, may be administered at two-month intervals, with resultant withdrawal flow two to seven days after the last pill. This treatment may not be indicated in the perimenopausal women. If no bleeding occurs, further evaluation is needed.

    For heavy bleeding at menarche
    1. An acute, profuse bleeding episode requires Premarin, 20 mg IV stat every two hours for a total of three doses.
    2. To reestablish endometrial development, combination oral contraceptive pills are started in conjunction with the first dose of Premarin for three to six cycles.
    3. D&C is rarely indicated for the adolescent patient.

    For heavy perimenopausal bleeding
    1. A D&C will remove accumulated abnormal endometrial growth. Normal endometrial function may return after this procedure.

2. For estrogen deficiency, Premarin, 0.625-1.25 mg/day, may be given from Day 5 to Day 25 of the cycle.
3. Hysterectomy may be performed in selected patients with other complications.
- Ovulatory cycles may be accompanied by dysmenorrhea, breast tenderness, and emotional lability.

    Follicular phase defect
    1. Stilbestrol 0.1 mg/day, is given orally from Day 1 to Day 14 of the cycle. Mechanical contraception should be used during this period.

    Luteal phase defect
    1. Patients desiring fertility: Progesterone vaginal suppositories (25 mg) are inserted twice daily after the temperature rise on the BBT (basal body temperature) calendar is noted, and are continued until the next menses.
    2. Patients not desiring fertility: Either of the following drugs are given.
        a. Norethindrone (Norlutin), 5 mg/day from Day 16 to Day 25 of the cycle for three to six cycles OR:
        b. Medroxyprogesterone acetate (Provera), 10 mg/day from Day 16 to Day 25 of the cycle for three to six cycles.

## Complications:

- Infertility
- Iron-deficiency anemia
- Post-treatment amenorrhea in the adolescent patient
- Hormone side effects
- Increased susceptibility to endometrial carcinoma with chronic anovulation

## Patient Teaching

- Explain to the patient that no organic pathologic process exists, and explain what is the cause, or probable cause, of her abnormal bleeding.
- Reassure the patient who is prescribed hormone therapy that it takes several months of treatment to establish regular cycles, after which normal function will probably resume. The exception may be in the perimenopausal woman.
- Explain the necessity of taking medication as directed. If hormone preparations are not taken each day as directed, vaginal bleeding will occur.

- Explain the use of oral contraceptives to control bleeding. Explain their effectiveness as a birth control measure, their method of use, and side effects.
- Counsel the teenage patient with bleeding problems in a straight-forward manner. She needs an interested and caring person to explain her problem, its treatment, and to answer her questions honestly. She may need close follow-up until her cycles become regular.
- Inform the patient to expect a heavy bleeding episode after initial treatment for anovulation or after a progesterone withdrawal test. (Explain this test to the patient, see Chap. 17.)
- Explain to patients anticipating D&C that it is being done to scrape away the thickened endometrial lining of the uterus. Often normal cycles will return after this treatment.
- Review dietary habits of the patient and stress the need for a diet high in iron-containing foods and for iron supplementation if prescribed.
- Stress the need for good personal hygiene during bleeding episodes to prevent odor or infection.
- Explore possible stress or sexual problems.

# DYSMENORRHEA

## Definition

Dysmenorrhea is a symptom, not a disease. *Primary dysmenorrhea* (intrinsic, essential, idiopathic, spastic) is painful menstruation occurring in the absence of pelvic disease with onset in young women three to five years post menarche. *Secondary dysmenorrhea* (extrinsic, acquired) is painful menstruation resulting from organic pelvic disease or an intrauterine device, which may occur at any time during the reproductive years. It is a separate entity from primary dysmenorrhea and its causes are multiple (see Differential Diagnosis) and will not be covered here.

## Etiology

Current theory suggests that primary dysmenorrhea may be due to chemical changes occurring in the reproductive tract. Increased production of prostaglandins, which are unsaturated fatty acids present in all human body cells, have been identified as responsible for increased activity of the uterine muscle. Prostaglandin concentration increases in the endometrial cells during the secretory phase of the menstrual cycle and reaches a peak during menstruation. The increased pressure of the uterine contractions causes decreased arterial blood flow to the myometrium causing ischemia of the muscle, resulting in pain to the patient. The average level of prostaglandin production may be seven times higher in the secretory endometrium of dysmenorrheic women than in nondysmenorrheic women.

Psychologic influences are a consideration but are no longer identified as the main causes of primary dysmenorrhea.

Primary dysmenorrhea, one of the most common gynecologic disorders, effects up to 50% of postpubescent women, and approximately 10% of this group is incapacitated for one to three days every month. It is the greatest single cause of school and work absences in young women, with an estimate of 140 million work hours lost each year.

## Clinical Features

### Symptoms

Symptoms seldom last more than two days and may include:
- Pain, which may be:
    Intermittent, sharp, or crampy, beginning before menses
    Most severe on the first day of flow and lasting 24-48 hours
    Strongest over the lower abdomen and radiating to the back
- Pelvic fullness and heaviness
- Nausea, vomiting, diarrhea, leg cramps
- Headache, fatigue, syncope
- Depression, irritability, inability to concentrate

### Signs

- Painful menses are rare during the first two to five years post menarche.
- Painful menses occur in ovulating women; the cause is unknown.
- Relief from painful menses after childbirth may be temporary.
- Pain in women over 20 years of age may be due to pelvic abnormalities (secondary dysmenorrhea).

## Differential Diagnosis

- Endometriosis
- Uterine fibroids or polyps
- Uterine malformations or malposition
- Psychogenic causes
- Cervical stenosis
- Pelvic infection
- Adenomyosis
- Pelvic masses
- Ovarian cysts
- Presence of IUD

## Diagnostic Studies as Clinically Indicated

- A careful, thorough history should be taken to determine the relationship of pain to the menstrual cycle and history of IUD use. Information about similar menstrual discomfort in the patient's mother or siblings may be pertinent.
- A psychosocial history should be taken.
- A physical examination is necessary to differentiate primary from secondary dysmenorrhea.
- Laparoscopy is indicated to rule out pelvic abnormalities.
- A Pap smear is done to rule out cervical dysplasia.
- A smear for gonococci is taken and a VDRL test is done to rule out venereal disease.
- A CBC and urinalysis are indicated.
- A hysterosalpingogram may be indicated for diagnosis of suspected organic problems.

## Management and Treatment as Clinically Indicated

- Consult or refer to a physician.
- Analgesia: Aspirin, 2 tablets orally every three to four hours, beginning one to three days before the expected onset of menses, is prescribed. Aspirin is a weak prostaglandin inhibitor.

- Prostaglandin inhibitors: These drugs are nonsteroidal anti-inflammatory agents originally used in the treatment of arthritis. Their inhibitory effects on prostaglandin synthesis was discovered empirically as a result of relief from dysmenorrhea in arthritic women using these drugs. They have not been approved by the FDA for use as analgesics.

   Naprosyn, 250 mg, is given orally twice a day for four days, starting two days before expected menses. The dosage may need to be increased to 500 mg twice a day, and the medication may have to be taken for several cycles to produce optimum results. This drug causes fewer complaints of GI upset than aspirin but may cause heartburn, nausea, dyspepsia, abdominal pain, or constipation. The dose may be adjusted if this occurs. *Treatment should be delayed until the onset of menses if there is any suspicion of early pregnancy.*

   Ibuprofen (Motrin), 300-400 mg, is given orally four times a day, beginning three days before the expected onset of menses and continuing through the first three days of menses. The total course should not exceed seven consecutive days. (Treatment is more effective if taken in this way, however, *it may be delayed until the onset of menses to avoid possible exposure of an early pregnancy*). Side effects may include a wide range of GI symptoms, skin rashes, dizziness, and dimmed vision. Its use is contraindicated in patients with nasal polyps, angioedema, and bronchospastic reaction to aspirin. The bleeding time is also prolonged in patients using this drug. Patients should report any of these symptoms immediately.

   Indomethacin (Indocin), 25 mg, is given orally three times a day, beginning three days before the expected onset of menses. Treatment should be delayed until onset of menses if there is a suspicion of early pregnancy. *Side effects may be severe in many patients.* These include dizziness, fatigue, GI toxicity, psychic disturbances, and eye problems. These symptoms should be reported promptly.

- Inhibition of ovulation: Combination low-dose oral contraceptive pills may be given to inhibit ovulation for three to six months. In postpubescent young women this treatment should be used only in patients who have regular menstrual periods and do not respond to analgesics.
- Exercise as a daily routine is beneficial for general good health.
- A heating pad to the lower abdomen may be comforting but may reinforce perception of "illness."
- Use of narcotics should be avoided.
- Alcoholic beverages to induce relaxation should not be recommended in order to avoid possible dependence.

## 228 PROBLEMS IN AMBULATORY OBSTETRICS AND GYNECOLOGY

- Surgical management

    Cervical dilatation is seldom used but may offer temporary pain relief to some patients.

    Presacral neurectomy interrupts the parasympathetic nerve supply to the uterus. It is only used after individual consideration in women with severely incapacitating dysmenorrhea not responding to conservative treatment. This procedure is used primarily in conjunction with conservative surgery for endometriosis.

## Patient Teaching

- Reassure the patient that she has no pelvic abnormalities, and that symptoms may subside with time. Normal fertility is not effected.
- Elicit from the patient how she has coped with menstrual pain in the past and what specific means of relief she has used. Explain possible causes of discomfort and what can be done for relief.
- Stress the importance of proper diet and routine exercise to maintain optimum health. Performing the pelvic rock exercise several times daily is helpful in alleviating backache.
- Suggest to patients not taking oral contraception to keep a menstrual calendar so assessment of ovulation can be made. For women on medication (i.e., naprosyn), which is taken before the onset of menses, the calendar could be used as a guide for starting medication premenstrually.
- Discuss drug side effects with those patients who are taking analgesics and prostaglandin inhibitors. Stress the need to inform the practitioner if they should occur.
- Explain to patients prescribed oral contraceptives that their use inhibits ovulation and causes cessation of cramps. Also discuss their reliability as a birth control method, their use, and side effects. Encourage patients to read the informational package insert.
- If psychosocial problems have been identified during the visit, explore these with the patient. If indicated, make an appointment for further counseling or refer to an appropriate resource.
- Inform the patient anticipating cervical dilatation that its benefit may be limited.
- Suggest frequent support visits for counseling and monitoring of treatment effectiveness as appropriate.

# THE PREMENSTRUAL SYNDROME
# (PREMENSTRUAL TENSION)

## Definition

The premenstrual syndrome is a condition that is characterized by a variety of somatic and psychologic symptoms that occur regularly during a particular phase of the menstrual cycle.

## Etiology

Causative factors of this syndrome are not clearly defined, nor are symptoms that occur in other than the premenstrual phase of the cycle. Premenstrual-like symptoms may also be associated with missed menses or menopause or may occur after a hysterectomy or oophorectomy. The incidence of premenstrual syndrome is difficult to assess but is thought to occur in 30-50% of women. Predisposing factors may include (1) increasing age—particularly a factor in women over 40 years of age, (2) living with a male partner, (3) history of a pregnancy complicated by pre-eclampsia, and (4) a history of premenstrual symptoms in the patient's mother.

Psychologic problems have been documented in some women with premenstrual syndrome. A positive correlation exists between the syndrome and higher rates of alcoholism, suicide, accidents, crime, and psychiatric, medical, and surgical hospital admissions. The effected group is also twice as likely to have a family history of severe depression than the general female population.

Hypotheses on the etiology and pathophysiology of the premenstrual syndrome include:

- Hypothalamic factors: Dalton (1977) suggests that the hypothalamus, which controls the release of hormones, has a faulty "progesterone feed-back pathway." This malfunction causes low progesterone levels during the luteal phase of the menstrual cycle and effects all systems of the body. This system-wide deficit may be responsible for many of the distressing symptoms of the premenstrual syndrome.
- Metabolic and endocrine factors:
  Sodium and water retention are responsible for generalized edema and weight gain. Redistribution of water and electrolytes in the body effects the physiologic and psychologic functions of all body systems.

Hyperaldosteronism has been implicated as a possible mechanism responsible for symptoms. High levels of aldosterone cause change in the sodium-potassium ratio, which occurs when progesterone levels are high enough to inhibit the renal action of aldosterone. Evidence does not support a direct effect on cortical function.

Imbalance between estrogen and progesterone secretion premenstrually may be an important factor in producing symptoms. High levels of estrogen and low levels of progesterone, with consequent generalized edema, may be an important factor in cerebral edema and may help to explain many of the somatic manifestations of the syndrome.

- Psychological factors: This theory suggests that women experiencing the premenstrual syndrome have underlying emotional conflicts resulting from an unsatisfactory relationship with their mother during menarche.
- A transient hypoglycemic factor: This theory suggests that hypoglycemia may be a contributing factor in acute episodes of symptoms premenstrually.

## Clinical Features

### Symptoms

Symptoms may occur as early as 7-10 days premenstrually, peak 1-2 days before menstruation, and subside 2-4 days after the onset of menstruation. The common factor to consider is the recurrence of symptoms with each menstrual cycle. These symptoms may be extremely diverse, may not be the same each cycle, and may effect any body system. The following symptoms according to their mechanism have been defined by Dalton (1977).

| *Mechanism* | *Symptoms* |
| --- | --- |
| Water retention | Bloatedness, weight gain, edema, backache, sinusitis, glaucoma, headache |
| Sodium and potassium imbalance | Tension, depression, irritability, lethargy |
| Hypoglycemia | Headache, epilepsy, fainting, panic, nausea, exhaustion, aggression |
| Allergy | Asthma, rhinitis, urticaria |
| Lowered resistance to infection | Upper respiratory infections, tonsillitis, acne, styes, conjunctivitis, boils, herpes |

## Signs

*Signs do not occur in anovulatory women.*

- Increased symptoms may occur in times of stress.
- More than one symptom may occur at one time, and common complications (not necessarily beginning together) include: (1) tension, headache, mastitis, (2) depression, nausea, backache.
- Symptoms most often occur four days before the onset of menses and during the first four days of menses.
- Symptoms may disappear with the onset of menses.
- Fluctuation of blood pressure and weight are common.
- Edema of the hands, face, and ankles may be evident.

## Differential Diagnosis

- Dysmenorrhea
- Psychoses

## Diagnostic Studies as Clinically Indicated

There are no tests to detect this syndrome. Diagnosis depends on history taking and the perception of the practitioner in assessing the cyclic recurrence of symptoms.

A practical system for definitive diagnosis of true premenstrual tension (Hall and Jacobi, 1978) is provided by the following four criteria.

- The presence of one or more of the following emotional changes:
    Sadness, blues, or depression serious enough to disrupt normal activities
    Tension or nervousness that adversely affects daily functioning
    Emotional lability accompanied by spontaneous weeping
    Diminished energy, apathy, agitation, and restlessness.
- One or more of the following physiologic changes:
    Swelling of the face, fingers, legs, or ankles
    Bloating of the abdomen
    Tenderness and engorgement of the breasts
    Weight gain of at least 3 lb preceding the onset of menses

- Subjective symptoms preceding menses that interfere with the patient's life to such an extent that normal interpersonal relations are disrupted.
- A report that others are able to recognize sudden behavioral changes when the patient is about to menstruate. These changes should abate abruptly with the onset of menses.

    *Note:* These symptoms must appear during a minimum of four successive menstrual cycles.

    Other information that may be collected by the patient to help her to recognize or to understand her symptoms may include:
- A menstrual calendar: This will help to determine the menstrual pattern and aid in dating the type and frequency of symptoms. Letters such as "H" for headache, "D" for depression, or "He" for herpes can be used to show a pattern over time. Clusters of symptoms will be evident before or during the menses, and other days of the month will be free of symptoms.
- A basal body temperature calendar: This will determine if there is a rise in temperature at ovulation, which indicates normal progesterone secretion. A drop in the temperature would indicate a deficient luteal phase of the cycle. If this does occur, it does not necessarily diagnose premenstrual syndrome but is another parameter that can be used in assessment.

## Management and Treatment as Clinically Indicated

- Treatment depends on the severity of premenstrual symptoms and their effects on the woman's life.
- Treatment of mild premenstrual symptoms may include:

    Limiting salt intake starting a week before the onset of menstruation

    Supporting the patient with information and counseling
- Treatment of moderate to severe symptoms may include:

    Limiting salt intake 7-10 days premenstrually

    Supporting the patient as above

    Prescribing a mild diuretic for salt and water retention

    1. Ammonium chloride, 1.0-2.0 g, is given orally four times a day for 7-10 days premenstrually. OR
    2. Chlorothiazide (Diuril), 250-500 mg, is given orally for the first two to three days of the menses. OR

    Advising the use of an oral contraceptive such as Norinyl 1+50 OR

    Giving progesterone, 25 mg, every other day from the midcycle to menses OR

Giving medroxyprogesterone acetate (Provera) 10 mg is given orally twice daily for seven days premenstrually
- Treatment of severe symptoms may include:

Any of the treatments above that provides relief, with the *cautious* addition of a tranquilizer for those women with symptoms of anxiety that interfere with their normal daily functions. Diazepam (Valium) or chlordiazepoxide hydrochloride (Librium) may be ordered and is to be used only during the week before menses. (Drowsiness may occur from use of these drugs.)

Referral for psychologic counseling of patients with severe personality changes.

## Complications

- Psychiatric disturbances

## Patient Teaching

- Review the menstrual calendar with the patient and explain how it can be useful in demonstrating clusters of symptoms and timing of drug use premenstrually.
- Stress the need for a good well-balanced diet and adequate exercise. Explain why salt restriction is necessary premenstrually so the patient will be more apt to comply with this difficult restriction.
- Explain that even though daily exercise is important, the patient also needs increased rest and relaxation during the period she is most symptomatic. Encourage the patient to tone down her life-style and to do less stressful or exhausting tasks and social activities at this time.
- Explore with the patient what her activities are and what interests she may have outside the job or home.
- Encourage the patient to bring in her partner, or other family member, for a joint discussion if this seems appropriate.

## REFERENCES

Chan W, Dagwood M, Fuchs F: Relief of dysmenorrhea with the prostaglandin synthetase inhibitor ibuprofen; effect on prostaglandin levels in menstrual fluid. *Am J Obstet Gynecol* 135:102, 1979.

Corson S, Bolognese R: Ibuprofen therapy for dysmenorrhea. *J Reprod Med* 20:247, 1978.

Dagwood M: Primary dysmenorrhea, Part I: Treatment. *The Female Patient* 14:80, 1979.

Dalton K: *The Premenstrual Syndrome and Progesterone Therapy.* Chicago, Year Book Medical Publishers, 1977.

Field P, Funke J: The premenstrual syndrome: Current findings, treatment and implications for nurses. *JOGN Nursing* 5:23, 1976.

Green T: Gynecology, *Essentials of Clinical Practice,* ed 2. Boston, Little, Brown and Company, 1971, pp 128, 175-177.

Halbert D, Demers L, Jones D: Dysmenorrhea and prostaglandins. *Obstet Gynec Sur* 31:77, 1976.

Hall R, Jacobi K: How to treat premenstrual tension. *The Female Patient* 3:59, 1978.

Hammond C, Judd H, Marshall J, et al: Forum: menstrual dysfunction. *The Female Patient* 3:90, 1978.

Keye W, Jaffee R: Hirsutism and dysfunctional uterine bleeding, in Glass R (ed): *Office Gynecology.* Baltimore, Williams & Wilkins Company, 1976, pp 219-225.

Koeske R: Premenstrual emotionality: Is biology destiny? *Women and Health* 1:11, 1976.

Kreutner A, Hollingsworth D: *Adolescent Obstetrics and Gynecology.* Chicago, Year Book Medical Publishers, 1978, pp 313-316.

March C: Management of dysfunctional bleeding. *The Female Patient* 2:54, 1977.

Reyniak J: Dysfunctional uterine bleeding. *J Reprod Med* 17:293, 1976.

Speroff L: Normal and abnormal menstruation, in Benson R. (ed): *Current Obstetrics and Gynecologic Diagnosis and Treatment.* Los Altos, Lange Medical Publications, 1978, p 112.

Speroff L: Amenorrhea, in Speroff L, Glass R, Kase N: *Clinical Endocrinology and Infertility* ed 2. Baltimore, Williams & Wilkins Company, 1978, pp 93-131.

Stewart F, Stewart G, Guest F, et al: *My Body, My Health.* New York, John Wiley & Sons, 1979, pp. 386-392.

Taymor M: Evaluation of anovulatory cycles and induction of ovulation. *Clin Obstet Gynec* 22:125, 1979.

Wentz A: Abnormal uterine bleeding. *Primary Care* 3:9, 1976.

# 11

# Endometriosis

## Definition

Endometriosis is a disorder resulting from the presence of functioning endometrium implanted at aberrant sites. This tissue is normally only found lining the uterus. More common implantation sites include the ovaries, uterosacral ligaments, uterovesicular peritoneum, posterior cul-de-sac, and the broad ligaments. Less frequent sites are the bladder, small bowel, appendix, umbilicus, pleura, lungs, and bones of the extremities.

## Etiology

The second most common gynecologic disorder after leiomyoma, endometriosis has been estimated to occur in 20–25% of women during their menstrual years. Women who delay childbearing until a later age seem to have greater susceptibility to the disease than women who bear children earlier. Aberrant endometrial tissue responds to hormonal stimulation in much the same way as uterine endometrium does. Monthly cyclic bleeding occurs with extravasation of blood into the implantation sites and infiltration of local tissue. This chronic local irritation leads to formation of adhesions, obstructions, or perforations of tissue.

- Theories of histogenesis

    Transplantation
    1. Transtubal migration by reflux of menstrual blood containing desquamated endometrial cells is carried into the peritoneal cavity where it may implant and grow.

2. Abdominal surgery involving entrance into the uterine cavity may transplant endometrium elsewhere in the abdominal cavity.
3. Postdelivery episiotomy sites and cervical or vaginal lacerations may grow endometrial implants.
4. Benign metastasis by vascular or lymphatic spread may explain endometriosis occurring in uncommon sites such as the lung and thigh.

Coelomic cell metaplasia: Remnants of embryonic cells with potential for developing into endometrium are thought to persist and function with the onset of ovarian hormonal stimulation at menarche.

- Predisposing factors

    Congenital anomalies such as obstructive lesions or malformations of the genital tract

    Prior surgical procedures, vaginal delivery, or injury to the lower genital tract

    Performance of tubal insufflation, hysterosalpingography, or cervical dilatation during menstrual flow

## Clinical Features

### Symptoms

Symptoms may occur in adolescence but usually begin in the early 20s and disappear after menopause. Twenty-five percent of the patients have no symptoms.

- Abnormal vaginal bleeding may occur from associated leiomyomas or endometriosis involving the ovaries and may result in dysfunctional bleeding.
- Unilateral or bilateral pain due to peritoneal irritation may occur from the presence of blood in the abdomen.
- Dysmenorrhea is especially significant if it occurs after years of painless menses. It usually begins premenstrually, becomes most severe when the flow is heaviest, and persists throughout the menstrual period.
- Constipation may increase around the menses and defecation may be painful.
- Urinary tract symptoms of dysuria, frequency, and occasionally hematuria may occur during menses.
- Dyspareunia may occur from pressure on the nodules of endometrial implants located in the posterior cul-de-sac or rectovaginal septum.
- Cyclic sciatica is an uncommon symptom that may occur during menses.
- Infertility may occur as a result of scarring and adhesions of pelvic structures.

*Signs*

- Severity of symptoms may not be consistent with the amount of disease present.
- Location of the symptoms may be a clue to the sites of endometrial implants.
- Palpable signs are many and varied and require careful evaluation. These may include:

    Increased sensitivity of lesions during menses

    An asymptomatic pelvic mass

    Irregular, moveable nodules on the external genitalia, vagina, cervix, or internal pelvic organs that enlarge and become painful preceding menstruation
    1. An enlarged, cystic, adherent ovary
    2. A retroverted, fixed uterus

    Nodular tender thickening of the posterior cul-de-sac and uterosacral ligaments felt on rectovaginal examination

    Fibrotic or cystic masses fixed to underlying tissue of the umbilicus or abdominal scars, with puckering of the skin

- Congenital deformities or variations of pelvic organs, such as hymenal occlusion or cervical stenosis, may be found.
- Endometriosis may frequently be associated with leiomyomas.

## Differential Diagnosis

- Primary dysmenorrhea
- Adenomyosis
- Leiomyoma
- Pelvic infection
- Pelvic adhesions
- Ectopic pregnancy
- Appendicitis, ulcerative ileitis
- Diverticulitis, intestinal malignancy

## Diagnostic Studies as Clinically Indicated

- A careful history taking of symptoms with a thorough abdominal, pelvic, and rectal examination should be done.

## 238 PROBLEMS IN AMBULATORY OBSTETRICS AND GYNECOLOGY

- Laparoscopy may be done for visualization and biopsy of suspicious lesions. For definitive diagnosis histologic findings need to identify two of the following: (1) endometrial glands, (2) endometrial stroma, and (3) hemorrhage.
- Barium enema or rectosigmoidoscopy are done during menses to identify lesions.
- Cystoscopy or urography are performed premenstrually or during menses.

### Management and Treatment as Clinically Indicated

The patient's age, parity, severity of symptoms, presence of other reproductive abnormalities, and interest in childbearing need to be considered before starting treatment. Consultation or referral of the patient to a physician is always necessary.

- Observation is indicated for the patient with no significant symptoms or physical findings who does not desire pregnancy. Analgesics may be indicated for minor pelvic discomfort.
- Analgesics may be ordered for mild or early painful symptoms.

    Aspirin, 10 gr, is given orally every four hours as needed, beginning one week before the expected onset of discomfort.

    Aspirin with codeine, 0.003–0.006 gr, may be given every four hours for more severe pain.

- Prostaglandin inhibitors are primarily used for patients with dysmenorrhea who have little success with or intolerance of other medications.

    Naprosyn, 500 mg orally, is given initially, followed by 250 mg every six hours for a maximum of five days. Medication should be started two days before expected menses to be most effective. Caution the patient about possible drowsiness, dizziness, vertigo, or depression. Common GI complaints from this medication include heartburn, nausea, dyspepsia, abdominal pain, constipation, stomatitis, diarrhea, or vomiting. The dose may be lowered if these symptoms occur. *Treatment should be delayed until the onset of menses if there is any suspicion of early pregnancy.*

- Hormonal therapy offers temporary benefit for the woman who has been diagnosed as having early or moderate surface endometriosis. It is not to be used if leiomyoma are present.

    Combination oral contraceptives are used to suppress ovulation and produce amenorrhea. A low-dose estrogen and high-dose progesterone combination pill such as Ovral, Demulen, or Norlestrin (2.5 mg) is effective. One tablet is given orally daily for three weeks, then 2 tablets daily for three weeks, followed by 3 tablets daily for six to nine months. Side effects of oral contraceptive pills need to be stressed with patients placed on this regimen.

Cyclic combination oral contraceptives such as Ovral, Demulen, or Norlestrin (2.5 mg) used as a contraceptive method, will help to relieve dysmenorrhea but probably will not effect the course of the disease.

Progesterone used alone offers relief to some patients

1. Provera 10 mg, is given orally three times a day for six to nine months.
2. Depo-Provera, 150 mg, is given IM every three months for nine months. Patients may experience breakthrough bleeding and may need to be counseled as with combination drugs. Bleeding may be disturbing to the patient but does not lessen the therapeutic effect of progesterone.

Antigonadotropin therapy renders the endometrial tissue inactive and atropic. It is to be used only for patients amenable to hormonal management who cannot tolerate or who are unresponsive to other drug therapy. A positive diagnosis of endometriosis must be made before using this medication.

Danazol is a synthetic androgen that suppresses FSH and LH secretion. Danocrine, 400 mg, is given orally twice a day as continuous therapy for three to six months, not exceeding nine months. Ovulation and cyclic bleeding usually return within 60 to 90 days after discontinuing the drug. This medication is an expensive form of therapy. *Its use is contraindicated in pregnant and lactating women and during episodes of undiagnosed abnormal genital bleeding.* Androgenic side effects may include acne, mild hirsutism, or edema. Hypoestrogenic effects such as flushing, sweating, vaginitis, and nervousness may be experienced.

- Surgical treatment: A thorough fertility workup should be done before surgical intervention.

  Conservative surgery is indicated for women who are under 35 years old who wish to retain or enhance their fertility.

  1. A laparotomy may be done to resect or fulgurate implants, to resect large implants, and to release adhesions. Pregnancy rates after this procedure have been estimated up to 63%. The recurrence rate after this treatment is 20 to 50%.
  2. A presacral neurotomy may be done at the time of laparotomy for patients who experience dysmenorrhea and for prevention of symptoms of recurrent disease. The usefulness of this procedure is questionable since it is of limited value to patients with more extensive disease and is not without operative risk.

  Semiconservative surgery may be performed for women in their 30s whose reproductive function is lost but in whom ovarian function is to be retained.

A hysterectomy will eliminate dysmenorrhea, abnormal bleeding, and the main source of ectopic endometrium. However, in patients with endometrial implants on the bladder, bowel, or ureter, this treatment is not indicated. The patient must also be informed of possible recurrence of the disease and the need for further surgery.

Radical or definitive surgery removes ovarian function. It is indicated in women who are over 35 years old with advanced disease or in women who have completed their families. A total abdominal hysterectomy, bilateral salpingo-oophorectomy, resection of peritoneal implants, and appendectomy are done.
- Irradiation by the use of x-ray therapy is limited to symptomatic women with recurrent disease who refuse surgery or who are at medical risk for surgery.

## Complications

- Infertility
- Pelvic adhesions, bowel or bladder obstructions
- Rupture of an endometrioma
- Postmenopausal malignant change

## Patient Teaching

- Assess the patient's knowledge of the disease and implications for symptoms, complications, treatment, and fertility.
- Describe drug therapy, its purpose, and the necessity to follow the prescribed regimen.
- Describe drug side effects and the need to report untoward effects (see section on prostaglandin inhibitors).
- Counsel patients with mild or moderate disease that with proper hormonal or surgical treatment 50-80% will have relief from pain and return of fertility.
- Explain or reinforce the physician's explanation of procedures to patients who are candidates for surgery.
- Allow the patient to express her fears and concerns about decision making regarding surgery or of the operative procedure.
- Reassure the patient anticipating radical surgery that this treatment is curative for most women.

- Prepare for the patient's physical well-being before surgery by stressing adequate diet.
- Encourage the patient to return when she is scheduled to do so or whenever she is anxious or feels the need for clarification or support.
- Refer the patient for psychologic support or nutrition counseling if necessary.
- Assess the home situation for surgical patients to ensure the presence of a support person postoperatively.

## REFERENCES

Cohen, M: Advances in endometriosis management. *The Female Patient* 3:77, 1978.

deAlvarez R: *Textbook of Gynecology.* Philadelphia, Lea & Febiger, 1977, p 27.

Falconer M, Patterson H, Gustafson E, et al: *Current Drug Handbook.* Philadelphia. WB Saunders Company, 1978–1980, p 227.

Ingram J: Endometriosis, in Benson R (ed): *Current Obstetrics and Gynecologic Diagnosis and Treatment.* Los Altos, Calif, Lange Medical Publications, 1978, p 323.

Mattingly R: *TeLinde's Operative Gynecology,* ed 5. Philadelphia, JB Lippincott Company, 1977, p 226.

Parsons L, Sommers, S: *Gynecology,* ed 2. Philadelphia, WB Saunders Company, 1978, p 957.

*Physicians' Desk Reference.* Oradell, NJ, Medical Economics Company, 1979, p 1716, 1845.

Speroff L, Glass R, Kase N: *Clinical Gynecologic Endocrinology and Infertility,* ed 2. Baltimore, Williams & Wilkins Company, 1978, p 356.

# 12

# Benign Breast Disease

Since breast cancer is the most common cause of death from cancer in women, breast lesions have become a major health concern of women today. With the current emphasis on breast self-examination women are discovering lesions earlier and are seeking medical care sooner than in the past. Although 80-90% of these lesions are benign, early recognition and identification is essential for the woman's future physical and mental well-being.

- Certain factors have been identified as associated with increased risk of breast cancer, which can alert the Nurse Practitioner to this group of women. The following factors need to be considered.

    Women over 40 years of age are most commonly effected, with postmenopausal women at highest risk.

    White women are at higher risk than other racial groups.

    Women who have never married have a 40% greater risk of being effected.

    A family history of maternal or sibling breast cancer increases risk three times.

    A medical history of cancer in one breast increases the risk sevenfold.

    Women with a history of an early menarche and late menopause, with the total menstrual years being greater than 30, are at higher risk.

    Environmental factors such as cigarette smoking, chemical carcinogens in drinking water, or exogenous estrogen intake are implicated in increased risk.

    Exposure to oncogenic factors such as viruses, foods, and obesity, may increase risk.

243

nplemented the following guidelines for

nd the report of any abnormal findings

qualified medical personnel

mammography only if the woman has a

nammography examination only if a woman
immediate relatives or a personal history of

phic examination may be considered.

ast is done to differentiate cystic from solid

ople discharge is performed. (*Note:* Phenothia-
ple discharge from increased prolactin levels.)
when:
in the breast or axilla
mpling, discoloration, puckering, or sudden nip-
rsion or discharge, occur
ize or shape occurs.
ied to extract fluid or tissue from a suspicious
tologic examination.
ned to collect tissue for histologic examination of

n of the breasts may reveal findings suggestive of

tary, unilateral lump
der lump
fixed to the surrounding tissue.
ion, erosion, elevation, or change in position of the

t.

5. Skin retraction over the lesion
6. Inflammation or edema of the tissue
7. An "orange peel" ("peau d'orange") appearance of the skin
8. Increased size or firmness of one breast
9. A lesion located in the upper outer quadrant of the breast
10. Axillary lymphadenopathy

## BENIGN LESIONS OF THE BREAST

The majority of breast lesions are benign. All must be examine malignancy, and many may require treatment. Only the more com their diagnosis and treatment, will be discussed here. See Table 2 fc of the common breast diseases.

## FIBROCYSTIC BREAST DISEASE (CHRONIC CYSTIC MASTITIS, CYSTIC DISEASE OF THE BREAST, MAMMARY DYSPLASIA)

### Definition

Fibrocystic breast disease is the formation of multiple cysts in the tern and acini of the breast.

### Etiology

Fibrocystic breast disease is the most common of all breast lesions, bu is unknown. It is thought to result from an exaggerated, or abnormal re breast tissue to cyclic hormone stimulation. This theory of estrogen de seems likely since women between 20 and 50 years of age are most su to develop the disease and it rarely occurs in postmenopausal women ( cents. Approximately, 1 in 20 women will develop palpable cystic disea their reproductive years.

**Table 2**
Common Breast Diseases

| | Fibrocystic Disease (30%) | Carcinoma (30%) | Fibro-Adenoma (12%) | Intraductal Papilloma (5%) | Mammary Duct Ectasia (5%) | Fat Necrosis (unknown) | All Others (10%) |
|---|---|---|---|---|---|---|---|
| > Median Age | 30 years | > 40 years | 20 years | 40 years | > 40 years | All ages | |
| Pain or tenderness | Pre-menstrual, menstrual | None | None | Moderate | Pain during inflammatory process | Initially with trauma | |
| Nipple discharge | Absent | Usually absent | Absent | Serous or bloody | Sticky, multicolored | Absent | |
| Retraction | Absent | Present | Absent | Absent | Present | Present | |
| Mobility | Mobile | Fixed | Mobile | Not palpable | Fixed | Fixed | |
| Delineation | Discrete | Non-defined | Discrete | Non-defined | Non-defined | Non-defined | |
| Consistency and number | Firm, multiple | Firm, usually single | Rubbery, usually single | Soft, usually single | Firm, single | Firm, single | |
| Unilateral or bilateral | Bilateral | Usually unilateral | Unilateral | Unilateral | Unilateral | Usually unilateral | |
| Etiology | Unknown | Unknown | Unknown | Unknown | Unknown | Trauma | |

## Clinical Features

### Symptoms

Symptoms, which depend on the number of cysts, their size, and growth rate may include:

- An asymptomatic lump
- Pain, tenderness, and enlargement of the cysts premenstrually
- Discharge from the nipple
- Tenderness to palpation
- Cyclic breast pain
- Fluctuations in the size of the cysts
- A transient breast lump

### Signs

- Firm, mobile, well-defined cysts
- Regression of cyst size after menstruation
- Multiple, and most often bilateral, involvement
- Dispersed, small cysts, which feel "shotty"
- Absence of a nipple discharge
- Regression of the cysts postmenopausally

## Differential Diagnosis

- Fat necrosis
- Fibroadenoma
- Carcinoma

## Diagnostic Studies as Clinically Indicated

- A complete medical history should be taken, and physical examination should be performed, taking into consideration the risk factors previously delineated.
- Breast palpation with careful examination of axillary lymph nodes should be performed.
- Biopsy of suspicious lesions should be done.

- Aspiration of a cystic mass with cytologic examination of the fluid may be done.
- Mammography or xerography may be helpful diagnostic aids.
- Transillumination of cysts may aid differential diagnosis.

## Management and Treatment as Clinically Indicated

- Physician consultation or referral is necessary.
- Aspiration of the cyst may be done to reduce its size and to alleviate symptoms.
- Surgical excision is controversial. (To prevent malignant change in moderate to severe polycystic disease, some physicians advocate prophylactic bilateral subcutaneous mastectomy with breast reconstruction.)
- Hormone therapy is controversial.
- Breast examination should be performed every two to four weeks for 3 months after initial diagnosis, then every 6 to 12 months. Visits should be scheduled at least every 6 months for women at risk for developing carcinoma.

## Complications

- Malignant change
- Sclerosing adenosis
- Intraductal hyperplasia
- Papillomatosis
- Recurrence of cystic breasts in menopausal women receiving estrogen therapy

## Patient Teaching

- Assess the patient's knowledge of the disease and supplement information as necessary. Explain that the incidence of carcinoma is twice as great in women with cystic disease. Allow the patient time and opportunity to express her feelings about the disease and her possible risk.
- Stress the importance of monthly breast self-examination after cessation of the menses and of reporting any new masses to the physician or nurse practitioner.
- Warn the patient against trauma to the breasts.

- Encourage the patient to wear a supportive, protective brassiere both day and night.
- Explain that pain and tenderness of the breasts may occur monthly during the premenstrual period. These symptoms subside after menopause.
- Explain to the patient that some women with benign breast disease who have eliminated coffee, tea, cokes, and chocolate from their diet have had resolution of palpable breast nodules, pain, and tenderness in one to six months. Common ingredients of these products, called methylxanthines, have been found to influence the development of fibrocystic breast disease. Some women may be interested in trying to eliminate these products from their diets.

## INTRADUCTAL PAPILLOMA

### Definition

Intraductal papilloma are epithelial tumors that occur within the ductal system of the breast and are the second most common benign breast lesions.

### Etiology

Papillomas can occur in any woman over 20 years of age, but they are more common in women over 40. These small, ductal tumors are usually single and are often nonpalpable. Ducts located in the subareolar area are the most commonly effected. Nipple discharge occurs when one of the papillomas grows into a major collecting duct, causing trauma and erosion of the fragile tissue. Diffuse disease is not common but is often associated with cystic breast disease.

### Clinical Features

*Symptoms*

- Unilateral, spontaneous, serous or bloody nipple discharge is the primary symptom.

- Moderate breast pain and tenderness may occur.

*Signs*

- A tumor mass may not be palpable, or a palpable, soft, and poorly delineated mass may be present.
- Nipple discharge may be present.
- Associated cystic breast disease may be present.

## Diagnostic Studies as Clinically Indicated

- Localization of the involved duct is done by applying systematic pressure over successive areas of the areola. The involved duct will produce a discharge from the nipple.
- Cannulation and injection of radiopaque dye into the discharging duct identifies the area for excisional biopsy.
- Cytologic examination of the nipple discharge is done. (False-negative results are obtained in 20% of the cases.)

## Management and Treatment as Clinically Indicated

- Consultation or referral to a physician is necessary.
- Solitary tumors are surgically excised.
- Repeated surgical excision of multiple tumors is done.

## Complications

- Recurrent intraductal papillomas
- Malignant change (rare)

## Patient Teaching

- Discuss the nature of the tumor and explain to the patient why the nipple discharge occurs.

- Reinforce or clarify the physician's explanation of the diagnosis and prescribed treatment.
- Discuss and demonstrate breast self-examination when necessary, and stress the need to report any breast changes to the physician or nurse practitioner.
- Reassure the patient that malignant change is rare.
- Stress the importance of regular follow-up visits for breast examination.
- Allow time for the patient to express her fears and concerns.

# FIBROADENOMA

## Definition

Fibroadenoma is a benign breast neoplasm consisting of proliferative ductal epithelium and fibrous stroma.

## Etiology

The etiology of the tumor is unknown, but it is primarily a disease of younger women (usually under 25 years of age) and is the most common breast lesion found in the adolescent female. Association of the tumor with estrogen stimulation is suspected since it occurs in young women, increases in size during pregnancy, and is rarely found after menopause. Black women develop this tumor more often and at an earlier age.

## Clinical Features

### Symptoms

- Asymptomatic tumors are usually discovered accidentally around the nipple or on the lateral side of the upper quadrant of the breast.
- Enlargement of the tumor may be rapid.

### Signs

- A discrete, round, rubbery and freely moveable mass is felt.

- Pain and tenderness is uncommon.
- The tumors are usually single, but in 20% of the patients they are multiple.
- The tumor is persistent and usually unilateral.
- Tumor growth rate is variable with an increase in size; they lactate during pregnancy and shrink after delivery.

## Differential Diagnosis

- Fibrocystic breast disease
- Fat Necrosis
- Carcinoma (rare)

## Diagnostic Studies as Clinically Indicated

- Mammography is indicated to aid diagnosis.
- Transillumination of the breast shows a semiopaque tumor.
- Excisional biopsy with histologic examination of the specimen may be done.

## Management and Treatment as Clinically Indicated

- Consultation or referral to a physician is necessary.
- The lesion is surgically excised.
- Conservative management of the adolescent patient includes frequent observation and palpation to assess the tumor growth rate. Premature surgery may interfere with normal breast development.

## Complications

- Cystosarcoma phyllodes (a benign fibroadenoma)
- Malignant change
- Contraction of massive fibroadenoma
- Postmenopausal development of fibroadenoma after estrogen therapy

## Patient Teaching

- Discuss and demonstrate the breast self-examination if necessary, and explain the need to report any breast changes to the physician or nurse practitioner.
- Reinforce or clarify the physician's explanation of the lesion, what the treatment will be, and its possible outcome.
- Reassure the patient that malignant change is rare.
- Warn the patient to avoid any trauma to the breast.
- Involve the mother of an adolescent patient in the counseling if possible. Talking to the mother and daughter separately also gives them the opportunity to express their individual concerns.

## MAMMARY DUCT ECTASIA (COMEDOMASTITIS)

### Definition

Mammary duct ectasia is a degenerative disease of the secretory epithelium lining the large ducts of the breasts.

### Etiology

The cause of mammary duct ectasia is unknown, but it is primarily a disease of older women and is found most commonly during the perimenopausal and menopausal years. The degenerative process that occurs causes atrophy and necrosis of the ductal secretory epithelium. The ducts, which lie beneath the areola and nipple, become clogged and tortuous causing a spontaneous discharge from the nipple. Small bluish-green discolorations which appear in the tissue at the base of the areola and nipple are evidence of these clogged ducts. As many as twenty ducts may be involved, and as they shorten and thicken, they cause nipple retraction. The walls of the ducts may become weakened and rupture, spilling their contents into the surrounding tissue causing irritation and infection. The body, in an attempt to wall off this chronic inflammatory process sets up a fibrous tissue response, resulting in the development of a firm, deep, mass beneath the areola.

Although there is no known association with malignancy, differentiating mammary duct ectasia from carcinoma is extremely difficult, and diagnosis may only be possible after histologic examination of the affected tissue.

## Clinical Features

### Symptoms

- A sticky, multicolored spontaneous nipple discharge from one breast
- Breast pain and tenderness
- Inflammation of the breast tissue

### Signs

- Nipple retraction.
- Bluish-green 3- to 5-mm discolorations at the base of the areola and nipple
- A fixed tumor mass of firm consistency felt centrally below the areola
- Unilateral involvement
- "Orange peel" ("peau d' orange") skin over the tumor
- Axillary lymphadenopathy

## Differential Diagnosis

- Fat necrosis
- Carcinoma

## Diagnostic Studies as Clinically Indicated

- Careful history taking with emphasis on the signs, symptoms, and progress of the breast lesion, correlated with physical signs, may permit a presumptive clinical diagnosis.
- Cytologic examination of the nipple discharge is indicated.
- Mammography, xerography, or thermography may be done to aid diagnosis.

## Management and Treatment as Clinically Indicated

- Consultation or referral to the physician is necessary.
- Surgical excision is performed. The tissue containing the dilated ducts is excised along with wide margins of normal tissue to ensure total removal of the effected tissue.

## Complications

- Breakdown and inflammation of the tumor mass
- Involvement of the entire breast in the disease process

## Patient Teaching

- Assess the patient's knowledge of her breast disease and supplement information as needed.
- Reassure the patient that malignant change of the tumor is rare.
- Explain to the patient the importance of performing a breast self-examination every month. Postmenopausal women are at higher risk of developing a malignant breast tumor.

## FAT NECROSIS

Although a rare lesion, fat necrosis is discussed briefly because it may be impossible to differentiate from cancer while performing a breast examination.

Injury to the breast may cause hemorrhage into the fatty tissue causing ecchymosis and tenderness. The patient may not know when the trauma occurred. During healing, the damaged tissue becomes hard and fibrotic; the mass resulting from this process becomes fixed to the skin, and nipple retraction may occur. These are classical signs of cancer and diagnosis is made by biopsy and histologic examination of the tissue. A mass resulting from fat necrosis may gradually regress, but generally surgical excision is necessary.

## REFERENCES

Greenwald L, Nasca L, Lawrence C, et al: Estimated effect of breast self-examination and routine physical examinations on breast-cancer mortality. *N Engl J Med,* 299:271, 1978.

Kreutner A, Reycroft D: *Adolescent Obstetrics and Gynecology.* Chicago, Year Book Medical Publishers, 1978, p 411.

Leis H, Pilnik S, Black M: Diagnosis of breast cancer. *Hospital Medicine,* November 1974, pp 33–65.

Minton J, Foecking M, Webster D, et al: Response of fibrocystic disease to caffeine withdrawal and correlation of cyclic nucleotides with breast disease. *Am J Obstet Gynecol* 135:157, 1979.

Mitchell G: The gynecologist and breast disease. *Clin Obstet Gynecol* 20:865, 1977.

Ochsner A: Diseases of the breast. *Postgrad Med* 57:77, 1975.

Parsons L, Sommers S: *Gynecology.* Philadelphia, WB Saunders Company, 1978, p 1223.

Regenie S, Russell L, Kirkman A: An educational resource breast disease. *J Nurs Midwife* 20:8, 1975.

Siegel A: Detection of breast cancer; a practitioner's viewpoint. *Primary Care* 4:755, 1977.

Study links fibrocystic disease to breast carcinoma. *Obstet Gynecol Observer,* June 1977, p 3.

*The Breast Cancer Digest. A Guide to Medical Care, Emotional Support, Educational Programs and Resources.* U.S. Department of HEW, Public Health Service, National Institute of Health, National Cancer Institute, Bethesda, Md. DHEW Pub. No (Nih) 79-1691, 1979.

Vorherr H, Messer, R: Breast cancer: Potentially predisposing and protecting factors. *Am J Obstet Gynecol* 130:335, 1978.

Wilcox P, Ettinger D: Benign breast disease: Diagnosis and treatment. *Primary Care* 4:739, 1977.

Zimmerman, D: How doctors are changing breast cancer treatment. *Woman's Day,* September 20, 1979.

# 13
# Urinary Tract Infection

Infection is the most common problem occurring in the urinary tract of women and is due to invasion of pathogenic organisms into the normally sterile urinary system. Upper tract infections involve the kidneys; lower tract infections involve the bladder and urethra. Women with lower tract infections constitute one-third of the gynecologic patient population. Twenty-five percent of women develop a urinary tract infection during their lifetime, and the incidence increases with age: 1 in 10 women over age 70 are affected.

Urinary tract infection is much more frequent in women than in men largely due to anatomic differences. Nearness of the urinary meatus to the vagina and rectum makes contamination of the urethra a common occurrence in women. Organisms inhabiting the perineum easily enter the urethra or bladder during sexual intercourse or are introduced into the urethra from improper hygiene practices. The female urethra is only one and one-half inches long (as compared with the male urethra, which is 4–5 inches). This permits infectious organisms to enter and to ascend through the connecting system from the urethra, through the bladder and ureters to the kidneys.

The body's first line of defense against pathologic organisms in the urinary tract is the acidity of the urine and the act of urination, which washes away bacteria. Conditions that may alter normal function and predispose to urinary tract infections are:

- Sexual intercourse or change in sexual pattern
- Poor perineal hygiene
- Pregnancy changes
- Oral contraceptive use

- Ignoring or resisting the urge to urinate
- Instrumentation, catheterization, or indwelling catheters
- Vesicoureteral reflux
- Neurogenic bladder
- Tissue effects of aging
- Sickle cell trait
- Bladder prolapse
- Surgical trauma
- Congenital anomaly of the system
- Incomplete emptying of a bladder cystocele
- Blockage of the system with stones, tumors, endometriosis, or pelvic infection

Specific information to be sought in the history taking of patients with suspected urinary tract infections includes:

- Age and socioeconomic status
- Family history of renal disease, hypertension, diabetes
- Childhood history of unexplained illnesses, temperature elevations, or urinary tract infections
- Presence of predisposing diseases such as hypertension, diabetes, sickle cell trait, or kidney disease
- Relationship of urinary infections to menstruation or sexual activity
- Sexual history
- Menstrual and obstetric history
- History of trauma to the pelvis or of abdominal or pelvic surgery
- History of oral contraceptive use
- History of drug allergy
- Presence of vaginal discharge or symptoms

Methods of urine collection to avoid contamination include:

- Clean-catch midstream voided specimen (The reported presence of epithelial cells indicates vaginal contamination. A damp cotton ball placed in the introitus may help eliminate this problem.): A carefully collected specimen is about 80% reliable, and reliability increases to 90% if a second consecutive clean-catch specimen is reported to contain the same number of bacteria.
- Catheterization ensures a clean specimen, but its use is controversial and individual specific protocols should be followed.
- Suprapubic aspiration of urine ensures a sterile specimen, and any reported bacterial colonization is significant.

- Evaluation of the urine specimen may include:

    A Dipstick examination to identify the presence of glucose, protein, or blood

    A microscopic examination of stained or unstained urine sediment to identify gram-negative or gram-positive cocci, white blood cells, or red blood cells. The finding of more than five white blood cells per high power field is significant. If the bacterial count of the urine specimen is $10^5$/ml (100,000) or more, the microscopic reliability may be as high as 80-90%.

    A urine culture, and sensitivity studies are done to identify the offending organism. The specimen should be refrigerated within 15 minutes of collection as bacterial growth in the urine doubles every 45 minutes, resulting in an unsatisfactory specimen. Culture results may be obtained within 48 hours. The finding of 100,000 ($10^5$) or more colonies of bacteria per milliliter of urine in a clean specimen indicates a urinary tract infection. If vaginal contamination is indicated by the results of the colony count, a new urine specimen should be collected and the tests should be repeated.

- Cystoscopy may be indicated.
- A fluorescent antibody test may be indicated (see Chap. 17).

# CYSTITIS

## Definition

Cystitis is an acute or chronic inflammation of the urinary bladder most commonly caused by poor hygiene practices, trauma, or contamination of the urethral meatus by sexual intercourse.

## Etiology

The most common site of urinary infection is the bladder with the most common offending organism being *Escherichia coli.* Other agents causing cystitis are other bacteria, parasites, fungi, and chemical or mechanical irritants.

Chronic cystitis is infection of the bladder that has been present over a period of months with continuous or intermittent symptoms of cystitis, with the exception of low-grade fever. The symptoms may be minor or debilitating, and the presence of upper tract infection or physiologic abnormality needs to be ruled out.

## Clinical Features

### Symptoms

- Dysuria with pain or burning on urination
- Urgency to void due to bladder spasticity
- Frequency of urination, usually in small amounts
- Nocturia which is a continuation of daytime frequency
- Pressure, cramps, or spasm (tenesmus) of the bladder
- Painful intercourse (dyspareunia)
- Tenderness in the suprapubic area
- Discharge from the vagina
- Low-grade fever and malaise

### Signs

- Presence of symptoms 24-48 hours after sexual intercourse
- Absence of flank pain, no costovertebral tenderness
- Slight suprapubic tenderness
- A temperature of less than 101°F (38.3°C)
- Occasional gross hematuria (Rule out blood in urine from other sources such as the rectum or vagina.)
- Abnormal vaginal discharge
- Presence of atrophic vaginitis
- Presence of foul smelling urine

## Differential Diagnosis

- Vaginitis, cervicitis
- Urethritis, urethrocele, urethral diverticulum
- Cystocele
- Salpingitis
- Pyelonephritis
- Abdominal disorder

## Diagnostic Studies as Clinically Indicated

- History taking (see p. 257)
- Physical examination with special attention to:
  Oral temperature
  Costovertebral tenderness
  Lower abdominal tenderness
  Pelvic examination to include:
  1. Inspection of the external urinary meatus for erythema, polyp, caruncle, or induration
  2. Inspection of anterior vaginal wall for evidence of infection
  3. Palpation of anterior vaginal wall from the anterior vaginal fornix to the external urinary meatus feeling for lesions and stripping the urethra to express discharge from infected Skene's glands
  4. Bimanual examination for identification of pelvic tumors, infection, pregnancy, or pelvic relaxation
  5. Rectovaginal examination for identification of tumors, rectocele, fistulas
- Pap smear and culture for *Neisseria gonorrhoeae*
- Wet mount to rule out vaginal infection
- Urinalysis, culture, and sensitivity
- Fluorescent antibody test (see Chap. 17). (Positive findings indicate an upper tract infection. False-negative findings may occur if the urinary tract infection is recent.)

## Management and Treatment as Clinically Indicated

- For patients with recurrent or chronic infections, complications, hypertension, diabetes, or other systemic illness, physician referral is necessary.
- For patients who are asymptomatic, urine culture and sensitivity results should usually be obtained before instituting antibiotic therapy.
- For patients who are symptomatic, antibiotic therapy is begun immediately with reassessment and change of therapy as necessary if the culture and sensitivity report indicates that the pathogen is insensitive to the prescribed drug.
- To dilute the bacterial count and to increase the washing action of urine, the patient is told to increase fluid intake. However, urinary dilution also decreases the content of the antimicrobial agent in the urine. Check with your physician about this practice.

- Antibiotics most commonly used include:

    Sulfisoxazole (Gantrisin): 1 g orally four times a day for 10 days after an initial loading dose of 2 g. *Check for sulfa allergy.*

    Ampicillin: 250 mg orally four times a day for 10 days. *Check penicillin allergy.*

    Tetracycline: 250-500 mg orally four times a day for 10 days. *Tetracycline is contraindicated in pregnant and lactating women. Milk or antacids should not be taken within one hour before or after an oral dose. They cause a 20-25% decrease in absorption of the drug.*

    Phenazopyridine HCl (Pyridium): 100 mg orally three times a day for two to three days. It acts as an analgesic and will relieve bladder spasms. *Inform the patient that her urine will turn bright orange.*

- To assure that treatment has been adequate urine culture should be obtained one week after completion of drug therapy and again at three and six months. Treatment failure of an infection caused by a sensitive organism may indicate urinary tract abnormality or renal infection.

## Complications

- Chronic, recurrent, or relapsing cystitis
- Asymptomatic bacteriuria
- Pyelonephritis
- Cystic cystitis

## Patient Teaching

- Reassure the patient that cystitis is common in women and is not a serious infection. Response to treatment is rapid, and symptoms should be relieved within a day or two.
- Stress the importance of taking all prescribed medications even though symptoms have disappeared. It is necessary to complete the entire course of medicine to prevent relapse or recurrence of the infection.
- Advise the patient with bladder spasms against the use of coffee, tea, alcohol, and spices until the infection has cleared since these stimulants can further irritate the bladder.
- Advise the patient to drink plenty of fluids to keep the urinary system flushed.

- Make sure the patient understands the necessity of returning in one week to obtain a repeat urine culture. Explain that if her symptoms persist after three days of treatment she should contact the practitioner.
- Preventive counseling

    Impress the importance of good perineal hygiene. After a bowel movement cleansing with tissue from the anus backward will prevent urethral contamination. A second piece of tissue should then be used to pat the urethra dry.

    Suggest drinking a glass of liquid before sexual intercourse and urinating shortly afterward to wash out any bacteria that may have entered the urethra.

    Advise the patient to urinate when the desire occurs and not try to "hold it." The ability to clear bacteria from an overdistended bladder is diminished.

    Maintain adequate fluid intake to decrease urine concentration and keep the bladder flushed.

## BACTERIURIA ASSOCIATED WITH SEXUAL INTERCOURSE ("HONEYMOON CYSTITIS")

There is no proven causal relationship between urinary tract infection and sexual intercourse. However, studies show a transient rise in bacterial counts in the urine of some women postcoitally, indicating introduction of bacteria into the urethra during intercourse. It has been suggested that some women may lack antibodies in the cervix and vagina to organisms that normally inhabit the bowel, the most common offenders in recurrent urinary tract infections.

Many sexually active women have recurrent infections that never become chronic. In women who experience chronic infections, each infection needs to be reevaluated by urinalysis, culture, and sensitivity studies. These chronic infections are probably the result of contamination by different organisms during sexual intercourse.

The signs, symptoms, and complications of bacteriuria associated with sexual intercourse are the same as those of cystitis.

### Management and Treatment as Clinically Indicated

If underlying abnormalities have been ruled out by intravenous pyelogram and recurrent infections have been established as related to sexual intercourse, prophylactic use of medication may reduce the frequency of such attacks. After successful treatment of acute infection in patients with more than three infections in a six-month period, the following prophylactic treatment should be considered:

- Cotrimoxazole (Bactrim Septra) is used for bacteria resistant to sulfonamides alone. One tablet is to be taken immediately after intercourse.
- Nitrofurantoin (Furandantin): one 50-mg tablet is to be taken immediately after intercourse. *Check for sulfa allergy* and for *G-6-PD deficiency. (Sulfa will cause hemolytic anemia.)* Tell the patient her urine will turn a brownish color.
- Follow-up: Women with two to three infections a year treated successfully, as evidenced by negative cultures, should be followed for asymptomatic bacteriuria every three months for a year, then yearly. The numbers of untreated women with urinary tract infections is significant. Exacerbation of chronic or low-grade infection may mean permanent kidney damage for some women.

## Patient Teaching

- Refer to the patient teaching section for cystitis.

## RECURRENT URINARY TRACT INFECTIONS

Recurrent urinary tract infections with significant bacteriuria (after underlying urinary tract abnormalities have been ruled out) are of two types: relapse, which is caused by a flare-up of a previous infection due to inadequate treatment, or reinfection, which is caused by the introduction of a different organism into the system. The following chart clarifies the two types of infections.

|  | *Relapse of Initial Infection* | *Reinfection* |
| --- | --- | --- |
| Cause | Treatment failure | New bacteria introduced |
| Pathogenic organism | Same | Usually different |
| Location of infection | Kidney | Bladder |
| Incidence | Less than 10% | More than 90% |
| Length of therapy | Usually six weeks | 10-14 days |
| Time of infection | Within three weeks of previous infection | More than three weeks after previous infection |

The frequency with which chronic urinary tract infection progresses to pyelonephritis has not been documented but is a serious problem. Methods of treatment of these infections is controversial at this time, and physician referral is mandatory.

# PYELONEPHRITIS

## Definition

Pyelonephritis is an acute inflammation of the ureters, renal pelvis, and kidneys.

## Etiology

The infection is most commonly caused by *Escherichia coli,* which ascends to the kidney from the lower urinary tract. Women in their childbearing years and girls under age 10 are the most frequently effected. It is a serious disease and if it becomes chronic may produce significant kidney damage. For predisposing factors (see page 256)

## Clinical Features

### Symptoms

- Temperature elevation, which may exceed 104°F (40°C)
- Symptoms of cystitis (see section on cystitis)
- Nausea, vomiting, anorexia
- Malaise, chills
- Unilateral or bilateral flank pain, which may radiate to the midabdomen
- Vaginal discharge

### Signs

- Tenderness to deep abdominal palpation in flank of effected area
- Suprapubic, costovertebral tenderness

- Hematuria
- Abdominal distention
- Hypotonic bowel sounds, rigid abdomen
- Enlarged kidneys, foul-smelling urine
- Cold, damp skin or dehydrated, warm and dry skin

## Differential Diagnosis

- Cystitis, pyelitis
- Back pain from other causes
- Acute bowel disease (appendicitis, diverticulitis, regional ileitis)
- Pelvic inflammatory disease
- Ectopic pregnancy

## Diagnostic Studies as Clinically Indicated

- See page 257 for history taking and page 260 for information on the physical examination.
- Urinalysis of clean-catch specimen shows clumps of WBCs, WBC casts, RBCs, or proteinuria.
- A urine culture is done to identify offending organisms.
- A Gram stain shows gram-negative bacilli.
- A CBC, $SMA_6$, and fasting blood sugar determination should be ordered.
- A wet mount is done to rule out vaginal infection.
- A fluorescent antibody test may be indicated (see Chap. 17).
- Radiographic kidney studies are done after the acute episode has cleared.

## Management and Treatment as Clinically Indicated

- Refer all patients to a physician.
- Bed rest or hospitalization may be indicated for patients requiring parenteral antibiotics.
- Antibiotic concentration needs to be achieved in the blood and kidney tissue as well as in the urine. The drug of choice is ampicillin, 500 mg orally every six hours for 14 days. *Check for penicillin allergy.* Further treatment or alter-

nate treatment would depend on the results of urine culture and sensitivity studies.
- For other treatment refer to the section on cystitis.
- Close follow-up is necessary. The patient should call if there has been no improvement after 48 hours of treatment.

## Complications

Chronic pyelonephritis is a serious progressive disease resulting from repeated episodes of acute disease or a long history of chronic cystitis. Scarring and fibrosis of the kidneys and tubular dilatations result from repeated healing processes. End-stage renal failure may result from this chronic destructive process.

## REFERENCES

Buckley R: Urinary tract infections related to sexual intercourse. *The Female Patient* 3:40, 1978.

Cimino J: Diagnosis and management of urinary tract infections. *Hospital Medicine,* October 1974, p 59.

Diddle A: Special medical and surgical considerations in gynecology, in Benson R (ed): *Current Obstetrics and Gynecologic Diagnosis and Treatment.* Los Altos, Calif, Lange Medical Publications, 1978, p 374.

Falconer M, Patterson H, Gustafson E, et al: *Current Drug Handbook 1978-1980.* Philadelphia, WB Saunders Company, 1978, p 27.

Freidlan G, McCue J, Perlman F, et al: Urinary tract infection and vaginitis, in Komaroff L, Winickoff R (ed): *Common Acute Illnesses: A Problem-Oriented Textbook with Protocols.* Boston, Little, Brown and Company, 1978, p 41.

Gleason, D: Female urologic disease, in Devine C, Stecker J (ed): *Urology in Practice.* Boston, Little, Brown and Company, 1978, p 208, 435.

Jeffcoate, SN: *Principles of Gynecology,* ed 4. London, Butterworth and Company, 1975, p 380.

Ledger, W: Infectious disease, in Romney S, Gray J, Little A, et al (ed); *Gynecology and Obstetrics The Health Care of Women.* New York, McGraw-Hill Book Company, 1975, p 442.

Marshall J, Judd G: Guide for the management of women with symptoms arising in the lower urinary tract: *Clin Obstet Gynecol* 19:2, p 247.

Rubinoff H: Urinary tract infections. *Primary Care* 4:617, 1979. Takahashi M, Loveland D: Bacteriuria and oral contraceptives. *JAMA* 227:762, 1974.

# 14

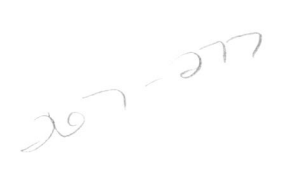

# Benign Pelvic Masses

This chapter does not discuss pelvic malignancy since the intent is to cover conditions that lend themselves to management by the Nurse Practitioner. Beginning with the most common benign lesions of the vulva, vagina, and cervix the chapter progresses to the more complex masses of these structures and the ovaries.

Patients with pelvic masses or lesions of questionable etiology should be referred to a physician.

## ADENOSIS (DES)

### Definition

Adenosis is the presence of benign, glandular epithelium, which is typically found in the endocervix, in the vagina or on the exocervix.

### Etiology

During the 1940s diethylstilbestrol (DES), a nonsteroidal estrogen believed to reduce fetal loss, was widely used in women with high-risk pregnancies (see Fig. 2). As many as two million women experiencing high-risk pregnancy were given this drug between 1941 and 1971. Daughters born to these women experienced vaginal and cervical changes as a result of exposure to DES in utero. Adenosis is

## MINOR BENIGN PELVIC LESIONS

| Lesion | Location | Description | Symptoms | Treatment |
|---|---|---|---|---|
| Intertrigo | Upper inner thighs, labial sulcus, inguinal folds | Intertrigo is a superficial chronic dermatitis of the external genitalia caused by friction between moist opposed surfaces. Red or brownish pigmentation occurs, and is usually seen in obese women during hot weather. | Burning and itching occurs. Vaginal discharge prolongs irritation. | Keep the skin clean, wash thoroughly with soap and water. Dry carefully, and apply cornstarch. Discontinue use of feminine hygiene sprays. Wear cotton underwear. Treat any vaginal infection. |
| Fibroma | Labia majora | Fibroma is a small or moderate-sized connective tissue tumor. It tends to become pedunculated with some reaching large proportions and producing ulceration of overlying tissue. | Asymptomatic until they enlarge and cause a sensation of heaviness and pain in the labia | Surgical excision |
| Hidradinoma | Labia majora | Hidradinoma is a rare tumor arising from apocrine sweat glands. It occurs almost exclusively in white women. It is a sharply circumscribed, elevated, subcutaneous nodule about 1 cm in cir- | Asymptomatic | Surgical excision, histologic examination |

| | | | |
|---|---|---|---|
| | | cumference. It is nonmalignant but may be mistaken for adenocarcinoma. | |
| Sebaceous cyst | Labia majora | The duct of a sebaceous gland becomes occluded and sebum is retained causing cystic enlargement of the gland. The cysts are single or multiple, 1–2 cm, and are moderately firm and moveable. | Asymptomatic unless infection occurs and it becomes tense, red, swollen, and painful | None, or aid spontaneous drainage with moist heat; incision and drainage if necessary |
| Gartner cyst | Vagina | Gartner cysts are congenital and are formed from blind pouches of embryonic epithelial remnants, which retain their glandular lining. Ducts in the lining persist and remain secretory giving rise to cystic tumors. Single or multiple cysts are localized on the lateral vaginal wall. They are soft and easily compressed to the side and are often found incidentally on vaginal exam. They are usually small but may enlarge to resemble a cystocele. Rarely do they become infected. | Asymptomatic; symptomatic when large causing dyspareunia, pain, bladder pressure, or labor dystocia | None, or surgical excision |

269

## MINOR BENIGN PELVIC LESIONS (continued)

| Lesion | Location | Description | Symptoms | Treatment |
|---|---|---|---|---|
| Inclusion cyst | Vagina | Tags of vaginal mucosa are buried beneath the submucosal tissue of the vagina as a result of delivery, trauma, or vaginal surgery. They become encysted and are usually small, multiple, and filled with cheeselike exudate. | Asymptomatic. If symptomatic they cause dyspareunia. | None, or surgical excision |
| Papilloma | Cervix | This lesion located on the portio vaginalis, is composed of connective tissue covered by squamous epithelium. A small, 1-cm, raised nodule is usually discovered on routine pelvic examination. It may be confused with condyloma acuminata or squamous cell carcinoma. In 95% of the patients it is benign. | None | Surgical excision by electrocauterization |
| Nabothian cyst | Cervix | Nabothian cysts occur during the process of squamous | Asymptomatic | None |

metaplasia, when mucus-secreting glands on the exocervix become occluded. The glands continue to secrete mucus, and become distended, producing nabothian follicles. These are silvery white or yellowish in color, 1–2 mm in diameter, and feel firm and raised to palpation.

**Figure 2**
DES-Type Drugs That May Have Been Prescribed to Pregnant Women

| Nonsteroidal Estrogens | | Nonsteroidal Estrogen-Androgen Combinations | |
|---|---|---|---|
| Benzestrol | Mikarol | Amperone | Teserene |
| Chlorotrianisene | Mikarol forti | Di-Erone | Tylandril |
| Comestrol | Milestrol | Estan | Tylosterone |
| Cyren A | Monomestrol | Metystil | |
| Cyren B | Neo-Oestranol I | | |
| Delvinal | Neo-Oestranol II | *Nonsteroidal Estrogen-* | |
| DES | Nulabort | *Progesterone Combination* | |
| DesPlex | Oestrogenine | | |
| Diestryl | Oestromenin | Progravidium | |
| Dibestil | Oestromon | | |
| Dienestrol | Orestol | *Vaginal creams and* | |
| Dienoestrol | Pabestrol D | *Suppositories with* | |
| Diethylstilbestrol dipalmitate | Palestrol | *Nonsteroidal Estrogens* | |
| Diethylstilbestrol diphosphate | Restrol | | |
| | Stil-Rol | AVC cream with | |
| | Stilbal | Dienestrol | |
| Diethylstibestrol dipropionate | Stilbestrol | Dienestrol cream | |
| Diethylstilbenediol | Stilbestronate | | |
| Digestil | Stilbetin | | |
| Domestrol | Stilbinol | | |
| Estilben | Stilboestroform | | |
| Estrobene | Stilboestrol | | |
| Estrobene DP | Stilboestrol DP | | |
| Estrosyn | Stilestrate | | |
| Fonatol | Stilpalmitate | | |
| Gynben | Stilphostrol | | |
| Gyneben | Stilronate | | |
| Hexestrol | Stilrone | | |
| Hexoestrol | Stils | | |
| Hi-Bestrol | Synestrin | | |
| Menocrin | Synestrol | | |
| Meprane | Tace | | |
| Mestilbol | Vallestril | | |
| Methallenestril | Willestrol | | |
| Microest | | | |

SOURCE: US Department of Health, Education and Welfare Information for Physicians: DES Exposure in Utero. Publication No (NIH) 76-1119, pp. 10-11.

**Figure 2.**
DES-type drugs that may have been prescribed to pregnant women. (From US Department of Health, Education, and Welfare, Information for Physicians: DES Exposure in Utero. Publication No. (NIH) 76-1119, pp 10-11.)

the most common manifestation but a number of less common structural abnormalities of the vagina and cervix have also been identified.

In Boston in 1971 seven cases of clear cell adenocarcinoma were reported in teenage girls. A study investigating this phenomenon documented association of the neoplasm with intrauterine exposure of the young women to DES. Gestation of pregnancy when DES therapy was initiated, the length of exposure, and the total dose of the drug given were found to be crucial factors in tumor formation. In most cases of documented malignancy, DES therapy was begun before 18 weeks' gestation, however, a few cases have been reported when treatment was started after 18 weeks.

Although adenosis is found in association with almost all vaginal clear cell adenocarcinomas, a direct transition from adenosis to cancer has not been identified. The risk of developing carcinoma from DES exposure is rare (about 0.1%). Long-term prognosis or the effect of subsequent estrogen exposure on the DES daughter, as well as on her mother, is not known.

## Clinical Features

### Symptoms

- May be absent
- Abnormal vaginal bleeding
- A mucoid vaginal discharge
- A feeling of heat in the vagina
- Dyspareunia

### Signs

- A normal pelvic examination and Pap smear
- Cervical and vaginal structural abnormalities or stigmata
- Firm 1- to 5-cm submucosal vaginal cysts, which may not be visible but found only by thorough, careful palpation of the entire vaginal mucosa
- Punctate patches or "sand granules" palpable on the vaginal wall
- Ectropion
- Positive areas of tissue, which are nonstaining with Lugol's solution on the cervix or vagina and which may indicate a premalignancy, malignancy, metaplasia, or denuded epithelium.

## Differential Diagnosis

- Clear cell adenocarcinoma
- Squamous cell carcinoma
- Squamous metaplasia

## Diagnostic Studies as Clinically Indicated

*Patient history should include:*

- A birth date after 1942
- A history of unusual vaginal discharge or bleeding
- A history of the mother having medical problems during pregnancy:
    Did she have diabetes, bleeding, premature births?
    Did she take hormones early in her pregnancy? (See Fig. 2)
    Are her medical records available to review for prenatal hormone ingestion?

*Examination of the population at risk includes:*

- Examination of premenarchial patients with unexplained vaginal bleeding or unexplained heavy discharge
- A screening pelvic examination at menarche, or at age 14 if not menstruating
- Careful inspection and palpation of the external genitalia, vagina, and cervix looking for structural or tissue abnormalities
    Cervical changes may include a total or partial cervical sulcus, an anterior cervical protuberance, a recessed perioral area resembling a patulous lower endocervical canal, a cervix that is totally covered with columnar epithelium, or a pseudopolyp near the external os.
    Vaginal changes may include surface adenosis, usually found in the upper one-third of the vagina, cystic adenosis, a conical constriction of the proximal vagina, or a fibrous band of tissue beneath the vaginal mucosa. These changes are more common than those found on the cervix but are considerably more difficult to detect and interpret.
    Miscellaneous changes have been identified but are considered rare. Any abnormal finding during observation or palpation of the cervix and vagina needs careful evaluation by a skilled physician.
- A four-quadrant Pap smear with Lugol's staining of the cervix and vagina (Nonstaining areas are suspicious.)
- Colposcopy
    During the initial visit if feasible

- Assess her knowledge, understanding, and emotional status regarding her diagnosis.
- Determine if she has talked with her mother about her feelings.
- Reinforce or clarify the physician's explanation of what changes have occurred in her body as a result of DES exposure and the possible implications.
- Reassure the young woman regarding the rare (0.1%) incidence of malignant change when appropriate.
- Reassure patients with diagnosed adenosis or structural changes of the vagina or cervix that her sexual function or fertility will probably not be effected, and that many DES-exposed daughters have successful pregnancies.
- Explore the patient's prior experience with pelvic examination, and teach and counsel as necessary.
- Explain the controversy concerning use of oral contraception or the morning-after-pill in DES exposed daughters and that most physicians will not prescribe hormone preparations for birth control. Discuss alternate methods of contraception.
- Explain the use of vaginal tampons to dilate a virginal or tight vagina in young patients before a return visit for a pelvic examination.
- Stress to the patient the need for close follow-up and the importance of keeping appointments.
- Keep communications open by offering support via telephone, extra visits to talk, or referral for counseling.
- Explore with the patient's mother her reactions and feelings regarding her daughter's DES problem. If necessary make a separate appointment to talk with her or refer her for counseling if appropriate.

*Counsel the DES Mother about:*

- Her possible increased risk of acquiring breast or pelvic cancer from her DES exposure while pregnant
- Informing her gynecologist of her DES exposure before hormones for birth control or menopausal symptoms are prescribed
- The importance of following scheduled routine screening for possible complications. The Department of Health, Education and Welfare, Office of the Assistant Secretary for Health in the *1978 Physician Advisory* on the health effects of DES recommends:
    Having an annual pelvic examination, including bimanual palpation and a Pap smear
    Undergoing a breast examination that follows current National Cancer Institute guidelines for breast cancer screening, which include:

BENIGN PELVIC MASSES

When a Pap smear is abnormal
When squamous metaplasia is present
In nonstaining areas of the vagina
- A biopsy on suspicious lesions

## Management and Treatment as Clinically Indicated

- Refer the patient to a DES physician specialist or center as indicated.
- Local destruction by excision, cautery, or cryosurgery of atypical or vasive neoplastic changes that have been identified histologically.
- Topical progesterone and acidic vaginal jellies have been used but generally accepted as beneficial or appropriate.
- Surgical intervention is indicated after diagnosis of clear cell carcin been made. Depending on the extent of tumor involvement, the surg include radical hysterectomy, vaginectomy, pelvic lymph node dissec vaginal replacement with skin graft.
- Follow-up schedule
  Reexamine annually when the initial examination is negative.
  When adenosis or ectropion are present an examination shoul formed two to three times a year. It should include:
  1. Inspection and palpation of the vagina and cervix
  2. Quadrant cytologic sampling of the vagina
  3. Lugol's staining of the vagina and cervix, with biopsy of suspic
  4. Colposcopic examination of the cervix and vagina when availa

## Complications

- Psychosocial problems
- Infertility
- Clear cell adenocarcinoma
- Squamous cell carcinoma

## Patient Teaching

- Question the young woman to ascertain when she first lear exposure.

1. Monthly breast self-examination, reporting any abnormal findings to the physician
2. Annual palpation of the breasts by a qualified medical professional
3. No mammography under age 35 for routine screening
4. Annual mammography between age 35 to 39 only if the woman has a personal history of cancer
5. Annual mammography between age 40 to 49 only if a woman has a history of breast cancer in immediate relatives (mothers and sisters) or a personal history of breast cancer
6. An annual screening mammography may be considered in women over age 50.
7. The Task Force is concerned about the use of X-ray mammography as a screening modality in DES mothers under 50 years of age. This concern relates to (a) lack of proven benefit of such screening in these younger women, (b) presumed risk of irradiation, and (c) experimental work suggesting an interaction between DES and radiation.

With any signs or symptoms suggestive of breast cancer, a diagnostic workup, which may include mammography, is indicated.

## CERVICAL POLYPS

### Definition

Cervical polyps are benign, pedunculated growths arising from the mucosal surface of the ectocervix or endocervical canal. They are usually small and may be single or multiple. The pedicle may enlongate causing the polyp to protrude through the cervical os.

### Etiology

The etiology of polyp formation is uncertain. They may be caused by a chronic inflammatory process or localized vascular congestion, or they may be related to hyperestrinism. (They are often found in association with endometrial hyperplasia.)

## Clinical Features

### Symptoms

- Often asymptomatic
- Thick leukorrhea (most common symptom)
- Menorrhagia, intermenstrual bleeding, postcoital bleeding, or vaginal bleeding after straining at stool or douching
- Postmenopausal bleeding
- Mucopurulent, blood-tinged vaginal discharge (with multiple endocervical polyps)

### Signs

- Polyps are pear-shaped, single or multiple, soft, pedunculated growths, which may protrude through the cervical os.
- Polyps are pink to bright red and are vascular and friable. They may be palpable or nonpalpable.
- They usually occur in parous and early postmenopausal women.
- Ectocervical polyps are pale and flesh-colored and may be rounded or pedunculated. They are less friable than endocervical polyps.
- Endocervical polyps may be more obvious during the preovulatory phase when the cervical os opens, and more concealed during the secretory phase by a tighter cervical os.

## Differential Diagnosis

- Submucous pedunculated myoma (firm, musclelike rather than soft)
- Endometrial polyps
- "Pill polyps," polypoid adenomatous hyperplasia related to oral contraceptive use (regress after stopping the pill but may be easily confused with adenocarcinoma of the cervix)
- Products of conception
- Pseudopolyp (extension of fibromuscular tissue in a DES-exposed daughter)

## Diagnostic Studies as Clinically Indicated

- Culture and sensitivity studies of the cervical discharge are indicated.
- A Pap smear and a smear for gonococci should be collected.
- Hysterography may demonstrate endocervical polyps, which can be the basis of infertility.
- A D&C may be performed for investigation of abnormal bleeding at which time polyps are found.
- Histologic studies should be performed on the excised polyps.

## Management and Treatment as Clinically Indicated

- Treatment of underlying cervical infection should be done after identification of the offending organism.
- Removal of the polyp by the physician as an office procedure may be done. The pedicle of the polyp is grasped with a hemostat and twisted until it is separated. Slight bleeding usually occurs.
- Electrosurgical excision of large or broad-based polyps may be necessary. Suturing may be needed to control bleeding, so hospitalization may be indicated for this procedure.
- A surgical D&C is performed when the cervix is soft, the polyps are large, and the pedicle is not visible.
- Broad-spectrum antibiotics should be given if the patient shows signs of infection after the polyps have been removed.

### Complications

- Iron-deficiency anemia from prolonged or heavy bleeding
- Exacerbation of pelvic infection from polypectomy or diagnostic instrumentation

## Patient Teaching

- Explain to the patient what polyps are and how they develop.
- Give an explanation of why the polyps have caused vaginal discharge or bleeding.

- Explain the importance of routine follow-up to assure chronic cervical infection is not present and to have a Pap smear done.
- Advise women taking birth control pills about the need to use an alternate contraceptive method. Polyps should regress with discontinuation of the Pill.
- Reassure patients that malignant change is rare (1%).
- Reassure the patient who is to have polyps removed that they seldom recur, especially when they are single.
- Advise the patient to take warm vinegar douches (1 tablespoonful of vinegar to a quart of warm water) after polypectomy to control inflammatory reaction. Prophylactic antibiotic therapy is not usually given.

## LEIOMYOMA OF THE UTERUS
## (FRIBROID, FIBROMA, MYOMA)

### Definition

Leiomyoma is a smooth muscle tumor of the uterus. It is the most common gynecologic tumor, effecting 20% of the female population.

### Etiology

Leiomyomas are composed of muscle and fibrous connective tissue and are discrete, spherical, and have a capsular covering making them easily enucleated from surrounding tissue. Originating in the myometrium, 98% of the tumors are found in the uterine body and 2% in the cervix. Rarely do they occur before menarche, and they do not develop after menopause. The majority are benign, asymptomatic, and slow growing. They may occur singly, but are usually multiple, and range in size from microscopic to masses of 50 pounds or more. With earlier and better diagnosis large tumors are rare today. The true etiology of the tumor is unknown, but four theories that attempt to explain its existence are:
- Genetic factors: In the United States leiomyomas are most frequently found in Jewish and black women. Fifty percent of black women develop the tumor.
- Estrogen stimulation: Tumor growth is increased with estrogen therapy or with pregnancy, and its growth decreases after menopause. Usually found in women over 35 years of age, the slow-growing tumor may need 20–25 years of estrogen stimulation to become palpable.

- Human Growth Hormone (HGH): This hormone may be a factor in growth of the tumor since its secretion is increased by estrogen stimulation and pregnancy.
- Contraction of uterine muscles results in stress along the myometrium and may cause tumors by proliferation of the tissue.

Three types of leiomyomas have been identified. These are:

- Submucous tumors lie just beneath the endometrium and may become pedunculated and appear or protrude through the cervical os. This type is called a fibroid polyp.
- Intramural or interstitial tumors are the most common type and are located within the uterine wall. They are encapsulated nodules of various sizes, and if extended laterally into broad ligament, are known as intraligamentary leiomyoma.
- Subserous or subperitoneal tumors grow outward from the serosal surface of the uterus toward the peritoneal cavity, and may also develop pedicles. These tumors have a large area in which to grow and may become larger than the uterus itself. If they acquire an extrauterine blood supply from the omentum, the pedicle may atrophy and resorb. The tumor is then said to be parasitic.

## Clinical Features

### Symptoms

Symptoms are more common with submucous and polypoid tumors and include:

- Abnormal uterine bleeding or hypermenorrhea with clot formation, which may result from:
    Hyperplasia surrounding the submucous-type tumor
    Large tumors causing greater vascular congestion
    Dilatation of the uterine cavity causing increased endometrial surface area
    Mechanical disturbance of vessels supplying the endometrium
- Pain, an uncommon symptom that may result from:
    Degeneration or torsion of a pedicle
    Contractile effort of the uterus to expel the tumor
    Large tumors causing pelvic heaviness and bearing-down sensation
    Pressure on nerves from large tumors
    Pressure of the tumor causing dyspareunia or dysmenorrhea
- Pressure from the tumor causing:
    Urinary frequency or urinary retention

Intestinal obstruction or constipation, decrease in the diameter of the stool
Increased abdominal size
Vaginal discharge, bleeding, dyspareunia
- Anemia from prolonged bleeding
- Infertility, which occurs in 25-35% of women with leiomyomas. (The patient is able to become pregnant but is unable to maintain it and may experience habitual abortion.

*Signs*

- Abdominal palpation reveals an irregular, nodular, firm tumor protruding through the abdominal wall. Small tumors may be felt at the level of the symphysis.
- Bimanual examination may reveal:
    Enlargement or distortion of the normal uterine contour
    Asymmetry of the uterus with submucous tumors
    A firm fundus with multiple, irregular, usually freely moveable nodules
    Subserous pedunculated tumors, which may be felt distant from the uterus and may be confused with adnexal tumors

## Differential Diagnosis

- Pregnancy, ectopic pregnancy
- Ovarian cysts or tumors
- Adenomyosis uteri
- Pelvic inflammation
- Subinvolution
- Congenital anomaly
- Malignancy
- Uterine hypertrophy

## Diagnostic Studies as Clinically Indicated

- A careful history should be taken, and physical examination should be done with special emphasis on the abdominal, vaginal, and rectal examinations.
- A pregnancy test will rule out uterine enlargement from pregnancy

- A CBC and urinalysis to rule out infection or anemia should be done.
- A Pap smear should be done.
- An x-ray film, hysterogram, or ultrasonogram will aid in the differential diagnosis.
- A D&C may be indicated for heavy bleeding or for collection of an endometrial sample for histologic studies.
- Culdoscopy or laparoscopy may be indicated for diagnostic purposes.

## Management and Treatment as Clinically Indicated

The type of treatment should depend on the age of the patient, general health, desire to conceive, severity of symptoms, future risk to the patient, or an association of leiomyoma with other lesions such as cystourethrocele or endometritis. Three types of treatment are conservative, surgical, and irradiation.

- Consultation or referral to a physician is necessary.
- Conservative treatment is nonsurgical and used in patients with few or no symptoms.

    Bimanual pelvic examination is done every three to six months to follow tumor growth rate. Palpation of the posterior cul-de-sac and uterosacral ligaments for nodules of endometriosis is important since they frequently coexist.

    A Pap smear should be done yearly.

    Treatment of iron-deficiency anemia may be indicated in patients with heavy bleeding
- Surgical treatment is indicated if:

    The uterine size exceeds that of a 12-14 weeks' gestation

    Growth rate of the tumor is excessive (except in pregnancy)

    The mass invades the cervix, broad ligament, or there is excessive encroachment into the uterine cavity

    The tumor is pedunculated

    There is excessive pressure, pain, or bleeding caused by the tumor
- Types of surgical treatment

    Myomectomy is used for patients wishing to preserve fertility

    Indications for its use include:

    1. Obstruction of the birth canal
    2. Severe irregularity of the uterine cavity
    3. Obstruction or angulation of the fallopian tubes

4. History of three or more spontaneous abortions have occurred.
5. Pedunculated lesions projecting into the external cervical os.

Hysterectomy is the most specific and effective form of treatment. A D&C with a frozen section of the uterus should precede surgery. Hysterectomy is indicated when nonsurgical treatment or D&C are inadequate or when myomectomy is contraindicated. It may also be indicated in the multiparous woman over 40 years of age. Advantages of hysterectomy include no risk of recurrence and removal of potential cancer-bearing tissue in the pelvis. Removal of the ovaries during the procedure is controversial.

- Irradiation is used rarely in symptomatic patients who are surgical risk.

## Complications

- Red degeneration (carneous) of the myoma (torsion or thrombosis of the pedicle)
- Hydroureter, hydronephrosis
- Endometrial polyps
- Leiomyosarcoma
- Polycythemia (rare)
- Pregnancy complications
    Abortion from atrophic changes of the endometrium
    Malpresentation or abortion from distortion of the uterine cavity
    Failure of fetal engagement
    Premature labor from increased uterine irritability
    Pain from torsion or degeneration of the tumor
    Dystocia or obstruction of the birth canal
    Postpartum hemorrhage from reduced uterine contractility

## Patient Teaching

- Determine from the patient what she knows about her "fibroids." Provide information as necessary (pictures of the different types of fibroids will be helpful).
- Reassure the patient that fibroids are very common in women and are almost always benign.

- Discuss her symptoms (if any) explaining why they occur and what treatment is planned.
- Tell her that fibroids do not disappear and may grow during the reproductive years when estrogen is being produced. They will shrink and possibly disappear after menopause. Many women have the tumor for years and never need more treatment than regular examinations to check rate of growth.
- Encourage women of reproductive age to use the diaphragm or foam and condoms for contraception. If the patient insists on oral contraception, and the tumor is not large and is slow growing, low-dose birth control pills may be given. However, close follow-up with bimanual examinations is necessary to assess tumor growth rate.
- Explain or reinforce information the physician has given the patient who is to have surgery. The procedure should be discussed with the physician so the patient will know what surgery will be done. Her partner (if appropriate) should be included in this discussion.
- Plan time with the pregnant patient who will need someone to share her concerns and offer support.
- Stress to all patients the need for regular follow-up.

## OVARIAN ENLARGEMENT

Ovarian enlargement is characterized by a palpable mass of neoplastic or cystic origin involving the ovaries. While generally benign, about 15-25% prove malignant. For this reason, consultation and referral to a physician is mandatory to determine the precise nature of the adnexal mass.

### General Considerations

Some factors to consider when assessing a patient with an adnexal mass are:
- During early development, benign and malignant ovarian neoplasms have similar growth patterns and physical findings, therefore, clinical differentiation is difficult.
- Benign ovarian neoplasms are usually cystic, mobile, and unilateral. Malignant neoplasms are usually fixed, bilateral and solid or semisolid.

## 286  PROBLEMS IN AMBULATORY OBSTETRICS AND GYNECOLOGY

- Unilateral, cystic, mobile, and/or asymptomatic adnexal masses in women of reproductive age most often are functional cysts (follicular or corpus luteum cysts).
- Women regularly using oral contraceptive pills rarely develop functional cysts.
- Further investigation of an adnexal mass is indicated when it is solid rather than cystic, is a cystic mass that has persisted longer than three months in a woman of reproductive age, or is greater than 10 cm.
- Discomfort or pain caused by ovarian masses may be difficult to differentiate from that due to appendicitis, ectopic pregnancy, or pelvic infection.
- Eighty to ninety-five percent of the ovarian tumors found in women between the ages of 20 and 40 are benign, whereas 50-70% of those occurring in women 40-70 years of age are benign.
- The rate of malignant ovarian neoplasms has increased 10% in the past 20 years.
- Metastasis has already occurred in four-fifths of malignant tumors when diagnosed.
- The patient may be unaware of a neoplasm until a complication arises from it. Symptoms are rare except in some functioning tumors.

This section focuses on common cystic ovarian masses but does not include the complex and lengthy classification of benign and malignant tumors. Included are:

- Follicle cysts
- Corpus luteum cysts
- Theca-lutein cysts
- Paraovarian cysts
- Dermoid cysts (cystic teratoma)
- Mucinous cystadenoma
- Endometrioma

## FOLLICLE CYSTS

These physiologic cysts develop in the graafian follicle and may be manifest at any age before menopause. A common cause of detectable ovarian enlargement, they develop from immature dominant follicles that do not ovulate but remain active or from less-stimulated follicles that fail to regress normally. If multiple, they rarely exceed 1.0-1.4 cm, but if single, may grow to 6-8 cm. They are translucent and contain clear, serous, estin-rich fluid. Most of these cysts produce no symptoms and regress or rupture spontaneously within one or two months.

## Clinical Features

### Symptoms

Symptoms usually occur from a large or ruptured cyst and may include:

- Acute or chronic lower abdominal pain
- Low back pain
- Dyspareunia (painful intercourse)
- Menstrual irregularities

### Signs

- A palpable cystic adnexal mass
- Slight tenderness to palpation

## Diagnostic Studies as Clinically Indicated

- A pregnancy test is done to rule out pregnancy.
- Sonography may be used to define the ovarian mass.

## Management and Treatment as Clinically Indicated

- A low-dose combination oral contraceptive pill, such as Norinyl 1/50, may be prescribed for 6-12 weeks to suppress follicular activity. This medication may have to be continued for three to six months. Reevaluation of ovarian size by bimanual examination is done after six weeks to assess patient response to the treatment.
- Cysts that grow, remain over 5 cm, or are bilateral need further evaluation.

## Patient Teaching

See p. 297.

## CORPUS LUTEUM CYSTS

These physiologic cysts are found only in ovulating women. They are more common than follicle cysts and are usually more symptomatic. They are formed when a mature corpus luteum persists with bleeding into its cavity. They are usually 5-10 cm in diameter, depending on the amount of hemorrhage. Corpus luteum cysts are difficult to differentiate from ectopic pregnancy, cause changes in the normal menstrual patterns, and usually regress spontaneously.

### Clinical Features

#### Symptoms

- Delayed menses followed by prolonged irregular bleeding
- Unilateral, dull, aching pelvic pain
- Symptoms similar to those of intraperitoneal hemorrhage, caused by rupture of the cyst

#### Signs

- A readily palpable, unilateral ovarian cystic mass, which occurs after ovulation
- Adnexal tenderness to palpation
- Spontaneous regression after two months
- Amenorrhea in some patients

### Diagnostic Studies as Clinically Indicated

- A pregnancy test should be done to rule out pregnancy.
- A sonogram may be done to define the ovarian mass.
- Bimanual adnexal examinations should be performed for one to three successive months at different times of the menstrual cycle to assess cystic growth.
- Laparotomy may be indicated for accurate diagnosis, but is rarely needed for treatment; oophorectomy is not indicated.

## Management and Treatment as Clinically Indicated

- Low-dose combination oral contraceptive pills, such as Norinyl 1+50, may be prescribed for six weeks to depress follicular activity. Reevaluation of ovarian size by pelvic examination is done after completion of the medication.

## Patient Teaching

See p. 297.

# THECA-LUTEIN CYSTS

These cysts are usually associated with trophoblastic tumors and are the least common of all the physiologic cysts. Stimulation or increased sensitivity to excessive levels of human chorionic gonadotropin (hCG) from a trophoblastic tumor appears to be the mechanism responsible for growth of thecal cells of the luteal follicle. The cysts are multiple, bilateral, pedunculated, and range in size from 1.5-30 cm in diameter. Torsion of the pedicle or ascites may result from the presence of these cysts, but they usually regress and disappear spontaneously after removal of the trophoblastic tumor.

## Clinical Features

### Symptoms

- Abdominal tenderness from rapid ovarian enlargement due to growing thecal cysts
- Acute suprapubic pain accompanied by vomiting (suggests torsion of the cyst pedicle)

### Signs

- Palpable bilateral cystic masses in the adnexa, which may be freely moveable
- Abdominal tenderness to palpation

### Diagnostic Studies as Clinically Indicated

- A pregnancy test is done to rule out pregnancy.
- A sonogram may be done to aid or to confirm diagnosis of cysts.

### Management and Treatment as Clinically Indicated

- Treatment is not indicated in the absence of complications.
- Laparoscopy for aspiration or correction of a twisted pedicle may be indicated.

### Patient Teaching

See p. 297.

## PAROVARIAN CYST

Although not a true ovarian mass, these cysts make up about 10% of all abnormal adnexal growths and are common in the 30- to 40-year age group. The cysts are located in the broad ligament between the fallopian tube and the ovary making them difficult to distinguish from ovarian neoplasms. They develop from embryonic remnants and are usually small 3-4 cm, contain clear fluid, and are not pedunculated. Rarely a paraovarian cyst may attain enormous size and fill the entire pelvis or abdomen. They are usually discovered during a routine pelvic examination.

### Clinical Features

#### Symptoms

- Symptoms are uncommon and are primarily due to secondary uterine displacement.
- Abdominal discomfort or increased urination caused by pressure from a large cyst are the most commonly occurring symptoms.

## Signs

- Small cystic masses may be palpated in the adnexa. They are not freely moveable.
- Abdominal or pelvic tenderness is absent.

## Diagnostic Studies as Clinically Indicated

- A pregnancy test is done to rule out pregnancy.
- A sonogram may be ordered to aid diagnosis.

## Management and Treatment as Clinically Indicated

- Surgical excision of the cyst is the usual treatment. Histologic examination of the excised tissue is necessary for verification of the diagnosis.

## Patient Teaching

See p. 297.

# DERMOID CYST
# (CYSTIC TERATOMA)

The dermoid cyst represents 10-15% of ovarian tumors occurring in women of any age and are the most common ovarian tumors of childhood. However, the majority (50%) are found in women between the ages of 30 and 50. The cysts are often multiple, and several may develop in the same ovary. Their size ranges from microscopic to large proportions, the average being 10-12 cm. Arising from the embryonic layers of the ectoderm, mesoderm, and endoderm, the cysts commonly contain hair, cartilage, teeth, and adipose and central nervous system elements. Usually unilocular and unilateral they are frequently pedunculated and lie close to the uterus. On palpation they feel soft and doughy and are often discovered when procedures such as abdominal x-ray studies or abdominal surgery are performed. The dermoid cyst is the most common ovarian neoplasm complicating pregnancy. Malignancy occurs in less than 1% of these cysts.

## Clinical Features

### Symptoms

The majority of patients with dermoid cysts are asymptomatic, but symptoms may result from complications such as:

- Torsion of a pedicle or rupture of the cyst. This will cause acute abdominal pain.
- A small rent in the tumor capsule allowing slow leakage of its contents into the abdominal cavity. This occurs over a period of months and low-grade peritoneal irritation and infection results causing progressive nausea, diarrhea, abdominal tenderness, and low-grade fever.
- Hemolytic anemia occurring rarely in conjunction with a dermoid cyst but disappearing after its removal

### Signs

- Palpation of single or multiple doughy masses lying close to the uterus on one side
- Absent abdominal tenderness when no complications exist

## Diagnostic Studies as Clinically Indicated

- Sonography should be done to aid diagnosis.
- A pregnancy test is done to rule out pregnancy.

## Management and Treatment as Clinically Indicated

- Management includes surgical resection of the cyst preserving as much ovarian tissue as possible. Investigation of the opposite ovary and histologic examination of the excised tissue specimen is necessary.

## Patient Teaching

See p. 297.

# SEROUS CYSTADENOMA

Serous cysts are the most common of all benign cysts of the ovary (20-40%), excluding the functional cysts. They may be single and multilocular but are most often bilateral. They are filled with serous fluid and may range from a small size to such large proportions that they fill the abdominal cavity. Pedunculated cysts, they lie free in the abdominal cavity making them easily displaced and able to occupy many positions. Torsion of the pedicle or implantation of the cyst on the serosal surface of abdominal viscera may occur. Malignancy occurs in 20-30% of these tumors.

### Symptoms

- None
- General deterioration of health and loss of weight when tumor enlargement has increased metabolic needs.
- Acute suprapubic pain accompanied by vomiting when torsion of a pedicle has occurred.
- Enlargement of the abdomen from the growing tumor producing pressure symptoms including:
  Bearing-down discomfort
  Edema of the lower extremities
  Urinary frequency
  Shortness of breath
  Engorged abdominal veins
  Varicosities, hemorrhoids
- Acute pain occurs when the tumor becomes impacted or there is restriction of its blood supply.

### Signs

- Palpation of small to large fluid-filled cysts that are moveable within the pelvis or abdomen
- Abdominal enlargement
- A generally debilitated-appearing patient
- Those signs accompanying the symptoms listed above.

### Diagnostic Studies as Clinically Indicated

- A pregnancy test is done to rule out an accompanying pregnancy.
- A sonogram is done to aid or confirm diagnosis.

### Management and Treatment as Clinically Indicated

Management may include:

- Laparotomy with excision of a unilaterally effected ovary. Bisection of the opposite ovary may be indicated.
- Total abdominal hysterectomy and bilateral salpingo-oophorectomy in women over 40 years of age when the cysts are implanted, bilateral, or are large and have destroyed all normal ovarian tissue. These tumors have a high incidence of recurrence.

### Patient Teaching

See p. 297.

## MUCINOUS CYSTADENOMA

The mucinous cystadenomas are less common than the serous cyst adenomas, representing about 20% of ovarian tumors. They usually occur postmenopausally and may attain enormous size, filling the entire abdominal cavity. Most of the large cystic tumors that are reported as medical curiosities are of this type. The tumors are most often unilateral and multilocular with compartments containing mucinous material, which tends to thicken and become gelatinous with increasing age of the patient. Malignant change occurs in approximately 6% of these tumors.

Pseudomyoma peritonei is a rare complication, which occurs when a mucinous cystadenoma ruptures. Spillage from the ruptured cyst contains secreting mucus cells that transplant and grow on the peritoneum causing intestinal obstruction, peritoneal adhesions, and possibly death.

## Clinical Features

### Symptoms

- None
- Abdominal enlargement
- Abdominal discomfort from the growing tumor
- Abdominal pressure symptoms (see the section on serous cystadenoma)

### Signs

- A palpable soft, unilateral pelvic or abdominal mass, particularly in a postmenopausal woman
- An enlarged abdomen

## Diagnostic Studies as Clinically Indicated

- A pregnancy test is done to rule out accompanying pregnancy in a sexually active premenopausal woman.
- A sonogram is done to aid or confirm diagnosis.

## Management and Treatment

Management may include:

- Examination of both ovaries for cystic involvement
- Unilateral oophorectomy when one ovary is involved in a young woman
- Total abdominal hysterectomy and bilateral salpingo-oophorectomy in women over 40 years of age

## Patient Teaching

See p. 297.

## ENDOMETRIOMA

This slow-growing cystic enlargement of the ovary results from cyclic hemorrhage of endometriosis implants on the ovary. It occurs during the reproductive years and is found most often in women between the ages of 25 and 40. In about 50% of patients with endometriosis the ovary is involved, and in 5% a mass will be palpable. Accumulation of old blood in the cysts may cause the ovary to enlarge to a diameter of 12-15 cm. These are the commonly known "chocolate cysts." The cysts are thin walled and often leak irritating contents into the abdominal cavity. Rupture usually occurs in the immediate premenstrual phase, and the resulting pain may range from minimal to acute, depending on the suddenness of rupture and the amount of spillage. Chronic dissemination of the endometrial tissue throughout the pelvis creates irritation with consequent formation of pelvic adhesions, which may greatly compromise fertility. Differentiating ectopic pregnancy, acute pelvic infection, and appendicitis from a ruptured endometrioma is a diagnostic challenge. Malignant change is rare.

### Clinical Features

Signs and symptoms may include (see also Chap. 11):

- Ovarian enlargement and tenderness
- Ovaries in a fixed position
- Cervical motion tenderness on bimanual examination

### Diagnostic Studies as Clinically Indicated

- Laparoscopic examination may be done to determine the presence of the cystic mass and the extent of endometriosis.

### Management and Treatment as Clinically Indicated

- Laparotomy with exploration and resection or fulguration of the endometrial implants and release of adhesions may be performed in young women

- Hysterectomy with bilateral salpingo-oophorectomy may be indicated in women over 40 years of age.

## Patient Teaching

- Review the anatomy of the pelvic organs and give a simple explanation of the menstrual cycle (using diagrams and charts) so the patient will understand what is happening.
- Explain to patient with ovarian enlargement that 75% of the enlargements are benign. Since many of these enlargements are difficult to diagnose on the first visit, further diagnostic tests such as a pregnancy test or sonogram may be necessary. Follow-up visits for bimanual evaluation of the cyst will probably be necessary.
- Explain to patients with functional cysts (follicle, corpus luteum cysts) how and why the cysts occur. Explain that they occur during the menstrual cycle and are fairly common in young women. The cysts are not treated but are followed with bimanual palpation for several months. This is to ensure that the cysts are regressing and not getting larger; they usually disappear spontaneously in two to three months.
- Birth control pills are often used to suppress activity of the ovary and cause the cyst to disappear. If menstruation has been delayed, a pregnancy test may be done to assure this is not the cause. Stress to the patient the need to return for follow-up assessment of the cyst.
- Explain or reinforce information given by the physician to patients with solid, persistent, enlarged, or symptomatic masses. They will need further diagnostic studies, which may include laparoscopy or laparotomy to obtain specimens for tissue examination.

    Explain that if lesions are benign the surgeon may be able to remove only the mass and leave the ovary. If the entire ovary must be removed, then the other ovary will produce enough hormones for the body's needs.

    Explain that if lesions are not benign, more extensive surgery will have to be performed. But regardless of the type of procedure necessary, the patient needs to be encouraged to discuss with the physician what the options for surgery might be.

- Encourage patients to bring their partners with them when they have scheduled visits so that both will be fully informed.
- Give patients the time and support necessary to allow them to express their concerns. Extra appointments may be necessary to do this, or referral for psychological counseling may be appropriate.

# POLYCYSTIC OVARY SYNDROME
# (STEIN-LEVENTHAL SYNDROME, SCLEROCYSTIC OVARIAN DISEASE)

The Stein-Leventhal syndrome criteria describing sclerocystic ovarian changes are currently considered inadequate. Polycystic ovarian syndrome (PCO) includes a wider scope of biochemical and physiologic defects. Recent studies have presented new insights into androgen metabolism and the hypothalmic-pituitary-ovarian system and their effects on this syndrome.

## Etiology

The etiology of PCO is not known but possibly originates from an adrenal disorder occurring in early menarche. It was formerly believed that the altered pattern of gonadotropin secretion, which occurs with this disease, was a result of dysfunction of the hypothalamic-pituitary system, or of an inappropriate feedback system from the polycystic ovary, or a result of both. Current thought suggests a disturbance in the function of androgen-estrogen conversion. The volume of estrogen secreted from extraovarian sources is such that the normal feedback mechanisms for gonadotropin release are overruled. (LH secretion is erratic or elevated and FSH secretion is decreased due to chronic inappropriate estrogen feedback.) Because of this mechanism, excessive androgens are converted to estrogen in the peripheral tissue resulting in anovulation and the PCO syndrome.

## Clinical Features

### Symptoms

- Menstrual irregularity with periods of amenorrhea
- Obesity
- Hirsutism
- Infertility
- Acne

*Signs*

- Bilateral enlarged, polycystic ovaries, which are palpable in 50% of patients. The ovaries feel oval, firm, nontender, and freely moveable.
- Slowly progressing hirsutism, which begins after menarche due to increased blood levels of androgen. The amount of excess hair does not correlate with amount of androgen excess.
- Obesity, which occurs in approximately 15% of patients
- Slight clitoral enlargement resulting from increased androgen secretion
- Underdeveloped breasts or uterus (uncommon findings)

## Differential Diagnosis

- Adrenal or ovarian tumors
- Congenital adrenal hyperplasia
- Hypo/hyperthroidism
- Cushings syndrome
- Pituitary or hypothalamic lesions
- Precocious menopause

## Diagnostic Studies as Clinically Indicated

- A careful menstrual history taking and pelvic examination may provide sufficient information for a presumptive diagnosis. According to Yen (1978) the following historical determinants have been associated with PCO:

    Mean age of menarche of 12.3 years

    Postmenarchial menstrual irregularity

    Excessive hair growth noticeable before or around menarche

    The patient is considered "overweight" by peers before menarche
- A bimanual examination may not demonstrate enlarged ovaries.
- Charting a basal body temperature may be helpful in assessing the menstrual pattern. Chronic anovulation is a major characteristic finding in PCO.
- Endometrial biopsy may be indicated to correlate the menstrual cycle with endometrial development.

- Diagnostic laparoscopy or ovarian biopsy may be performed.
- Sonography may be ordered to aid diagnosis.
- Serum LH and FSH assays are done to assess the levels of these hormones. An elevated LH/FSH ratio is significant.

## Management and Treatment as Clinically Indicated

- Physician referral is necessary.
- Medical treatment (An anovulatory workup should precede medical treatment in patients desiring pregnancy).

    Clomiphene citrate (Clomid), is a nonsteroidal anti-estrogenic orally active agent whose primary site of action is the hypothalamus, is given.
    1. The usual dose is 50 mg/day orally for five days, beginning the fifth to eighth day after an induced, or natural, vaginal bleeding period. If ovulation does not occur during the first cycle, the amount of drug is doubled and given daily for five days. If ineffective, the dose may be increased in this manner to a maximum of 200 mg/day for five days. If ovulation occurs, the same effective dose is given for six menstrual cycles.
    2. During Clomid administration, monthly pelvic examinations should be performed to determine if enlarged ovaries result from the use of this medication. The examination should be performed immediately before each course of therapy. A basal body temperature calendar is used to follow the patient's response to the drug.
    3. The patient should be told of possible side effects of Clomid therapy, which include visual disturbances, hot flashes, abdominal discomfort, breast tenderness, and dryness or loss of hair. The medication should be stopped and the physician should be notified if any of these symptoms occur.

    Human chorionic gonadotropin (hCG) may be used in conjunction with Clomid to improve the midcycle LH surge when there is failure to ovulate with a 200 mg Clomid dose, or with a demonstrated short luteal phase. *This treatment is controversial.*

    Human menopausal gonadotropin (hMG) contains gonadotropins extracted from the urine of postmenopausal women. This drug is rarely used since serious side effects may occur.

    For patients not desiring pregnancy the following regimen may be used:
    1. Medroxyprogesterone acetate (Provera), 10 mg/day for five days, may be used to produce periodic sloughing of the endometrium every five to eight weeks OR

2. Oral contraceptives may be used in patients with hirsutism in order to suppress ovarian androgen production.

## Complications

- Ovarian hyperstimulation
- Endometrial hyperplasia, dysplasia, carcinoma
- Breast carcinoma
- Infertility

## Patient Teaching

- Explain the process of the disease to the patient after determining her knowledge of it.
- Review the prescribed treatment with the patient and assess her understanding of how the drug should be taken and her possible compliance.
- Explain to patients desiring pregnancy the need to keep an accurate basal body temperature record to assess the menstrual cycle and ovulation, and explain its use.
- Explain to patients who desire pregnancy and for whom Clomid has been prescribed they have about a 50-70% chance of becoming ovulatory and about a 40% chance of becoming pregnant.

    Explain the side effects of Clomid to the patient.

    Advise the patient to have intercourse every other day for one week beginning five days after taking the last dose of medication.

    Explain the need for monthly pelvic examination to assess ovarian size, and possible conception, before initiating a subsequent treatment cycle.

    Reassure the patient that the risk of congenital defects in pregnancies resulting from Clomid treatment is not increased.

    Explain to patients concerned about multiple births that the incidence of multiple births in patients taking Clomid is approximately 8% and is usually twins. This percentage is now decreasing with standardization of therapy.
- Explain to women scheduled for ovarian wedge resection that successful results are almost always permanent. There is an 80% chance of restoring menses after this procedure, and the pregnancy rate is about 63%.
- Allow time for patients to express their fears and concerns about their disease, its treatment, or possible infertility.
- Express your concern for the infertile patient who desires pregnancy.

## REFERENCES

Anderson B, Watring W, Edinger D, et al: Development of DES-associated clear-cell carcinoma: The importance of regular screening. *Obstet Gynecol* 53:293, 1979.

Barclay D: Diseases of the vulva, in deAlvarez R (ed): *Textbook of Gynecology.* Philadelphia, Lea & Febiger, 1977, p 383.

Green T: *Gynecology, Essentials of Clinical Practice,* ed 2. Boston, Little, Brown and Company, 1971, p 287, 353.

*Guidelines for the Management of DES-Exposed Daughters 1978.* State of California Health and Welfare Agency, Department of Health Services.

Health effects of the pregnancy use of diethylstilbestrol, *Physician Advisory,* Department of HEW, Office of the Assistant Secretary for Health, October 4, 1978.

Herbst A: Ca and exposure to stilbestrol in utero. *Contemp Obstet Gynecol,* 5:19, 1975.

Herbst A, Scully R, Robboy S: Vaginal adenosis and other diethylstilbestrol related abnormalities. *Clin Obstet Gynecol* 18:185, 1975.

Herbst A, Scully R, Stanley J: Diethylstilbestrol-exposed females, in Glass R (ed): *Office Gynecology.* Baltimore, Williams & Wilkins Company, 1976, p 133.

Kern G: *Gynecology.* Chicago, Year Book Medical Publishers, 1976, pp 281, 298, 506.

Kreutner K, Hollingsworth D: *Adolescent Obstetrics and Gynecology.* Chicago, Year Book Medical Publishers, 1978, p 492.

Mattingly R: *Telinde's Operative Gynecology,* ed 5. Philadelphia, JB Lippincott Company, 1977, p 810.

McLennan C: Disorders of the uterine corpus, in Benson R (ed): *Current Obstetric and Gynecologic Diagnosis and Treatment.* Los Altos, Calif, Lange Medical Publications, 1978, p 214.

O'Brien P, Noller K, Robboy S, et al: Vaginal epithelial changes in young women enrolled in the national cooperative diethylstilbestrol adenosis (DESAD) project. *Obstet Gynecol* 53:300, 1979.

Parson L, Sommers S: *Gynecology,* ed 2. Philadelphia, WB Saunders Company, 1978, p 537, 1005.

Spanso W: Preoperative hormonal therapy of cystic adnexal mass. *Am J Obstet Gynecol* 116:4, 1978, p 551.

Speroff L: Anovulation and hirsutism, in deAlvarez R (ed): *Textbook of Gynecology.* Philadelphia, Lea & Febiger, 1977, p 135.

Stewart F, Stewart G, Guest F, et al: *My Body, My Health.* New York, John Wiley & Sons, 1979, p 420.

Yen S, Jaffee R: *Reproductive Endocrinology Physiology, Pathology and Clinical Management.* Philadelphia, WB Saunders Company, 1978, p 306.

# 15

# Pelvic Relaxation

The pelvic organs including the uterus, bladder, and rectum, are supported by the pelvic bones, the endopelvic fascia, and perineal muscles. Normally these structures maintain the proper position of the pelvic organs even during such periods of abdominal stress as lifting or coughing, for example. Pelvic relaxation occurs however, when stress weakens or damages the supporting structure. This results in the organs descending when the muscular or fascial tissue fails to maintain the position of the organs. Relaxation progresses over time and may cause problems years after the initial insult. Common conditions resulting from pelvic relaxation discussed in this chapter are uterine prolapse, urinary stress incontinence, cystocele, and rectocele.

### General Considerations

Stressors in the etiology of pelvic relaxation are:

- The birth process, affected by:
  Birth of a large baby
  Bearing-down efforts of the patient or extraction of the baby before the cervix is fully dilated
  Pressure of a prolonged second stage of labor
  Vaginal stretching and compression of its supporting tissue during labor
- The withdrawal of estrogen support to pelvic tissue during menopause and postmenopause, creating atrophic tissue changes
- The erect human posture, which causes a funneling effect and downward pressure to the pelvic organs. Added intra-abdominal pressure resulting from

conditions such as obesity, chronic respiratory disease, ascites, and abdominal tumors or physiologic functions such as straining at stool, coughing, sneezing, laughing, and running increase the downward thrust to the pelvis.
- The inherent weakness of the endopelvic fascia that supports tissues of the uterus and vagina (viewed as a probable cause for pelvic relaxation in the nulliparous woman.)

## URINARY STRESS INCONTINENCE

### Definition

Stress incontinence is the involuntary loss of urine in women resulting from increased intra-abdominal pressure on damaged pelvic musculature. It is the most common cause of involuntary loss of urine in women, representing 75% of all the cases of urinary incontinence.

### Etiology

Urinary stress incontinence occurs secondary to damage of muscular support to the bladder neck and proximal urethra during childbirth. Involuntary leakage of urine is brought on by coughing, lifting, or running or by similar stresses when the patient is in the upright position. This leakage occurs regardless of the amount of urine present in the bladder. A common occurrence in multiparous women, stress incontinence is not usually seen in nulliparous women. If present, it is usually a result of poor pelvic muscle tone or congenital weakness or innervation to the muscle supports of the bladder. The female bladder and urethra arise from common embryonic tissue; thus, inner and outer muscular layers are identical. The inner muscular layer runs horizontally, while the outer muscular layer forms a circular coat around the organs. Circular plus horizontal muscular support is the basis for the resting pressure of the urethra. With normal muscular support to the bladder neck and urethra, the urethra is maintained as an intra-abdominal structure because pressure within the structure is greater than that within the bladder. Normally when intra-abdominal pressure is increased by coughing or lifting, the stress is distributed equally in the bladder and upper urethra and no involuntary loss of urine occurs. When an alteration of this anatomic relationship between the bladder and urethra occurs as a result of an old obstetric injury, two things may happen: (1) the posterior urethrovesical (PU-V) angle becomes obliterated, causing the upper urethra to become an extension of the bladder with loss of its resting pressure (Fig. 3) and (2) a change in the urethral axis (angle of inclination of the proximal two-thirds of the urethra) causing loss of sphincter control during stress. If no stress occurs, the intraurethral pressure will maintain continence. But a sudden increase in abdominal pressure causes urine leakage from bladder pressure on the weakened urethrovesicular angle and sphincter. These two factors are the most crucial in the etiology of stress incontinence (Fig. 4).

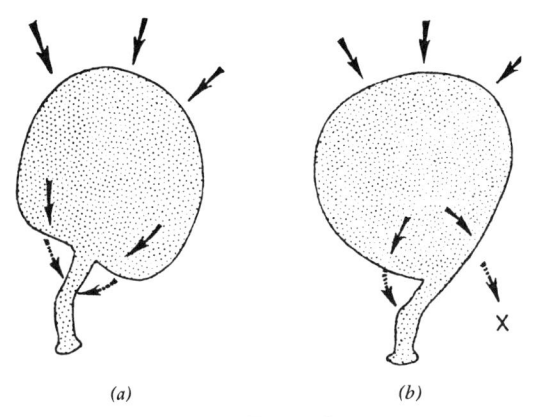

**Figure 3.**
Diagrams illustrating the inherent importance of the posterior urethrovesical (PU-V) angle to the continence mechanism. As shown in A, the presence of a normal PU-V angle permits maximal transmission (indicated by the arrows with dotted bases), on all sides of the proximal urethra, of sudden increases in intra-abdominal pressure. In this way intraurethral pressure is maintained higher than the simultaneously elevated intravesical pressure, which preserves the competency of the vesicle neck sphincter mechanism and prevents loss of urine with the sudden stress. In contrast, as shown in B, loss of the PU-V angle results in displacement of the vesicle neck to the most dependent portion of the bladder, the point of maximum hydrostatic pressure. This anatomic funneling effect also renders impossible the equal transmission of sudden elevations of intra-abdominal pressure to the lumen of the proximal urethra via its walls and their supports. (The arrow with a dotted base at X serves to indicate the impossibility of any effective transmission of pressure to the posterior aspect of the proximal urethra as well as the tendency for the "internal urinary meatus" at the level of the vesicle neck to be forced open.) Intravesical pressure in the region of the vesicle thus rises considerably more than intraurethral pressure just beyond it, and stress incontinence occurs. (From Urinary stress incontinence by TH Green in *Obstet Gynecol Survey,* copyright 1968 by The William & Wilkins Co., Baltimore. Reprinted by permission of the author and publisher.)

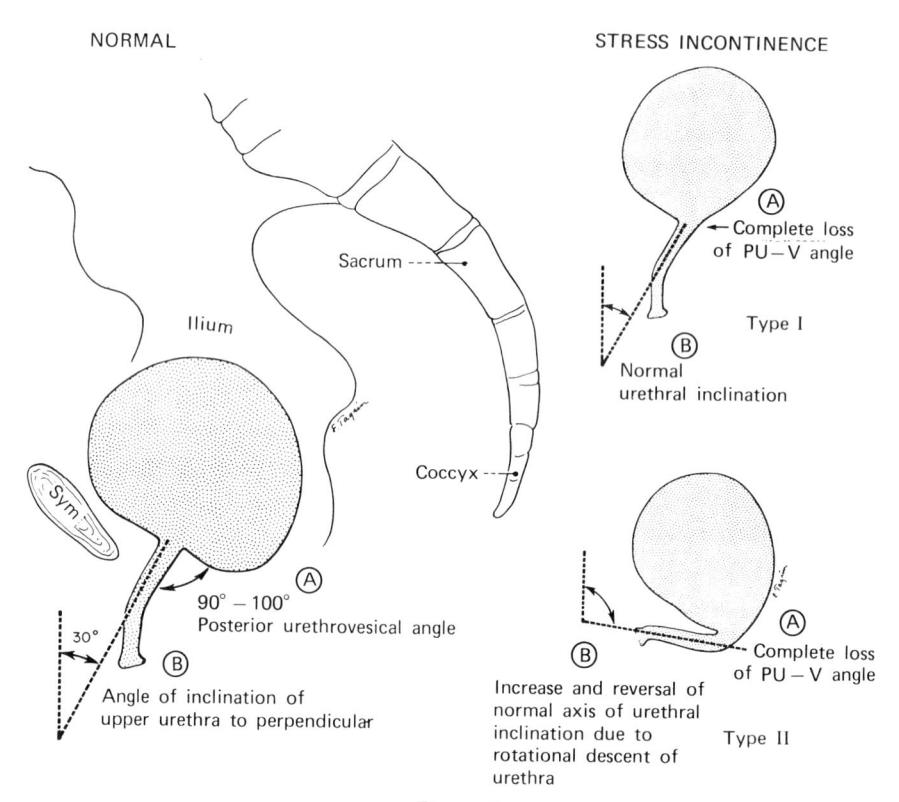

**Figure 4.**
The two basic types of anatomic configuration encountered in patients with stress incontinence as revealed by the lateral standing-straining view of the urethrocystogram. In both type I and type II, the posterior urethrovesical (PU-V) angle is lost, but in Type II there is, in addition, an increase in the angle of inclination of the urethral axis, the latter varying from 45° to 120°, depending on the amount of rotational descent of the urethra. The typical lateral straining urethrocystogram found in continent women with normal support is shown for comparison. (From *Gynecology Essentials of Clinical Practice,* ed 2 by TH Green Jr. Copyright 1971 by Little, Brown & Company, Boston. Used with permission of the publisher and author.)

To clarify diagnosis, Green (1975) has classified two types of stress incontinence:

- Type I includes patients in whom the anatomic defect causes complete or nearly complete loss of the PU-V angle.
- Type II includes patients who, in addition to the above, have a backward and downward rotational descent of the bladder and urethra. The angle of inclination to the vertical of the urethral axis is greater than 45° (Fig. 4).

Patients with type II stress incontinence experience the most severe symptoms, are difficult to treat, and tend to have higher rates of surgical repair failure.

## Clinical Features

### Symptoms

- Involuntary urine loss
- Sudden urgency
- Frequency, nocturia
- Emotional and social stress

### Signs

- Multiparity (stress incontinence is rare in nulliparous patients)
- Atrophic pelvic changes in aging women
- Lack of pain
- Leakage of urine in spurts
- Leakage occurring simultaneously with stress
- Leakage occurring only in the upright position
- Cystocele usually absent
- Urethral meatus pointing upward when the patient is in the lithotomy position

## Differential Diagnosis

No one factor is responsible for urinary incontinence. The physiologic mechanisms are poorly understood. Causes of incontinence may include physiologic problems, emotional disturbances, or systemic disabilities. Definitive diagnosis is difficult because of possible overlapping symptoms in patients who have multiple problems. Green (1977) has identified five causes of urinary incontinence, in addition to true stress incontinence, involving loss of urine:

- Pure urgency incontinence (atrophic vaginitis, trigonitis, urethritis, cystitis, trichomoniasis, moniliasis)
- Bladder neuropathies (diabetes, syphilis, multiple sclerosis, neurologic disorders, or injuries causing overflow incontinence)
- Congenital and acquired urinary tract anomalies (ectopic ureter, urethral diverticulum, urethra less than 2.0 cm, urethral and bladder fistulas)

- Psychogenic incontinence (unconscious, involuntary loss of urine, which occurs rarely)
- Detrusor dyssynergia (involuntary detrusor activity causing incontinence 10-20 seconds after stress). *This is the second most common cause (after stress incontinence) of urinary incontinence in women.*

## Diagnostic Studies as Clinically Indicated

Diagnostic studies must be carefully carried out to prove the presence of true stress incontinence and to rule out other causes of abnormal urine leakage. Inappropriate management of incontinence may cause the patient unnecessary surgery and may make her symptoms worse.

- A complete medical and psychosocial history should be taken. Special emphasis should be placed on the history of the voiding pattern. Information necessary to obtain in differentiating true stress incontinence from detrusor dyssynegia includes:

| *True Stress Incontinence* | *Detrusor Dyssnergia* |
|---|---|
| Leakage of urine | Voids rather than leaks |
| Small amounts of urine lost | Large amounts of urine lost |
| Leakage occurs simultaneously with stress | Voids 10-20 seconds after stress |
| Leakage only occurs in upright position | Loss of urine occurs in any position or change of position |
| Nocturia | Nocturia absent |
| Voiding can be stopped voluntarily | Voiding cannot be stopped voluntarily |

- Complete physical examination, including a neurologic examination and careful evaluation of pelvic floor relaxation, should be done.
- Consultation and/or referral to a physician should be done before diagnostic studies are ordered.
- Wet smear
- Urinalysis and culture
- Catheterization post voiding to measure the amount of residual urine
- Cystoscopy
- Intravenous pyelogram
- Urethroscopy

- Cystometrogram

(*Note:* The above studies are all normal in patients with true stress incontinence.)
- Vesicle neck elevation test
- Chain urethrocystogram

## Management and Treatment as Clinically Indicated

- Medical management is indicated for the patient with mild stress incontinence or who is unwilling or physically unable to have surgery. Although less effective, these methods may be beneficial to the patient in maintaining some degree of continence.

    Estrogen cream for atrophic vaginal changes in the postmenopausal woman (for specific creams see the section on atropic vaginitis)

    Kegel's exercises: If these pelvic muscle toning exercises are performed correctly and consistently, they will help strengthen the pubococcygeus muscle and restore some urinary control.
- Surgical management is most effective for true stress incontinence. Surgical repair elevates the urethrovesical junction above the lowest level of the bladder base at the time of stress. Factors that determine the type of surgery performed include (1) the degree of patient disability, (2) the physical condition of the patient and the condition of her pelvic tissue, and (3) the type of incontinence she is experiencing.

    The physician selects the method of surgery based on the specific type of urethrovesical anatomic abnormality. There are a number of procedures but most involve repair by a vaginal approach with an anterior colporrhaphy or by a suprapubic approach with a urethrovesical suspension.

    The immediate and long-term surgical outcome for the patient depends on (1) the condition of the tissues, (2) the type of anatomic abnormality being corrected, (3) the choice of surgical procedure, and (4) the skill of the surgeon. Depending on these factors, the cure rates may be as low as 3% and as high as 97%.

## Complications

- Vulvar dermatitis
- Psychologic and social stress

- Surgical complications or failure to maintain long-term continence

## Patient Teaching

- Help the patient to understand the anatomic abnormality that causes the incontinence and why the incontinence has occurred.
- Ascertain how well the patient is able to cope with the psychologic stress and physical discomfort that results from sporadic urine leakage.
- Discuss ways that symptoms can be minimized. Suggest that she:

    Urinate frequently and whenever the urge is felt to avoid an overdistended bladder

    Empty the bladder as completely as possible at each urination

    Perform Kegel's exercises faithfully and regularly. If done while urinating, the exercises not only strengthen the muscles but assure the patient she is doing them correctly by her ability to decrease or stop the urinary stream (Fig. 5).

    Keep the vulva as clean and dry as possible. Use of a sanitary napkin or mini pad to absorb the urine will help prevent embarrassment if leakage is excessive. Frequent change of pad is necessary to prevent odor.

- Explain the use of estrogen cream prescribed for the patient with atrophic changes. Warn that the cream should be used only as directed, and that if vaginal bleeding occurs to seek immediate attention.
- Assess the patient who has been identified for surgical repair by determining:

    What she has been told about her anticipated surgery and how well she understands what is involved

    How she feels about having surgery performed and if she needs someone to talk to about it

    Whether she has a support system to care for her during the postoperative period and if not, what the alternatives are for her care

    Her nutritional status. Encouraging and helping her to determine her nutritional needs before surgery may help optimize her recovery. Is the patient obese? The need for weight loss should be stressed. The success of a surgical repair is significantly decreased in patients with excessive fatty tissue.

    How much she smokes and if she has a chronic cough as a result. Encouragement needs to be given to reduce or discontinue the use of cigarettes. The pressure on the pelvic organs resulting from chronic cough is extreme and may compromise a surgical repair and affect the long-term success rate.

# UTERINE PROLAPSE (DECENSUS)

## Definition

Uterine prolapse is the descent of the uterus through the pelvic floor.

## Etiology

Etiologic factors include (1) obstetric trauma to the levator ani muscles and pelvic ligaments, (2) effects of aging with atrophic changes of the pelvic tissue, and (3) the erect posture with its downward gravitational pull. Signs and symptoms of uterine prolapse develop slowly. They are not usually evident until the middle years, the peak incidence occurring at age 50. In the United States, obese, white, multiparous women are most often affected. It occurs rarely in black women. Uterine prolapse is seen in three degrees of descensus (1) the cervix has descended halfway into the vagina, (2) the cervix has descended to the introitus, and (3) the entire uterus protrudes through the introitus with inversion of the vaginal canal (procidentia).

## Clinical Features

### Symptoms

- Awareness by the patient of the "womb dropping," causing heaviness and a bearing-down sensation in the lower abdomen
- Low backache, which results from pressure of the relaxed organs on posterior pelvic structures (a common complaint)
- Urinary tract symptoms, such as frequency, incontinence, or need of the patient to push the bladder up through the anterior vagina wall in order to void
- Dyspareunia, due to a shortened vaginal canal as the uterus descends. During sexual intercourse the penis forcefully strikes the descended cervix causing pain.
- Discomfort with walking or sitting when the uterus protrudes through the introitus in procidentia

*Signs*

- The vaginal outlet appears relaxed and gaping.
- The cervix or uterus is visible at the introitus.
- The cervix is palpable in the vagina.
- A cystocele and rectocele are usually visible.
- Edema of the vagina results from pressure of the descending uterus and causes vascular congestion.
- In procidentia the vaginal epithelium is thick, smooth, and dry, resulting from exposure of the tissue to the air. Chronic ulcers occur on the cervix and may bleed.
- Cervical protrusion usually recedes when the patient is lying down but will descend with bearing-down efforts.

## Differential Diagnosis

- Cervical hypertrophy
- Pelvic or abdominal tumors

## Diagnostic Studies as Clinically Indicated

Diagnosis is made clinically by:

- Inspection of the vulva and vagina
- Palpation of the uterus descending into the vagina when the patient bears down
- Palpation of a perineal hernia (Outline the uterus in order to rule out diagnosis of a hypertrophied cervix.)
- Traction from a tenaculum placed on the cervix brings the uterus down when the patient is in a lying or standing position

## Management and Treatment as Clinically Indicated

Management is influenced by the patient's desire for fertility, her age, the severity of symptoms, and the degree of prolapse.

- All patients should be referred to a physician who will determine the mode of treatment.

- Nonsurgical measures

    For patients desiring pregnancy who demonstrate a first- or second-degree prolapse with minimal symptoms, no treatment is indicated. Yearly follow-up should be encouraged.

    Use of pessaries for uterine prolapse is infrequent but may be selected as a temporary measure in symptomatic patients desiring pregnancy, or as long-term therapy for elderly patients in whom surgery is contraindicated. A pessary is a hard rubber or plastic ring used to maintain the normal position of the uterus in the pelvis. If it fails to do this, it is an inappropriate form of therapy. *Placement of a pessary.* While there are many types of pessaries, the one used most often is the Smith-Hodge. The uterus is first pushed into position by bimanual manipulation. The Smith-Hodge pessary is inserted into the vagina and placed so that the ring fits behind the pubic arch in the front and against the posterior fornix and uterosacral ligaments in the back. In this position it supports the vagina and acts as a cradle for the cervix. It should not cause discomfort nor interfere with sexual intercourse. It must be removed, cleaned, and replaced every two to three months because it can irritate or erode the vaginal epithelium, increase leukorrhea, and predispose to infection.

    Estrogen therapy: Local estrogen therapy is indicated only in the postmenopausal woman.

- Surgical measures: Before surgical repair can be considered, the following factors need to be assessed:

    The age and general health of the patient

    Desire of the patient to preserve fertility

    Degree of uterine prolapse

    Condition of the uterus and cervix

    The presence and degree of cystocele, rectocele, or enterocele

    Many surgical procedures are available to the surgeon for repair of pelvic relaxation. The most commonly used are:

    1. Vaginal hysterectomy with anterior and posterior colporrhaphies
    2. Manchester-Fothergill operation, which consists of anterior and posterior colporrhaphies with amputation of the cervix. It is usually performed in older patients who are at surgical risk for prolonged surgery or in the markedly symptomatic younger woman.
    3. Le Fort operation, which involves partial closure of the vagina. It is used as a last resort in elderly patients when nonsurgical methods have not proved efficacious.

## Patient Teaching

- Question the patient about her knowledge and understanding of the pelvic relaxation process and her particular diagnosis. Use diagrams and pictures to demonstrate anatomic changes.
- Advise the patient who has first- or second-degree prolapse who desires pregnancy to maintain a regular follow-up schedule of appointments for assessment of change in uterine position. Suggest she avoid straining at stool or running because these produce increased intra-abdominal pressure and additional stress to pelvic organs.
- Advise the patient who wears a pessary that its use does not cure the problem but may keep it from getting worse.

    Stress the importance of regular two- to three-month visits for removal, cleaning, and replacement of the pessary. Some women may learn to do this themselves, but for many it is too difficult.

    Review with the patient the symptoms that may occur from pessary use, which may include:
    1. Leukorrhea from vaginal irritation or possible infection
    2. Loss of the pessary because it is too small
    3. Urinary retention, which may occur when the device is too large. Pressure on the bladder and urethra from the device may necessitate immediate removal and replacement.

# CYSTOCELE

## Definition

A cystocele is a prolapse of the posterior bladder wall through a defect in the upper anterior vaginal wall usually resulting from trauma of childbirth.

## Etiology

Laceration of supporting fascial tissue may occur during the birth of a large baby, multiple births, or prolonged labor. Cystoceles may range in size from small, causing minor symptoms, to large, causing discomfort and urinary symptoms. Usually found in conjunction with other signs of generalized pelvic relaxation, their size and consequent symptoms increase with time and usually become problematic pre- or postmenopausally.

## Clinical Features

### Symptoms

- A bearing-down sensation in the pelvis, which may be aggravated by vigorous activity
- Urinary frequency, urgency, tenesmus, and occasionally incontinence
- Low backache, resulting from general relaxation of the pelvic organs and vasocongestion
- Difficulty in completely emptying the bladder. The patient may use her finger to apply pressure to the bulging anterior vagina to complete voiding.

### Signs

- Relief of urinary symptoms during the night when the patient is in the recumbent position
- A relaxed vaginal outlet with visible bulging of the anterior vaginal wall. If bulging is not obvious when the patient is lying flat, it will become visible as the patient bears down or coughs.
- Uterine prolapse in conjunction with a cystocele may occur.
- Symptoms increase in amount and severity over time.

## Differential Diagnosis

- Gartner duct cyst
- Urethrocele
- Urethral diverticulum
- Enterocele

## Diagnostic Studies as Clinically Indicated

- Clinical observation reveals bulging of the anterior vaginal wall.
- Palpation reveals a thin-walled, smooth mass bulging from the anterior vaginal wall.

- Catheterization of the patient after voiding is done to collect and measure residual urine.
- A urinalysis and urine culture are done to rule out urinary tract infection.
- Cystoscopic examination is performed for visualization of abnormal tissue or masses within the bladder.

## Management and Treatment as Clinically Indicated

- Nonsurgical Measures

    Kegal's exercises are prescribed to promote strengthening of the muscles of the pelvic floor for added support (see Fig. 5).

    Double voiding: The patient should repeat voiding two to three minutes after the first voiding to help empty the bladder of residual urine.

    Oral estrogen treatment in selected postmenopausal women is given to improve the tone and vascularity of the supporting tissue. Diethylstilbestrol, 0.25 mg/day orally, may be used.

    Local estrogen therapy with Premarin or Dienestrol cream, 1 applicatorful intravaginally at bedtime for one to two weeks may be given for relief of atrophic vaginitis symptoms. For maintenance, the dose is decreased to two to three times a week.

    As a temporary measure the use of a pessary is especially helpful in a postpartum patient with a retroverted uterus in conjunction with a cystocele. It can be used to maintain vaginal support until involution is complete. Its use is also helpful in older symptomatic patients in whom surgery is contraindicated, but who demonstrate adequate muscle tone to support its use.

- Surgical measures: Surgical repair should be appropriate for the patient's basic pelvic relaxation problem. A single procedure for cystocele repair is not usually indicated since further pelvic relaxation may occur and require additional surgery.

    A small or moderate-sized cystocele may not require immediate repair, especially in young women desiring children. Unless the patient is experiencing recurrent urinary tract infections or rapid enlargement of the cystocele with distressing symptoms, treatment should be postponed until childbearing is complete. Labor and birth, after a surgical repair, stretches or tears the pelvic tissue causing break down of the repair.

    For symptomatic patients who have completed childbearing the most common surgical procedure used to correct general pelvic relaxation is an anterior vaginal colporrhaphy in conjunction with vaginal hysterectomy and posterior colpoperineorrhaphy.

## Complications

- Chronic or recurrent cystitis
- Acute urinary retention

## Patient Teaching

- Determine what the patient knows about her problem and its treatment and supplement information as necessary. Allow her time to express her fears and concerns.
- Reassure the patient who requires no immediate treatment that her symptoms, although annoying, are not the result of a serious illness.
- Inform the patient that, in time, her symptoms may increase and surgical repair may be indicated in the future.
- Discuss the use of Kegal's exercises to help maintain the tone of her pelvic muscles (see Fig. 5).
- Discuss the use of a pessary in appropriate patients (see the section on management and treatment of uterine prolapse)
- Discuss estrogen use and its side effects when prescribed for patients. Explain that, although estrogen cannot correct the problem, it may help to increase the tone of the pelvic tissues. Advise patients to call immediately if vaginal bleeding occurs (See the section on management and treatment of menopause in Chapter 16 for information on the use of estrogen.)

# RECTOCELE

## Definition

A rectocele is a prominent bulging of the posterior vaginal wall as a result of trauma to the fascia and levator ani muscles which support a portion of the lower bowel.

## Etiology

A rectocele occurs only after previous injury to the perineum, particularly a traumatic childbirth. During labor the descent of the baby's head stretches or tears the fascia and muscles of the pelvic floor causing weakening of the rectovaginal septum. Complete tearing of the sphincter ani muscles and perineal body may occur during delivery leaving only a weak layer of perineal connective tissue. The rectocele develops slowly and activities such as straining at stool, heavy lifting, or pregnancy increases weakening of the perineal supports. Symptoms become most troublesome after menopause. Rectocele is usually found in conjunction with a cystocele, a grade I or II uterine prolapse, and perineal laceration.

## Clinical Features

### Symptoms

- Difficult defecation with the patient using a finger to apply downward pressure on the posterior vaginal bulge while bearing down to aid complete defacation
- Constipation or rectal fullness, due to interruption of the normal defecation process
- Hemorrhoids, resulting from increased pressure on the blood vessels of the rectum
- Sensation of fullness and pressure in the vagina, resulting from bulging of the posterior vaginal wall

### Signs

- A healed laceration of the perineal body
- Bulging of the posterior vaginal wall
- A thin-walled rectovaginal septum

## Differential Diagnosis

- Enterocele
- Tumors of the rectovaginal septum

## Diagnostic Studies as Clinically Indicated

- Diagnosis is made clinically by:
    Inspection of the posterior vaginal wall, which will show the amount of bulging present without added stress
    Palpation for a rectocele performed with the examiner's index finger placed in the vagina and the middle finger placed in the rectum while the patient is bearing down. A bulging upward from the rectum to the vagina is felt over the area of the rectal sphincter.
- Proctoscopic examination is performed to rule out colonic lesions.

## Management and Treatment as Clinically Indicated

- Referral to a physician is necessary.
- Nonsurgical measures
    Rectocles that are small may need no treatment.
    Fecal impactions require digital extraction.
    Kegel's exercises performed regularly may help strengthen pelvic muscular support.
    Diet counseling is needed to encourage increased intake of fluids and bulk foods to help reduce constipation. Regular bowel habits should be encouraged.
    Stool softeners or laxatives for patients with chronic constipation may be needed until regular bowel habits are established.
- Surgical Measures
    Posterior colpoperineorrhaphy may be done when the rectocele interferes with normal evacuation of the stool.
    Vaginal hysterectomy with posterior wall repair is performed when general pelvic relaxation is present in conjunction with involvment of other organs.

## Complications

- Chronic constipation
- Psychologic problems

## Patient Teaching

- Question the patient about her knowledge and understanding of her problem and its treatment. Supplement information as needed, and answer her questions.
- Be sensitive to the patient's concerns, and allow her time to express them.
- Discuss the use and benefits of performing Kegal's exercise regularly (see Fig. 5).
- Stress the importance of avoiding activities that place heavy strain on the perineal supports such as heavy lifting, straining at stool, or running.
- Explain to patients desiring pregnancy that surgical repair usually is not done until childbearing is completed. The trauma of childbirth could cause breakdown of surgically repaired tissue.
- Reassure patients anticipating surgical repair of a rectocele that it is most often curative.

**Figure 5.**

All about "Kegel's" for women.

These exercises were originally developed by Dr. Arnold Kegel (Kay-gill) to help women with problems controlling urination. They are designed to strengthen and give you voluntary control of a muscle called pubococcygeus (pew-bo-kak-se-gee-us), or P.C. for short. The P.C. muscle is part of the sling of muscle stretching from your pubic bone in front to your tail bone in back. Since the muscle encircles not only the urinary opening but also the outside of the vagina, some of Dr. Kegel's patients found that doing the exercises had a pleasant side effect—increased sexual awareness.

### Why Do Kegel Exercises?

Learning Kegel exercises

- can help you be more aware of feelings in your genital area;
- can increase circulation in the genital area;
- may help increase sexual arousal started by other kind(s) of stimulation;
- can be helpful after childbirth to restore muscle tone in the vagina.

**Figure 5.** *(Continued)*

### Identifying the P.C. Muscle

Sit on the toilet. Spread your legs apart. See if you can stop and start the flow of urine without moving your legs. That's your P.C. muscle, the one that turns the flow on and off. If you don't find it the first time, don't give up; try again the next time you have to urinate.

### The Exercises

Slow Kegels:
 Tighten the P.C. muscle as you did to stop the urine.
 Hold it for a slow count of three. Relax it.
Quick Kegels:
 Tighten and relax the P.C. muscle as rapidly as you can.
Pull in-Push out:
 Pull up the entire pelvic floor as though trying to suck water into your vagina. Then push out or bear down as if trying to push the imaginary water out. (This exercise will use a number of "stomach" or "abdominal" muscles as well as the P.C. muscle.)

At first do ten of each of these exercises (one "set") five times every day. Each week increase the number of times you do each exercise by five (15, 20, 25, etc.). Keep doing five "sets" each day.

- You can do these exercises any time during daily activities which don't require a lot of moving around: driving your car, watching television, doing dishes, sitting in school or at your desk or lying in bed.
- When you start you will probably notice that the muscle doesn't want to stay "contracted" during "Slow Kegels" and that you can't do "Quick Kegels" very fast or evenly. Keep at it. In a week or two you will probably notice that you can control it quite well.
- Sometimes the muscle will start to feel a little tired. Not surprising. You probably haven't used it very much before. Take a few seconds rest and start again.
- A good way to check on how you are doing is to insert one or two lubricated fingers into your vagina.
- Remember to keep breathing naturally and evenly while you are doing your Kegel's!

(Reprinted with permission from Human Sexuality Program, University of California-San Francisco School of Medicine.)

## REFERENCES

Green T: *Gynecology Essentials of Clinical Practice* ed 2. Boston, Little, Brown and Company, 1971, p 407.

Green T: Urinary stress incontinence: differential diagnosis. *Am J Obstet Gynecol* 122:368, 1975.

Hodgkinson C: Urinary incontinence in the female, in Caplan R, Sweeney W (ed): *Advances in Obstetrics and Gynecology*. Baltimore, Williams & Wilkins Company, 1978, p 519.

Marchant D: Urinary incontinence, in deAlvarez R (ed): *Textbook of Gynecology*. Philadelphia, Lea & Febiger, 1977, p 443.

Mattingly R: *TeLinde's Operative Gynecology* ed 2. Philadelphia, JB Lippincott Company, 1977, p 493, 599.

Nichols D: Effects of pelvic relaxation on gynecologic urologic problems. *Clin Obstet Gynecol* 21:759, 1978.

Novak E, Jones G, Jones H: *Novak's Textbook of Gynecology,* ed 8. Baltimore, Williams & Wilkins Company, 1970, p 268.

Parsons L, Sommers S: *Gynecology* ed 2. Philadelphia, WB Saunders Company, 1978, p 1451.

Slate W: Parturitional injuries and alterations of pelvic support, in deAlvarez R (ed): *Textbook of Gynecology*. Philadelphia, Lea & Febiger, 1977, p 491.

Symmonds R: Relaxations of pelvic supports, in Benson R (ed): *Current Obstetrics and Gynecologic Diagnosis and Treatment*. Los Altos, Calif, Lange Medical Publications, 1978, p 239.

Ulfelder H: Disorders of pelvic supporting structures, in Romney R, Gray J, Little A, et al (eds): *Gynecology and Obstetrics the Health Care of Women*. New York, McGraw-Hill Book Company, 1975, p 900.

# 16

# Problems During Menopause

*The climacteric* is the term used to describe the period of approximately 15 years during which a woman's body and mind are preparing for the cessation of menses. Climacteric means "rung of the ladder," clearly indicating a developmental stage in the life cycle of women. Also called menopause, it is a milestone in the progression of many physical and emotional events that occur during the transitional years from middle age to old age—the change of life.

The life span of women has increased by 25 years since the beginning of the century, so we are seeing more women in the climacteric years. Menopausal symptoms have for many years received a wide variety of interpretations, most of them "old wive's tales." Although defined by many physicians as an estrogen-deficiency disease, menopause is, in fact, a normal developmental life process.

The average age of women experiencing menopause is increasing and is now reported to be between 50 and 52 years. Factors contributing to this pattern of later onset stem from better nutrition, planning for parenthood, less hard physical labor, and better health care. Heredity also plays an important role in this event, with women following the pattern of their mothers. There is no relationship between the weight of the patient and the onset of menopause; just as there is no relation between the age of menarche and the age when menstruation ceases.

The menopausal years are years of change. Women undergo physiologic changes with accompanying symptoms and changes in physical appearance. They may also experience stress related to separation from children or older parents and readjustment of their marriage or life-style. Psychologic stress may also occur from feelings of lost femininity, loss of youthful attractiveness, loss of childbearing ability, and for some, a "loss of purpose" in their lives.

Research has centered on the changing physiologic processes that occur during menopause. This information has been invaluable to our understanding of changing body function and its relationship to aging. But we do not yet know enough about the cultural, social, and psychologic impacts of menopause and how women respond to this oftentimes stressful period.

# MENOPAUSE

## Definition

Menopause is the cessation of menses and is considered complete when no menstrual bleeding has occurred for one year. Artificial menopause is the abrupt termination of ovarian function by surgical removal, irradiation, or radium therapy. Premature menopause is cessation of ovarian function before the age of 40 years and occurs in 10% of the female population.

## Etiology

On a continuum, from perimenopause to late menopause, women go through three physiologic stages, (1) decreased fertility, (2) menopause, and (3) progressive tissue atrophy and aging. As early as the mid-30s, the frequency of ovulation begins to decrease. The graafian follicles of the ovary—responsible for estrogen secretion—become gradually depleted and are less sensitive to gonadotropin hormone (FSH and LH) stimulation. Estrogen production decreases and irregular menstruation results, one of the earliest signs of approaching menopause. Complete cessation of menstrual periods occurs when the ovarian function of estrogen secretion has ceased.

During postmenopause, low levels of estrogen are produced in peripheral body fat from adrenal and ovarian androgen precursors. The extent to which this androgen-estrogen conversion takes place is proportional to the age and total body weight of the woman and accounts for the majority of estrogen (estrone) produced. In women who experience postmenopausal bleeding, or in those who develop endometrial cancer, the amount of estrone produced by peripheral conversion is greater than in women who do not experience these problems.

Menopause and the aging process interrelate. With decreasing ovarian function, and consequent loss of estrogen, all systems of the body are affected and changed. The change in adrenal secretion of androgens from an anabolic process to a catabolic process is manifested by a wide variety of physical and psychologic effects. The most common are listed below.

- Genital tract changes resulting from ovarian failure include:
    Atrophy of estrogen target organs
    1. Shrinking of the ovaries with disappearance of the ova and graafian follicles
    2. Reduction in size of the labia majora, with loss of cutaneous fat and disappearance of the labia minora
    3. Loss of elasticity of vulvar tissue, with pubic hair becoming coarse and brittle
    4. Shrinking of the clitoris and tissue of the urethra
    5. Thinning and dryness of the vaginal epithelium
    6. Shrinking of the uterus and cervix (Leiomyoma do not disappear, but become smaller.)
    7. Atrophy of the endometrium (It is still able to respond to estrogen stimulation by bleeding.)
    8. Relaxation of muscles and ligaments of the pelvic organs and floor
- General body changes resulting from ovarian failure include:
    Atrophy and drooping of the breasts from replacement of adipose tissue by connective tissue
    Hair growth of the upper lip, chin, and overstimulation of sebaceous glands in the skin of the nose and face (These changes occur from increased androgen sensitivity)
    Increased skin pigmentation or depigmentation—poikiloderma of Civatte (Low estrogen levels cause disturbed melanocyte stimulation from the pituitary and adrenals.)
    Loss of adipose tissue causing the skin to become loose and flabby
    A tendency to become obese
    Changes in body contour with fat deposited on the back, abdomen, buttocks, and hips, with less fat deposited elsewhere
    An increased incidence of hypertension, hypothyroidism, diabetes, and osteoporosis in late menopause
- Psychogenic disturbances: These symptoms may not be directly related to ovarian failure but may result from:
    Prior psychologic problems
    Belief in "old wives tales"
    The role model of the mother

Current cultural or social stresses

Change in family structure (children gone, husband busy)

Real or imagined inadequacies

Change in body image

The constitutional make-up of the individual, inherited familial characteristics, culture, associated disease, and the psychologic effects of aging all have an impact on how the woman responds to myriad changes occurring during this period.

## Clinical Features

### Symptoms

Symptoms of estrogen withdrawal begin early in the climacteric and may produce problems of varying severity keyed to the rate of estrogen withdrawal. With rapid estrogen withdrawal, symptoms are usually more severe than with gradual hormone decline. Approximately 65% of menopausal women experience some symptoms, and 20% of these seek medical care.

- Vasomotor symptoms: The etiology of hot flashes (flushes) and sweats is not known but is related to decreased estrogen production, which causes instability between the hypothalamus and the autonomic nervous system. This symptom begins with a sensation of heat over the chest which moves to the neck and face. Flushing of the face may be visible. The number of hot flushes may vary from an occasional warm flush, to as many as 10-15 severe flushes daily with extreme sweating and chilling. The severity of the symptom provides a rough index to the degree of estrogen depletion.
- Atrophic vaginitis and urinary symptoms: Symptoms develop after general atrophy of genitourinary tissue. Vaginal dryness and infection, vulvar pruritus, dyspareunia, urinary frequency, and dysuria may be experienced (see the section on atrophic vaginitis in Chap 9).

The following symptoms relate to, or are coincident with, estrogen depletion of menopause, changes in the central nervous system, psychologic adjustment to the aging process, or to some combination of these factors.

- Back pain from osteoporosis (see the section on osteoporosis)
- Fatigue from metabolic disturbances, decreased thyroid function, decreased basal metabolic rate, increased blood cholesterol, or depression
- Weight gain from decreased physical activity, increased food intake, or decreased thyroid function

- Headache due to allergies, sinus infections, hypertension, or emotional tension
- Psychologic symptoms from social and emotional stresses that occur at this time of life (nervousness, insomnia, forgetfulness, irritability, depression, chronic tiredness, anxiety, and aggravation of prior psychologic problems
- Increased or decreased libido and sexual activity

*Signs*

- Changes in the menstrual cycle during the preimenopausal period
- Genital tract and general body changes resulting from ovarian failure (see p. 325).

## Differential Diagnosis

- Abnormal vaginal bleeding from other causes
- Pregnancy
- Endometrial carcinoma
- Psychologic problems
- Thyroid abnormalities
- Pituitary lesion
- "Post-Pill syndrome"

## Diagnostic Studies as Clinically Indicated

- A thorough medical history should be taken, and physical examination, including a breast and pelvic examination, needs to be done. A presumptive clinical diagnosis may be made. Depending on the patient's symptoms, further studies may be necessary.
- A Pap smear is indicated. A maturation index (MI) may also be done at this time (see Chap 17).
- Blood studies may include: A CBC, $SMA_{12}$, triglyceride determinations, $T_3$ and $T_4$ assays, and serum gonadotropin level measurements. (FSH levels may be increased to 15-fold, and LH levels may be increased five-fold in menopause.)
- Endometrial sampling before initiation of estrogen therapy is controversial at this time.
- Endometrial biopsy is indicated when abnormal uterine bleeding is present. OR

- A diagnostic D&C may be done for irregular bleeding to rule out malignant changes. This procedure may restore a more normal pattern of menses to some perimenopausal women.
- A progesterone withdrawal test may restore a more normal bleeding pattern after an endometrial biopsy has ruled out malignancy.
- A mammography in women over 50 years may be done to obtain baseline data for comparison in future breast studies.

A glucose tolerance test is indicated in women with a family history of diabetes or history of gestational diabetes.

## Management and Treatment as Clinically Indicated

Treatment of the menopausal patient is difficult. No definitive data exist on the risk-benefit rates of treatment for this group of women.

- Estrogen replacement therapy (ERT): There are currently two schools of thought on estrogen therapy. One school feels that treatment is only necessary when symptoms are severe; and the lowest possible dose of hormone should be given for the shortest possible time in order to minimize possibility of endometrial carcinoma. The second school favors long-term estrogen treatment maintained at the lowest dose to effectively control symptoms of estrogen deprivation.

    Although estrogen therapy for treatment of menopausal symptoms is controversial, its use in selected, *symptomatic* patients is warranted under certain circumstances. These are (1) when serum estrogen levels are low, (2) when no contraindication for its use exists, and (3) when the patient has been fully informed about possible side effects and complications and consents to its use.

    *Contraindications to estrogen use:* The Federal Drug Administration lists the following contraindications to estrogen therapy:

    1. When there is known or suspected cancer of the breast, except in appropriately selected patients under treatment for metastatic disease
    2. When there is known or suspected estrogen-dependent neoplasia
    3. When there is known or suspected pregnancy
    4. When undiagnosed, abnormal bleeding exists
    5. When active thrombophlebitis or thromboembolic disorders exist
    6. When there is a past history of thrombophlebitis, thrombosis, or thromboembolic disorders associated with previous estrogen use

Additional contraindications include:
1. Active liver disease
2. Porphyria (an inherited metabolic disease that occurs more commonly in women—abdominal pain is the primary symptom)
3. Malignant melanoma
4. Leiomyomata of the uterus
5. Migraine headache

Other considerations
1. Use of parenteral or subcutaneous pellets of estrogen probably should not be used. If complications arise, immediate withdrawal of the drug is not an option.
2. Oral contraceptive pills should not be used for menopausal symptoms since their dose is excessive and unnecessary.

Indications for estrogen therapy include:
1. Premenopausal surgical removal of the ovaries
2. Severe vasomotor symptoms
3. Atrophic changes of genitourinary tissue
4. Beginning signs of osteoporosis

For these conditions, estrogen should be given in the lowest dose, and for the shortest duration of time that offers symptom relief. It should be given cyclically with added progestin to prevent unopposed estrogen stimulation to the endometrium, which increases the risk of endometrial carcinoma. The dose of estrogen should be sufficient to alleviate symptoms yet not cause excessive uterine bleeding.

Ideally, before estrogen replacement therapy is started, endometrial biopsy should be performed to assess its estrogen effect, and to rule out malignancy. This procedure is repeated every 6-12 months throughout the treatment period. This regimen is recommended but is not a common practice.

For women with no contraindications, the following estrogen preparations are available:
1. Premarin is given on a cyclic basis, either three weeks on and one week off or from the first through the twenty-fourth day of each month. For the last seven days of estrogen treatment, a daily 10-mg dose of medroxyprogesterone acetate (Provera) is added. Premarin, a conjugated estrogen, is supplied in tablets of 0.3, 0.625, 1.25, and 2.5 mg. For early menopausal symptoms, where considerable endogenous estrogen is still present, the 0.625-mg dose is probably sufficient. In late menopause, where endogenous estrogen is low and symptoms are present a 1.25-mg dose may be appropriate. OR

2. Ethinyl estradiol, a synthetic estrogen, may be given in the cyclic fashion described above. It is supplied in tablets of 0.02, 0.05, and 0.5 mg. The dose is regulated according to the symptoms.
3. Diethylstilbestrol is a synthetic estrogen supplied in tablets of 0.1, 0.25, 0.5, 1.0, and 5.0 mg. The usual dosage is 0.2-0.5 mg/day, in a cyclic fashion. Spotting or bleeding occurring in patients taking estrogens requires evaluation. If bleeding is caused by estrogen withdrawal, consider reducing the dose.

After 12 months of estrogen therapy, a trial period without exogenous estrogen should be attempted. Weaning the patient from the drug (except those diagnosed as having osteoporosis) is important in preventing endometrial and breast malignancies.

- For vasomotor symptoms in women who have contraindications to estrogen therapy, medroxyprogesterone acetate (Depo-Provera) may be effective in relieving symptoms. A starting dose of 150 mg IM every three months is given. Its mode of action is unknown at this time.

  When hormonal therapy is contraindicated, vasomotor symptoms may be relieved by Bellergal. This drug is a combination of phenobarbital, ergotamine, and belladonna and is given four times daily (1 tablet in the morning, 1 at noon, and 2 at bedtime). This drug should not be given over a prolonged period, and the dose should be gradually decreased and withdrawn. Side effects may include blurred vision, dry mouth, flushing, or drowsiness.

- Treatment of abnormal bleeding in the perimenopausal period

  D&C: This procedure will resolve 40-70% of the cases of abnormal bleeding. Histologic studies are done on the curetted specimen to rule out abnormal changes. If bleeding does not resume in six months and there is no evidence of adenomatous hyperplasia on the endometrial sample, estrogen therapy can be started if indicated. If bleeding recurs after six months, a repeat curettage and histologic examination is needed.

  Endometrial biopsy may be performed as an office procedure to obtain a specimen for histologic study for symptoms of spotting or bleeding.

  Medical curettage (only done after endometrial sampling): Medroxyprogesterone acetate (Provera), 10 mg, or norethindrone acetate (Norlutate), 5 mg, is given orally daily for 7-10 days. This will cause the endometrial hyperplasia to be sloughed from the effect of the progesterone.

- Treatment of atrophic changes

  Estrogen replacement therapy as described may be used on a continuous basis for the patient with severe atrophic changes in tissues of the genitourinary system. For less severe atrophic changes, topical estrogen creams may be used to cause thickening of the tissue and decrease pruritus.

1. Premarin cream: One applicatorful is inserted into the vagina at bedtime for one to two weeks for symptom relief, then one to two times a week for maintenance.
2. Dienestrol cream: One applicatorful is inserted into the vagina at bedtime for 7-10 days, then one-half applicatorful one to two times a week.

    These creams must be used as sparingly as possible because systemic absorption can stimulate uterine bleeding or cause nausea and other side effects.

    *Note:* The use of topical estrogen creams in patients for whom estrogen is contraindicated is now under scrutiny. A recent study by Martin et al (1979) confirms previous studies that show "estrogens applied locally in the vagina are absorbed systemically with rapidity and efficiency. Within 12 hours of the first vaginal cream application, serum estrogen reached levels that are normal for the follicular phase in ovulating women." It would appear that contraindications to estrogen be considered before using topical estrogen creams.

- Treatment for osteoporosis (see p. 337).
- Contraception for the perimenopausal woman

    A method of birth control should be used by perimenopausal women until menstrual periods have stopped for one full year.

    After 35 years of age, women (especially those who smoke) should not use oral contraception. Risk of myocardial infarction and pulmonary emboli is greatly increased at this time due to the estrogenic component of the Pill. After age 40, the death rate in women who smoke and use the Pill is higher than if no contraceptive method were used.

    A woman over 35 years who elects to use the Pill should be aware of the higher risk, especially when additional factors such as diabetes, smoking, hypertension, and obesity are present. These diseases cause circulatory problems leading to increased early mortality.

    Alternate methods of contraception include:
    1. Surgical sterilization of either partner
    2. The diaphragm and jelly
    3. Foam and condoms
    4. Abortion back-up for method failures
- Sedative drugs and tranquilizers: These drugs may be used cautiously on a temporary basis for women who are anxious, depressed, or experiencing insomnia. For more severe emotional problems a psychiatric referral may be necessary.

    Sedatives (may cause drowsiness or withdrawal symptoms)

1. Phenobarbital, 0.25-0.5 gr. orally two to three times a day
2. Chlordiazepoxide (Librium), 5 mg orally one to three times a day (This drug may make a depressed patient even more depressed.)
3. Diazepam (Valium), 2.5-10 mg orally three to four times a day

Antidepressants
1. Amitriptyline HCl (Elavil), 10 mg orally three times a day
2. Imipramine hydrochloride (Tofranil), 25 mg orally two to three times a day (One to three weeks of treatment may be necessary before therapeutic effects are evident.)

- Treatment of hypothyroidism is indicated only when substantiated by laboratory data. Sodium levothyroxine (Synthroid), 0.1-0.2 mg/day, is given orally (may cause nervousness tachycardia or weight loss).
- Nutritional counseling or referral is necessary for those women whose diet has been identified as inadequate. If funds to buy food are inadequate, referral to a social worker may be necessary.

## Complications

- Osteoporosis
- Atrophic changes of the genitourinary tissue (atrophic vaginitis, adhesive vaginitis, cervical stenosis, urethral caruncle, cystitis, dyspareunia)
- Endometrial cancer (increased 5-14 times in women on unopposed estrogen replacement therapy, and 3-9 times in obese women)
- Acne rosacea—also called bottle nose, brandy nose, toper's nose, brandy face, rosy drop (caused by congestion and telangiectasis of the tissue of the face and is often accompanied by acne and seborrhea)
- Involutional depression in women with past psychologic problems
- Hyperlipidemia

## Patient Teaching

Women are likely to have received misinformation about the menopause with resulting misconceptions about what is really happening. What is needed is accurate information to help dispel fears about what may be perceived as a negative experience by some women. There is much support and information needed, but so little time to spare in a busy practice. An ideal mechanism for more efficient and effective counseling is the use of ongoing groups. In addition to

offering information to numbers of women, the group process also provides improved patient learning through sharing of information and peer support.
- Reassure patients that menopause is a normal life process that can be a positive experience. Related discomforts are probably temporary and will pass with time. Also give reassurance that sudden aging or personality change will not occur.
- Explore the patient's knowledge of menopause, what "myths" are believed, and what information is needed.
- Explain the physiologic processes occurring during menopause (audiovisual materials are helpful), why these changes occur, and possible symptoms that may be experienced.
- Explore the stresses and concerns verbalized by the patients. Much of what is discussed in a group will apply to many women, and it is an opportunity for those unwilling, or unable, to share their concerns to get answers.
- Focus on positive elements in the women's lives that can bring satisfaction and rewards. These may be social organizations, grandparenting, their sexual partner, community activity, religious affiliations, or special activities shared with their partners.
- Discuss the use of estrogen in the treatment of menopausal symptoms. This can be a stressful subject for many participants depending on what they believe the value of this therapy to be. Individual discussion may be necessary.
- Suggest avoiding overwork and fatigue. The need for routine, daily exercise (which will help to encourage sleep) is important for physical and mental health.
- Stress the importance of an adequate diet for general health and sense of well-being.
- Advise women who smoke (especially those on an estrogen replacement regimen) to stop smoking if possible. If they are unable to do so, decreasing the number of cigarettes per day will be beneficial. Refer interested women to a "stop-smoking" group.
- Reassure women experiencing hot flashes that these will probably decrease and stop within a year. They may temporarily readjust their lives by (1) wearing layered clothing, which allows removal of outer layers, (2) keep a jug of ice water handy to drink when they feel a flush coming on, and (3) keep covers on the bed to a minimum to maintain warmth without overheating.
- Recognize that loss of reproductive capacity may be felt keenly in women who have not had children. These women may experience grieving and need individual or group support.
- Reassure patients that although their sex life may gradually change, it should

continue to be an extremely satisfying experience. The following information may be helpful.

Lubrication of the vagina may decrease after menopause. The use of lubricant such as saliva, oil, or K-Y gel may be necessary for comfort.

As the male partner ages, it may take him longer to reach erection (although it can be maintained longer). This is a normal physiologic process and should not be cause for concern. In fact it may become a positive experience for the woman since it may also take longer for her to reach climax.

Women who continue regular sexual activity will maintain vaginal tone and secretions to a later age. Kegel's exercises are also helpful to maintain vaginal tone (see Fig 5).

Chronic or acute illness and some drugs may decrease the desire for sex. Drugs decreasing sexual activity include antihypertensives, antidepressants, antihistamines, barbiturates and methadone.

# OSTEOPOROSIS

## Definition

Osteoporosis is a major orthopedic disorder occurring in aging women, which causes a reduction in the quantity of bone mass resulting in structural fragility of the skeletal system.

## Etiology

It is unclear whether osteoporosis is a process of estrogen deprivation, a function of aging, or a combination of both these factors. In women between 35 and 45 years of age, bone mass remains at a relatively constant rate with daily bone formation and bone resorption in steady balance. At about 45-50 years of age, bone mass in the female skeleton begins to decrease, representing bone loss coincidental with menopause. It is not clear whether estrogen is an inhibitor of bone resorption or whether it decreases skeletal sensitivity to parathyroid hormone action. With decreased estrogen secretion, a state of physiologic hyperparathyroidism may exist, with the rate of bone resorption exceeding that of bone formation. Increased plasma calcium levels and urinary concentration of calcium, which have been mobilized from bone, results in a negative calcium balance. (These findings are reversed after treatment with estrogen.) Bone loss is greatest in the weight-bearing bones causing compression of vertebrae, kyphosis, and loss of height. The femur neck and distal radius (wrist) are frequent sites of fractures. Resorption of bone may also be influenced by (1) level of physical activity (2) calcium intake, and (3) the amount of calcium absorbed by the body. Bone loss is gradual and, if it remains untreated, the loss becomes critical. With advancing age serious fractures, deformities, and pain may result.

Statistics on osteoporosis reveal the following:

- Women at greater risk are slender, small-boned, and of European extraction; less prone are women who are black, tall, or obese. (Obese women are protected by the increased amount of estrogen produced in adipose tissue.)
- Osteoporosis is a universal process in postmenopausal women and varies only in the degree of bone lost.
- No corresponding process exists in men (bone resorption begins about 65 years of age).
- Twenty-five percent of untreated postmenopausal women have symptoms of osteoporosis.
- After physiologic menopause, symptoms appear in 5-10 years. After artificial menopause, symptoms appear in 2-5 years in 95% of the women.
- Fractures are 8-10 times more common in women than in men.
- Of an estimated 10,000 deaths per year associated with hip fractures, 80% occur in postmenopausal women.
- Fracture of the wrist is 10 times more frequent in women between the ages of 45 and 60 than in men in this age group.
- Oophorectomy causes earlier loss of bone mass, especially if surgery is performed before age 40.
- Bone lost postmenopausally occurs at an average rate of 1% of the total bone mass per year. By age 65-75, the bone mass of the female skeleton has decreased 15-20%.
- Pain associated with progressive osteoporosis is relieved by treatment with estrogen.
- Women who drink milk have more long bone fractures than milk nondrinkers. "There are no definitive studies clearly showing that dietary calcium deficiency is an important cause of osteoporosis" (Saville, 1973, p. 177).

## Clinical Features

### Symptoms

- Back pain

    Pain may be localized at the site of vertebral compression, radiating from the midline to the flank; it becomes worse with movement, and may be mild to severe. OR
    Severe pain with spasms of spinal muscles may be felt the length of the spine.

- Bone fractures of the spine, femur, and wrist are the most common.

### Signs

- Loss of height (humpback from shortening of the spine)
- Loss of weight

## Differential Diagnosis

- Multiple myeloma
- Immobilization
- Intestinal malabsorption
- Metastatic cancer
- Hyperparathyroidism
- Cushing's syndrome
- Rheumatoid arthritis
- Sustained corticosteroid excess
- Alcoholism
- Scheuermann's disease (juvenile vertebral epiphysitis, which occurs at puberty and causes humpback)

## Diagnostic Studies as Clinically Indicated

- Patient history and physical examination
- X-ray examination, radiogrammetry (measures the thickness of cortical bone of the second metacarpal)

- Measurement of serum levels of:

    Estrogen

    Calcium and phosphorus (normal values exclude hyperparathyroidism)

    Alkaline phosphatase (never elevated in osteoporosis, but elevated in metastatic cancer)
- Measurement of urinary calcium concentration
- Sedimentation rate (to rule out rheumatoid arthritis)

## Management and Treatment as Clinically Indicated

- Estrogen replacement therapy: There is no evidence that estrogen therapy will prevent the onset of osteoporosis, but it may delay bone resorption for 10-15 years.

    Conjugated estrogen (Premarin, Ovest, Genisis), 0.6 mg/day, is given orally. (Refer to the section on menopause for contraindications, side effects, and patient teaching information)

    Relief from pain occurs about three weeks after estrogen therapy is started.

    *Note:* The federal court ruled in 1975 that the FDA had to decide if estrogens were effective for treatment of osteoporosis. In 1977 the Endocrine Metabolic Advisory Committee and the OB/GYN Advisory Committee of the FDA agreed that estrogen does prevent postmenopausal bone loss, and that its benefits outweigh the risks.
- Treatment of women in whom estrogen therapy is contraindicated

    Calcium carbonate, 2.6 g/day, may be given orally. (Calcium gluconate or calcium glycerophosphate are ineffective and should not be used.) Although dietary calcium absorption is questionable, calcium supplementation does prevent bone loss.

    Tums are a good source of calcium and contain 250 mg of calcium per tablet. However 9-10 tablets per day are needed and may be expensive for the patient.

    Vitamin D is useful in treatment of osteoporosis and usually given in amounts three times the daily recommended allowance (RDA: 400 units). Excessive amounts may cause nausea, vomiting, diarrhea, lassitude, and urinary frequency. This vitamin is slowly metabolized and widely distributed in the body. Close supervision of patients who are taking this vitamin is necessary.

    Fluoride treatment is only used if there is rapid development of the disease (controversial).

Routine daily exercise should be advised, taking into consideration the capabilities and resources of the patients.

Severe back pain may be treated with bed rest and codeine, 1 gr every four to six hours as needed.

## Complications

- Compression fractures of the vertebrae
- Fractures of the wrist and femur neck
- Deformities and invalidism

## Patient Teaching

- Discuss with the patient the relationship of menopause and aging to the development of osteoporosis. (Refer to the section on menopause for further information.)
- Explain to the patient that osteoporosis occurs in all women, but that some women are more effected than others. Give reassurance that there are ways to halt further bone loss.
- Describe methods of treatment, either with estrogen (see the section on menopause) or with supplementary calcium. Since calcium may cause constipation, the diet of patients on this regimen should contain increased fiber (bran cereals, fruits, vegetables), and fluid intake should also be increased.
- Explore with the patient the type of physical activity she performs regularly. If her activity level is low, suggest exercise that would be appropriate. Depending on the health and ability of the patient, exercise could range from walking, performing a regular exercise routine, bicycling, swimming, or an activity the patient enjoys that is within her limits. Stress the importance of starting out slowly with gradual increase of activity as strength builds. Warn the patient against activity that causes strain or fatigue.
- Encourage good eating habits. If the diet is determined to be inadequate, referral for dietary counseling is appropriate.

# POSTMENOPAUSAL VAGINAL BLEEDING

## Definition

Postmenopausal bleeding is a symptom, not a disease. It is bleeding from the genital tract occurring six months or more after the last menstrual period. The amount of bleeding is variable but is likely to be slight.

## Etiology

Bleeding in the postmenopausal woman is usually organic in origin since menstrual dysfunction is absent after the age of 60. The most common cause of vaginal bleeding is prolonged administration of exogenous estrogen, which results in endometrial hyperplasia. The second most common cause is endometrial or cervical cancer. Two-thirds of the women who experience bleeding two to three years post menopause have a malignancy.

## Clinical Features

### Symptoms

- Spotting rather than diffuse bleeding
- Clear, watery discharge, which may precede frank bleeding of cancer by two to three months
- Pain or lower abdominal pressure after heavy exercise or defecation

### Signs

- Brownish or red blood in the vagina or cervix
- Atrophic vaginitis with or without trauma
- Change in size, shape, or pliability of uterus and pelvic floor
- Ovarian enlargement
- Lesions on the vulva, urethra, vagina, or cervix
- Hemorrhoids
- Obesity
- Inguinal adenopathy

## Differential Diagnosis

- Excessive exogenous estrogen
- Pelvic carcinoma
- Estrogen-producing functional ovarian tumor
- Cervical or endometrial polyps
- Urethral caruncle
- Atrophic endometrium
- Atrophic vaginitis and/or trauma
- Hemorrhoids
- "Unexplained"

## Diagnostic Studies as Clinically Indicated

- Complete medical, obstetric, and menstrual history with particular attention to questions about estrogen therapy, use of face, body, vaginal creams, or health food tablets containing estrogen
- General physical examination, paying particular attention to the breasts and pelvis (for lesions or masses) during observation and palpation
- Rectal examination and guaiac test on stool
- Sounding of uterus to determine the pathway of the cervical canal and depth of the uterine cavity
- Pap smear (only 50% effective in detecting endometrial cancer) Maturation index
- Endometrial biopsy
- Dilatation and fractional curettage
- Laparotomy
- A CBC, postprandial blood sugar test, urinalysis
- Wet mount if infection suspected

## Management and Treatment as Clinically Indicated

- Physician consultation is necessary
- Discontinuation of exogenous estrogen therapy until a diagnosis is made may be appropriate.
- Dilatation and curettage may stop the bleeding.

- A progesterone withdrawal test to determine the presence of endogenous estrogen may be indicated.
- Local estrogen therapy after ruling out malignancy may be indicated for atrophic vaginitis

    Premarin cream: One applicatorful is inserted into the vagina at bedtime for one to two weeks for symptom relief, then two to three times a week for maintenance of vaginal mucosa.

    Dienestrol Cream: One to two applicatorfuls are inserted into the vagina at bedtime for 7-10 days, then one-half applicatorful once or twice a week.

    AVC/Dienstrol Cream or Suppositories: One applicatorful or one suppository is used intravaginally once or twice a day.
- Systemic estrogen therapy after ruling out malignancy may be indicated for atrophic changes of the vagina, vulva, endometrium, and bladder.

    Premarin, 1.25 mg/day, is given cyclically: three weeks on, then one week off. Reassessment of dose level downward should be considered at least yearly.

    Diethylstilbestrol, 0.5-2 mg/day orally is given cyclically as above. (See the section on menopause for contraindications and patient teaching information.)
- Hysterectomy

## Patient Teaching

- Explain in detail to the patient the physiologic changes that have occurred during the climacteric to help her understand her particular problem.
- Explain to the patient (and significant other if appropriate), or reinforce the physician's explanation of the probable, or diagnosed, problem and the treatment required.
- Allow the patient time to express her concerns.
- Reassure the patient about her care and the need to report future abnormal physical or psychologic symptoms.
- Stress the importance of using prescribed oral or vaginal hormone preparations as directed, and to report any side effects promptly.
- Informed consent is necessary when prescribing estrogen. Use of the package insert included with estrogen preparations describing what the patient should know about its use and side effects could be one way of sharing and explaining this information to the patient.
- If surgery is indicated, assess the patient's knowledge of her diagnosis and

need for surgical intervention. Clarify or reinforce the physician's explanation of the procedure
- Prepare for the patient's physical well-being before surgery by stressing adequate diet.

    Adequate protein reserves are needed for the surgical and postsurgical periods for optimum wound healing and prevention of infections.

    Calories are needed for glycogen stores and to spare protein. If time permits, there is need to increase food intake if the patient is underweight and decrease it or change it if she is overweight.

    Vitamins and mineral stores are needed for increased metabolism of carbohydrates and protein postoperatively.

    The patient needs increased iron intake to correct iron-deficiency anemia and balanced electrolytes for an optimum postoperative course. Vitamins C, B, and E are especially useful in wound healing.

## URETHRAL PROLAPSE

### Definition

Urethral prolapse is a protrusion of the urethral mucosa through the urethral meatus, which appears as a rosette.

### Etiology

Urethral prolapse is precipitated by coughing, crying, or straining at stool and is most common in young women under 18 years of age and in women during the postmenopausal years. In the latter group it is associated with atrophic vaginitis, which reflects diminished estrogen production. It is usually a chronic problem, but when it occurs acutely, the onset is sudden with heavy bleeding as the primary symptom. The entire circumference of the urethral mucosa becomes prolapsed and may strangulate to form a circular purple tumor.

## Clinical Features

*Symptoms*

- Pain, dysuria and frequency

*Signs*

- Inspection reveals a circumferential pouting rosette or a circumferential purple tumor arising from the urethral meatus when strangulation has occurred.

## Differential Diagnosis

- Acute urethrocele
- Urethral caruncle

## Diagnostic Studies as Clinically Indicated

- A cytologic smear or biopsy is obtained to rule out carcinoma or sarcoma botryoides.

## Management and Treatment as Clinically Indicated

- Consultation with a physician
- Hot packs or sitz bath for symptom relief
- Topical estrogen cream for tissue atrophy in older women

    Premarin cream: One applicatorful is placed intravaginally at bedtime for one to two weeks for symptom relief, then two or three times a week for maintenance. OR

    Dienestrol Cream: One to two applicatorfuls is placed intravaginally at bedtime for 7-10 days, then one-half applicatorful is used once or twice a week for maintanance. OR

    AVC/Dienestrol Cream or Suppositories. One applicatorful or one suppository is inserted intravaginally once or twice a day.

- Surgical excision of the prolapsed epithelium
- Ligation of extruded tissue over a catheter may be done and the tissue allowed to slough.

## CHRONIC URETHRAL PROLAPSE

Chronic urethral prolapse is common postmenopausally. Atrophy of the urethral mucosa occurs causing the external meatus to gape and the lining of the posterior urethral rim to project as a small tumor. Usually no symptoms occur except when there is infection of the exposed tissue.

Treatment is not required unless symptoms exist.

## REFERENCES

Cancer risk and estrogen use in the menopause, editorial. *N Engl J Med* 293: 1199, 1975.

Gordon G, Genant H: Postmenopausal osteoporosis is a preventable disease. *Contemp Obstet Gynecol* 11:47, 1978.

Green T: *Gynecology Essentials of Clinical Practice,* ed 2. Boston, Little, Brown and Company, 1977, p 565.

Hammond C: Understanding and treating the climacteric. *The Female Patient* 2:16, 1977.

Hatcher R, Stewart G, Stewart F, et al: *Contraceptive Technology,* ed 10. New York, Irvington Publishers, 1980-81, p 46.

Hussey H: Osteoporosis among women who smoke cigarettes. *Jama* 235:1367, 1976.

Jaffee R: The menopause and perimenopausal period, in Yen R, Jaffee R: *Reproductive Endocrinology, Physiology, Pathophysiology and Clinical Management.* Philadelphia, WB Saunders Company, 1978, p 261.

Kempers R: The menopause, in deAlvarez R (ed): *Textbook of Gynecology* Philadelphia, Lea & Febiger 1977, p 209.

Kistner R: The menopause, in Caplan R, Sweeney W (ed): *Advances in Obstetrics and Gynecology.* Baltimore, Williams & Wilkins Company, 1978, p 551.

Lichten, E: Estrogen and alternative therapy of the menopausal patient. *Primary Care:* 5:607, 1978.

Martin P, Yen S, Burnier A, et al: Systemic absorption and sustained effects of vaginal estrogen creams. *JAMA* 242:2699, 1979.

Mattingly, R: *TeLinde's Operative Gynecology,* ed 5. Philadelphia, JB Lippincott Company, 1977, p 786.

McGuire L, Sorley A: Understanding and preventing the menopause crisis. *Nurse Practitioner* 3:15, 1978.

Overstreet E: Menopause and postmenopausal syndrome, in Benson R (ed): *Current Obstetrics and Gynecologic Diagnosis and Treatment.* Los Altos, Calif. Lange Medical Publications, 1978, p 498.

Parsons L, Sommers, S: *Gynecology.* Philadelphia, WB Saunders Company, 1978, p 1470.

Saville P: The syndrome of spinal osteoporosis. *Clin Endocrinol Metabol* 2:177, 1973.

Speroff L, Glass R, Kase N: *Clinical Gynecologic Endocrinology and Infertility,* ed 2. Baltimore, Williams & Wilkins Company, 1978, p 302.

Stewart F, Stewart G, Guest F, et al: *My Body, My Health.* New York, John Wiley & Sons, 1979, p 476.

Takaki N: Weight loss may reduce risk of endometrial and breast cancer. *The*

Williams, S: *Nutrition and Diet Therapy;* St. Louis, C.V. Mosby Company, 1969, p 43.

# Section III

# Diagnostic Procedures and Laboratory Values

# 17

# Diagnostic Procedures and Laboratory Values in Obstetrics and Gynecology

History taking in conjunction with clinical evaluation allows accurate diagnosis of a majority of patient problems. Special diagnostic procedures aid in confirming questionable diagnoses and are helpful in diagnosing abnormalities that cannot be inspected, palpated, or ascultated. Numerous diagnostic modalities are available, ranging from the simple to the most complex. This chapter provides information on those procedures that the Nurse Practitioner uses most commonly in her practice, or which will aid in explaining tests or test results to patients.

## AMNIOCENTESIS

Amniocentesis is performed on pregnant women to obtain amniotic fluid for study. A needle is inserted through the abdomen into the uterus, and fluid is drawn from the amniotic sac to be used for diagnostic studies. Amniocentesis can be performed only after 15 weeks' gestation when sufficient fluid has been produced to supply an adequate specimen (10 ml). Before the procedure sonography is indicated to localize the placenta and to reduce complications from injury by needle puncture to the fetus or placenta. Indications for use of amniocentesis can be either diagnostic or therapeutic.

Diagnostic indications:

- Prenatal diagnosis of congenital disorders or infections (for women who have had a previous child with birth defects or a family history of birth defects or for women over 35 years old)
    Chromosomal disorders (e.g., Down's syndrome)
    Enzyme deficiencies (e.g., Tay-Sachs disease)
    Sex-linked disorders (e.g., hemophilia)
    Metabolic disorders (e.g., cystic fibrosis)
- Studies of fetal well-being
    Estriol determination (high-risk pregnancies)
    Color of fluid (meconium-stained)
    Bilirubin determination (hemolytic disease)
- Estimation of fetal maturity
    Cytologic staining of fat cells
    Creatinine concentration
    Bilirubin (in the absence of hemolytic disease, it should decrease as pregnancy progresses)
    Osmolarity: Increased fetal urine in the amniotic fluid causes the fluid to become hypotonic.

Therapeutic indications:

- Relief of hydramnios
- Intrauterine transfusion
- Therapeutic abortion (second trimester)

Complications

Although many complications are possible, the risk of these occurring is 1%:

- Maternal complications
    Hemorrhage and hematoma formation from puncture of a uterine vessel
    Uterine contractions and premature labor
    Amniotic fluid leak (usually benign)
    Syncope from supine hypotension
- Fetal complications
    Fetomaternal bleeding with potential isoimmunization (sensitization of an unsensitized Rh negative patient)
    Infection
    Spontaneous abortion
    Hemorrhage (puncture of fetal vessel or placenta)
    Fetal puncture

## BASAL BODY TEMPERATURE (BBT)

Basal body temperature (BBT) is the temperature of the body when at complete rest. The oral or rectal temperature is taken for two to five minutes immediately on awakening in the morning, before any activity has occurred. (Any type of activity will cause an elevation of the base temperature.)
Indications

- Infertility workup (to assess ovulatory status)
- Natural family planning method (to calculate fertile days)
- As an indicator for initiation of drugs in treatment of dysmenorrhea

A BBT thermometer is used for easy reading since it has larger numbers to indicate degrees of temperature than a regular oral or rectal thermometer. The early morning body temperature is recorded on a BBT calendar every day (Fig. 6). Notations should be made on the calendar when illness, menses, coitus, or use of medications have occurred. The body temperature drops slightly 24-36 hours after ovulation, then rises abruptly. Progesterone, produced by the ovary after ovulation (luteal phase), causes an elevation of the basal body temperature of 0.5-0.7 degrees. This temperature elevation continues until the end of the menstrual cycle and indicates ovulation. The BBT calendar should be kept over a period of months to demonstrate a temperature pattern. A biphasic curve usually indicates ovulation and can be helpful in predicting when ovulation will occur. A monophasic curve usually indicates anovulatory cycles.

## BIOPSY

A biopsy is the removal of a small portion of tissue for histologic examination.

### Cervical Biopsy

Indications:

- Suspicious-looking area on the cervix
- Abnormal Schiller's test
- Abnormal area of tissue identified by colposcopy

Cervical biopsy may be done as directed by the Schiller's test, or by the four-quadrant method with specimens collected at the 12, 3, 6, and 9 o'clock positions on the cervix. Samples should include tissue from the squamocolumnar

## INSTRUCTIONS FOR KEEPING TEMPERATURE RECORD

1/ Insert date at top of column in space provided for date of month.

2/ Each morning, upon awakening, but *before* you get out of bed, place thermometer under tongue for at least two minutes. Do this every morning, even during menstruation. Be sure not to eat, drink or smoke before taking temperature.

3/ Accurately record temperature reading on the graph by placing a dot in the proper location (see example below) Indicate days of coitus (intercourse) by a down-pointing arrow (↓) in the space provided.

4/ The first day of menstrual flow is considered to be the start of a cycle. Indicate each day of flow by blocking the square indicated (■) on the graph, starting at the extreme left under the first day of cycle.

5/ Any obvious reasons for temperature variation such as colds, infection, insomnia, indigestion, etc., should be noted on the graph above the reading for that day.

6/ Ovulation may be accompanied, in some women, by a twinge of pain in the lower abdomen. If you notice this, indicate the day it occurred on the graph.

7/ Start new cycle on next graph.

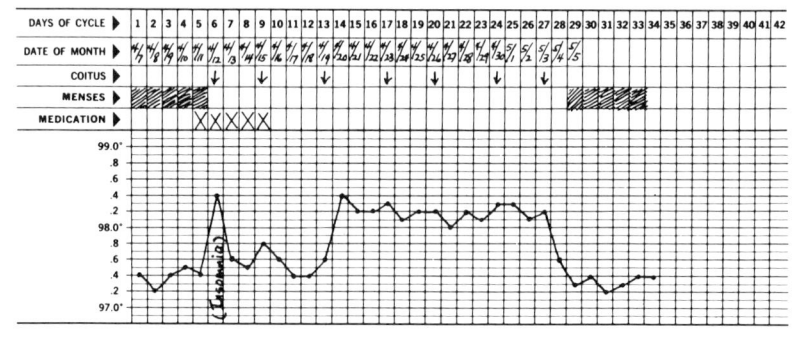

**Figure 6.**
Basal body temperatures record. (Reprinted with permission from Merrell-National Laboratories, Cincinnati, Ohio.)

junction of the cervix, which is the most common site of malignancy. Endocervical scrapings should also be collected.

No anesthesia is used routinely (the cervix has few nerve endings), but there may be some discomfort to the patient. Bleeding from the site is controlled by cautery with a silver nitrate stick and placement of a tampon in the vagina.

## Endometrial Biopsy

Indications:

- Ovarian dysfunction

Figure 6. (continued)

- Infertility (to assess endometrial effects of estrogen and progesterone)
- Perimenopausal bleeding (to rule out malignancy)

The procedure may be performed with an endometrial biopsy curet or by use of a suction instrument. No anesthesia is used, and the patient may feel cramping when the sound is passed and when the samples are collected.

It is important to provide menstrual data on the accompanying laboratory slip. If menstrual disturbances are being evaluated the pathologist needs this information when identifying proliferative or secretory endometrium and in dating the progestational phase of the sample.

## BUCCAL SMEAR

The buccal smear is commonly used for determining a person's nuclear sex chromatin pattern. The buccal smear technique is more efficient than either the blood smear or skin biopsy.

Indications:

- Primary amenorrhea
- Ambiguous genitalia
- Prepubertal girls who are excessively short in stature
- Male infertility
- Mental retardation/psychotic or antisocial behavior
- Aggressive, antisocial behavior in males of excessive height

Recognition of a sex chromatin body in the cell nucleus is the basis of this test. Sex chromatin bodies are more commonly found in a much larger proportion of female cells than male cells. The percentage of sex chromatin bodies present in the cells of either sex gives an indication of possible genetic abnormality. Further chromosomal analysis is done for more definitive information on abnormal buccal smears. Special collection and handling techniques are needed for these smears.

## CHAIN URETHROCYSTOGRAM

The chain urethrocystogram is a method of x-ray evaluation of the bladder in women with possible stress incontinence.

Indications:

- To confirm the diagnosis of true stress incontinence
- To rule out pseudostress or other types of incontinence
- To measure the degree of anatomic change of the urinary tract
- As an index to the type of corrective surgical repair necessary

The procedure is performed by the placement of a metallic, beaded chain through a catheter into the bladder. For optimum visualization of the vesicle neck, a warm iodized oil solution is instilled into the bladder, then x-ray films are taken with the patient in various positions. The films aid in diagnosis of true stress incontinence when they show loss of the posterior urethrovesical angle, rotational descent of the urethra and bladder neck, and a change in the axis of inclination of the urethra.

## COLPOSCOPY

Colposcopy is examination of the cervix and vagina by means of a colposcope, which is an optical instrument with a magnification of 10-20 times. It enables three-dimensional visualization of areas of cellular dysplasia or vascular abnormalities on the cervix or in the vagina.

Indications:

- Evaluation of cytologic abnormalities
- Examination of the cervix when there is suspicion of malignancy but no obvious lesion
- Evaluation of abnormalities detected on clinical examination
- To guide biopsy of suspicious lesions
- Evaluation and follow-up of DES-exposed daughters

Early identification and treatment of abnormal lesions is possible with the magnification of the cervical and vaginal tissues afforded by the colposcope, the cytologic sampling of cells, and the biopsy of suspicious lesions. A precise and accurate diagnosis of the nature and extent of a malignant lesion can be made with the help of a colposcope in 85% of patients who have been identified as being at risk by cytologic or pelvic examination. In many cases, the trauma and expense of a cone biopsy can be avoided.

Normal colposcopic findings include:

- Squamous epithelium
- Squamous metaplasia (transformation zone)
- Columnar epithelium

Abnormal colposcopic findings include:

- Leukoplakia or "white epithelium"
- Mosaicism (thickened epithelium with a patchy appearance)
- Punctation (thickened areas with different levels of tissue and punctiform vessels)
- Atypical transformation (thickening of squamous epithelium, overgrowth of columnar epithelium, and irregularity of the blood vessels.

*Note:* At times colpomicroscopy is performed to evaluate the tissues of the cervix and vagina in situ. The colpomicroscope has higher powers of magnification (up to 400 times) than the colposcope.

## COLPOTOMY (CULDOTOMY)

Colpotomy is surgical incision through the posterior vaginal fornix into the rectouterine pouch.
Indications:

- To visualize the pelvic structures
- To perform surgical procedures on the tubes or ovaries
- To allow intraperitoneal palpation for diagnostic purposes.

Colpotomy requires general anesthesia and hospitalization. In some patients it may not be anatomically possible to get sufficient expansion for visualization or performance of palpation or surgery with this procedure.

## CONE BIOPSY (CONIZATION)

Conization of the cervix is the surgical excision of a cone of cervical tissue surrounding the external os with the apex of the cone extending into the endocervical canal. A dilatation and curettage (D&C) is usually performed in conjunction with this procedure.
Indications:

- When a deep-seated cervical infection exists
- When a significant discrepancy exists between the cytology report, the colposcopic findings, or the biopsy report
- When the limits of a lesion cannot be seen colposcopically
- When a significant lesion exists and the squamocolumnar junction cannot be visualized
- When microinvasive cancer is present or suspected
- When patient follow-up may be difficult

Hospitalization is necessary for this procedure. Cone biopsy may be avoided in 90% of the patients with abnormal cytologic smears. When a colposcopic examination with a guided cervical biopsy followed by a D&C are performed, diagnosis can usually be made, rendering a cone biopsy unnecessary.

## CRYOSURGERY (CRYOTHERAPY)

Cryosurgery is a method of treatment for benign lesions, which causes local tissue destruction by the application of subfreezing temperatures. Diagnosis of the lesion must be made before the use of this technique because treatment of invasive cancer with cryosurgery will have serious consequences. Genital lesions treated by cryosurgery include condyloma and chronic cervicitis.

Cryosurgery is performed by passing liquid refrigerant, such as nitrogen, Freon 22, carbon dioxide, or nitrous oxide, through a hollow probe that is placed on the effected tissue and left until the desired amount of freezing occurs. The use of anesthesia is usually unnecessary. The frozen tissue sloughs as healing takes place and new epithelium is formed. Postoperative bleeding is uncommon, and no scarring of the tissue occurs during healing. The patient will experience profuse leukorrhea for two to three weeks after treatment from continued sloughing of tissue. Complete healing takes place within six weeks.

## CULDOCENTESIS

Culdocentesis is aspiration of fluid from the rectouterine pouch by means of a needle inserted through the posterior vaginal fornix. This procedure may be done on an outpatient basis.

Indications:

- To evaluate acute upper abdominal disorders
- To identify peritoneal fluid, pus, or blood in the pelvis
- To drain an abscess in the cul-de-sac

Culdocentesis is of limited value, and its use may not provide a diagnosis. When the absence of fluid (normal), or the nature of the fluid present is determined, it may prove of diagnostic value when integrated with other clinical findings.

## CULDOSCOPY

Culdoscopy is direct visualization of the pelvis, pelvic viscera, and surrounding structures by means of an endoscope inserted through the posterior vaginal fornix.

It is indicated as a diagnostic tool in:

- Unexplained acute or chronic pelvic pain
- Suspected ectopic pregnancy
- Pelvic masses of unknown nature
- Endocrine problems (ovarian disease)
- Endometriosis
- Tubal patency
- Peri-adnexal adhesions

This procedure requires anesthesia and hospitalization. Culdoscopy is preferred over laparoscopy by some physicians because, in addition to providing good visualization, it is felt to be easier to perform and safer for the patient.

## ESTRIOL MEASUREMENT IN PREGNANCY

The purpose of estriol measurement in pregnancy is to establish the physiologic state of the fetoplacental unit. Estriol is the principle estrogen of pregnancy, with precursors for its production located in the fetal liver and adrenal glands. The measurement of estrogen in the pregnant woman reflects the state of this maternofetoplacental unit and is useful for early detection of possible problems. Estriol levels (serum or urinary) may vary from day to day in pregnant women, which necessitates serial measurements to establish a baseline trend in pregnancies at risk. Levels that drop suddenly are usually associated with fetal distress.

Although samples for measuring serum estriol are easier to collect than those for determining urinary levels (because the latter requires a 24-hour specimen), only the measurement of urinary estriol concentration will be discussed since this is the only method available in some settings. (For normal values for serum estriol see the chart of blood chemistry values at the end of this chapter.)

Indications:

- Diabetes
- Toxemia

- Intrauterine growth retardation, post maturity, small for gestational age (SGA)
- Rh incompatibility
- Chronic hypertension/renal disease

Ideally urinary estriol levels are measured every 48 hours in late pregnancy for optimum information about fetal well-being. The patient begins the test in the morning on arising, discarding the first morning urine specimen, and noting the time. She then collects *every* urine specimen for the next 24-hours including the first-voided specimen the next morning, again noting the time. The 24-hour collection bottle should be kept refrigerated to prevent bacterial growth. It is important that *all* urine is collected over the 24 hours, otherwise the test result is inaccurate.

Urinary estriol levels range from 3 to 40 mg/24 hr depending on the week of gestation. A lower-than-normal estriol level for the week of gestation in a properly collected and assayed specimen indicates fetoplacental problems.

## FERN TEST
## (CERVICAL MUCUS ARBORIZATION TEST)

The fern test is a microscopic slide test of endocervical mucus used to qualitatively assess estrogen secretion in a patient. Ferning of the mucus (a fernlike pattern on a dried smear) occurs during the early proliferative phase of the menstrual cycle and reaches maximum at ovulation when estrogen peaks.

Indications:

- To determine the presence or absence of ovulation
- To determine the time of ovulation
- To monitor the induction of ovulation
- To assess corpus luteum function (progesterone secretion)
- To be used as one parameter of an infertility workup

For the test, endocervical mucus is spread on a glass slide and allowed to dry for 10-20 minutes. The slide is then examined microscopically to assess arborization (fernlike configuration) of the mucus. A positive test shows ferning and crystallization, indicating a predominantly estrogenic effect. (Maximal ferning is indicated when crystal formations are at four right angles to each other). A negative test shows no ferning or crystallization, indicating little or no estrogenic effects (or estrogen suppression from progesterone activity). Within 24-72 hours after ovulation ferning disappears due to the effect of the progesterone.

## FLUORESCENT ANTIBODY TEST (FA)

The fluorescent antibody test is useful in differentiating upper from lower tract urinary infection. When a urinary tract infection is suspected, examination by fluorescent microscopy of bacteria from the urine that have been stained with a fluorescent dye may reveal antibody-coated bacteria, which exhibit fluorescence. The finding of antibody-coated bacteria constitutes a positive FA test and indicates that infection is in the kidney. A negative FA test is an indication that infection is in the bladder. A false-negative finding may occur if the urinary tract infection is recent.

## GLUCOSE TOLERANCE TESTS (IN PREGNANCY)

Controversy continues over the use of oral vs intravenous glucose tolerance tests. The test used depends on the setting, the physician, and/or the laboratory who makes the decision. The oral glucose tolerance test (OGTT) is currently the test of choice. Either test is unnecessary in patients with fasting blood glucose levels above 90 mg/dl, in whole blood, or 105 mg/dl. in plasma since the patient is overtly diabetic.

Indications:

- Family history of diabetes
- History of a large baby (over 4,000 g)
- Previous stillbirth or infant with anomalies
- Obesity
- Consistent glycosuria
- Recurrent urinary tract infection

In preparation for an OGTT the patient should have a minimum of 200-250 g of carbohydrate for three days before the test. The patient should fast for 10-12 hours, but no more than 16 hours, before the test. Salicylates, nicotine, and some diuretics diminish glucose tolerance and should be omitted three days before testing.

On the morning of the test blood is drawn to determine the fasting blood sugar level. A 100-g oral glucose load is given, and blood specimens are drawn one, two, and three hours after the glucose load.

Normal Blood Sugar Values

| Hour | Whole Blood | Plasma | Serum |
|---|---|---|---|
| 0 | 90 mg/dl | 103 mg/dl | 110 mg/dl |
| 1 | 165 | 188 | 200 |
| 2 | 145 | 165 | 150 |
| 3 | 125 | 143 | 130 |

Abnormal values in any two specimens constitute a positive oral glucose tolerance test. A normal OGTT in the first trimester may become abnormal later in pregnancy and should be repeated if predisposing factors for diabetes exist.

## GRAPHIC STRESS TELETHERMOMETRY (GST)

This method for screening women for breast lesions is currently under study. It will function as a breast cancer risk indicator and is intended for use in conjunction with breast examination and mammography. It uses the principle of determining "warm" spots, similar to thermography. However, rather than defining hot areas, a computer records temperature change in the breast and assigns a risk score from 1 to 99. Scores of 40 or below indicate low risk; scores of 41 to 70, above average risk; and scores over 70, high risk. Women who score 70 and above need close follow-up. Mammograms or other diagnostic measures are indicated in these women.

## HYSTEROSALPINGOGRAM

Hysterosalpingogram is an outpatient radiologic procedure used for obtaining films, while allowing immediate visualization of the endocervix, uterine cavity, and fallopian tubes by monitoring under fluoroscopy.
  Indications:
- Evaluation of tubal patency
- Identification of congenital anomalies or deformities of the genital organs

- Identification of polyps, leiomyomas, hydatidiform moles, and extrinsic pressure

The test is most commonly used during fertility workup to provide more explicit information than can be collected in other ways (i.e., sonography). The greatest weakness of the test is that it does not show the condition of the frimbriae and peritubal area. The test is performed one week after a menstrual period to prevent reflux of endometrial cells into the tubes and peritoneum. Sedation may be necessary for some patients, and if severe pain occurs, the procedure should be discontinued.

To perform the test, 1-10 ml of contrast medium is instilled into the cervix in small increments under low pressure. Films are taken after each injection, at 45 minutes after completion of the test to assess spillage of the medium into the peritoneum (indicating tubal patency), and in 24 hours to evaluate peritubal adhesions. Fluoroscopic viewing of the contrast medium entering the cervix and uterus at the time of the procedure may give the physician more immediate data.

Complications:

- Pain
- Hemorrhage, shock
- Endometriosis (peritoneal reflux of endometrial cells)
- Allergic reaction to the medium
- Injection of the medium into the bloodstream

# LAMINARIA

*Laminaria digitata* is a species of seaweed, which is hygroscopic. Its ability when dried to expand as it draws fluid from its surroundings makes it useful for slow dilatation of the cervix before first or second trimester therapeutic abortions.

One or two small sticks of compressed *L. digitata* are placed in the cervical canal 6-12 hours before a procedure is to be performed. The gradual cervical dilatation resulting from the expanding *Laminaria* is less traumatic to the endocervical canal than is the use of metal cervical dilators.

# LAPAROSCOPY

Laparoscopy is an endoscopic procedure performed to permit visualization of the abdominal and pelvic organs and is the second most commonly performed surgical procedure for gynecologic diagnosis.

## Indications May Be Diagnostic or Therapeutic

- Infertility workup
- Evaluation of:
  Genital malformations
  Possible ectopic pregnancy, adnexal mass
  Pelvic pain, endometriosis, pelvic infections, appendicitis, pelvic masses
  Postsurgical complications (uterine perforation)
- Biopsy
- Aspiration of physiologic ovarian cysts
- Lysis of peritubal adhesions
- Extraction of an IUD located in the abdomen

The laparoscope, which has a telescopic lens, is introduced through an umbilical stab incision into the abdomen after creation of a pneumoperitoneum. The instrument provides a 180° view of the abdominal and pelvic organs. Ancillary instruments for performing biopsy, tubal ligations, lysing of adhesions, and for photographing the structures can be used by their insertion through the cannula of the laparoscope. Hospitalization and general anesthesia are necessary for performing laparoscopy.

# LECITHIN-SPHINGOMYELIN RATIO (L/S RATIO)

The lecithin-sphingomyelin ratio (L/S ratio) is a test done on amniotic fluid during pregnancy to monitor fetal lung maturity to aid in the prevention of respiratory distress syndrome (RDS) in the neonate. Pulmonary surfactant, which normally prevents collapse of the alveoli in the lungs, contains lecithin and sphingomyelin. Measurement of the ratio of these two substances in the amniotic fluid surrounding the fetus gives an indication of lung maturity in the fetus. In high-risk pregnancies where optimum fetal well-being is desired, early delivery may be necessary. Before this can be attempted the state of the fetal lung needs to be assessed. An amniocentesis is performed to obtain an amniotic fluid sample for L/S ratio and other tests.

High-risk pregnancies that may need early delivery include:

- Erythroblastosis fetalis
- Maternal diabetes
- Toxemia of pregnancy
- Hypertension

Test interpretation:

- An L/S ratio greater than 2 to 1 or higher signifies fetal lung maturity.
- An L/S ratio of 1.5 to 1.9 indicates possible mild or moderate RDS.
- An L/S ratio of 1.0 to 1.49 indicates immaturity of the fetal lungs with moderate to severe RDS.
- An L/S ratio of less than 1.0 predicts severe RDS.

## MAMMOGRAPHY

Mammography is a soft tissue x-ray examination of the breast and is used as an early detection screening device for breast tumors.

Indications:

- To aid in the diagnosis of palpable lumps in the breast and axilla, or when skin, nipple, and breast size changes have occurred
- To differentiate fibrocystic breast disease
- To follow postmastectomy patients for examination of the remaining breast
- To detect early, nonpalpable lesions
- To be used as a baseline for future comparative studies, especially in women over 50 years of age

When both breasts are examined by mammography the total radiation exposure is 2 rads. However, since rads are cumulative over time, to minimize unnecessary exposure to radiation in women the National Institutes of Health (NIH) have developed the following guidelines for its use.

- Mammography screening should be available for screening women over 50 years of age. (*Note:* When combined with breast self-examination, mammography is beneficial in reducing death by 40% in this age group. Below the age of 50, no differences in mortality have been found.
- Mammography should be performed only on women between 40 and 49 years who have had previous cancer or a family history of cancer.
- Mammography should be used only in women between 35 to 39 years when they have had previous cancer in one breast.
- Mammography is never to be used to screen women under 35 years of age.
- Thermography should not be used.

*Note:* When a breast lump or other suspicious changes are identified, mammography is indicated at any age.

## MATURATION INDEX (MI)

The maturation index is a qualitative index of estrogenic activity. It is determined by microscopic examination of a stained smear of the upper midvaginal mucosa. Used most commonly in assessment of the relative estrogen status of menopausal women, it measures the percentage of vaginal mucosal cells, which are parabasal, intermediate, or superficial in that order. A greater percentage of superficial cells indicates good estrogen effect, while a greater percentage of parabasal and intermediate cells indicates decreased estrogen effect.

Examples of MIs (these are not standard measurements) are:

- 100/0/0: Indicates all parabasal cells and absent estrogen (menopause)
- 0/40/60: Characterizes the proliferative phase of the menstrual cycle and adequate estrogen
- 0/70/30: Characterizes menstrual phase of the cycle with deceased estrogen
- 0/95/5: Indicates progesterone dominance, as in pregnancy

This test does not indicate absolute levels of estrogen and indicates a rough estimate of its presence. It should be used only as one parameter of diagnosis in conjunction with patient history, physical examination, and clinical signs and symptoms.

## NONSTRESS TEST

The nonstress test is done in late pregnancy to evaluate the activity of the fetal heart rate as it relates to fetal movements. The result of the test is an indication of the health of the baby and how well the stresses of labor will be tolerated.

Indications:
- Post-term pregnancy (over 42 weeks)
- Hypertension, pre-eclampsia
- Small for gestational age
- Previous problem pregnancy
- Diabetes, anemia, kidney disease.

To perform the test, two monitoring leads are attached to the pregnant woman's abdomen. One monitor measures uterine contractions while the other monitors the baby's heart beat; both are recorded simultaneously on a graph. The baby must be awake for the test to be performed since the heart rate should increase with fetal movements.

Test interpretation:

- Reactive fetus

    At least four fetal movements in 20 minutes with acceleration of the fetal heart rate of at least 10 beats per minute

    Long-term variability amplitude of at least 10 beats per minute

    Baseline rate within normal range

    This test result is associated with survival of the fetus for one week in more than 99% of the cases.

- Nonreactive fetus

    No fetal movements or no accleration with fetal movement

    No long-term variability

    Baseline rate may be outside (or within) normal range

    This test result is associated with poor fetal outcome in approximately 20% of the cases. Because of the 80% false-positive rate, it needs to be followed immediately by an oxytocin challenge test* (which has approximately a 2-50% false-positive rate).

- Unvertain reactivity

    Less than four fetal movements in 20 minutes, or with acceleration less than 10 beats per minute

    Long-term variability amplitude decreased below 10 beats per minute

    Abnormal baseline rate

    This test should be followed immediately by an oxytocin challenge test* or should be repeated within one to three days at the physician's discretion.

## OXYTOCIN CHALLENGE TEST OCT (CONTRACTION STRESS TEST)

The purpose of the oxytocin challenge test is to determine fetal oxygen reserve before labor by evaluation of the fetal heart rate response to induced labor contractions. This test has largely been replaced by the nonstress test, which does not use medication to induce contractions and is equally as reliable.

Indications

---

*Unless oxytocin is contraindicated (e.g., previous classical cesarean sections, risk of premature labor, placenta previa).

- Hypertension
- Diabetes
- Postterm pregnancy (over 42 weeks)
- Pre-eclampsia
- Suspected intrauterine growth retardation

The procedure is performed by administering sufficient amounts of IV oxytocin to the pregnant woman to produce uterine contractions. If the oxygen reserve of the placenta is marginal, the fetus becomes compromised during contractions. A fetal heart pattern of late deceleration occurs indicating placental insufficiency.

Test interpretation:

- Negative: The fetal heart rate is stable without evidence of periodic decelerations.
- Positive: Uniform late decelerations, or the onset of deceleration at or beyond the peak of the contraction, occur.
- Suspicious: Late decelerations of the fetal heart rate are not repetitive, and excessive uterine activity is present.

## PAPANICOLAOU SMEAR

The Pap smear is used for the cytologic screening of cells collected from the cervix of women, specifically for detection of cervical cancer. It is an inappropriate screening procedure for endometrial or ovarian cancer.

### Considerations Before Specimen Collection

- The optimum time for collecting a Pap smear is five days after the last menstrual period.
- The patient should not have douched or used a vaginal medication within the previous 24 hours.
- The smear should not be collected during menses; the presence of red blood cells makes cytologic interpretation difficult.
- Lubricating jelly distorts the cells and should not be used on the speculum before insertion. Tap water is used to lubricate the speculum.

## Specimen Collection

The diagnostic value and accuracy of the Pap smear is greatly influenced by the method of obtaining the specimen and preparing the slide. Each clinical setting has its own method of specimen collection usually dictated by the cytology laboratory, and this method should be followed. One method of Pap smear collection is as follows:

- Two slides are prepared by labeling in waxed pencil the patient's last name, the date, and source of the specimen:

    Slide 1: "V" for vaginal

    Slide 2: "C" for cervical and "E" for endocervical.

    If placed in solution, a paper clip applied to the end of one slide will prevent them from sticking together. This is not necessary when cardboard holders are used.
- The Pap smear is collected after the specimen for culture of *Neisseria gonorrhoeae* is taken, and before the bimanual examination.
- A sponge stick is used to remove any material on the cervix such as mucus, blood, or discharge that might obscure the cells.
- Speed of specimen collection and use of a fixative is essential to prevent drying and distortion of the cells.
- A Q-tip is inserted into the endocervical canal and rotated several times to moisten. Withdraw the Q-tip and role the specimen on one-half of the "C and E" slide.
- Firmly rotate a spatula twice around the cervical os, or where the squamocolumnar junction is visible, and smear a thin specimen of the material obtained on the other half of the "C & E" slide and drop immediately into the fixative or spray with fixative. This should be done quickly to prevent drying of the slide.
- Using the spade end of the spatula, take a sample of vaginal material from the posterior vaginal fornix and smear it on the slide marked "V" and drop into fixative or spray with fixative and place in a cardboard container.

## Classification of Pap Smear Results

These classifications will differ depending on the laboratory reporting the results.

- Class I: Negative—Only normal cells are present
- Class II: Negative—Some atypical cells are present (may be stated as "inflammatory changes" if a chronic infection exists).

- Class III: Doubtful—Atypical cells suggestive of malignancy are present.
- Class IV: Positive—Atypical cells are present.
- Class V: Positive—Numerous atypical cells or cell groups are present.

## PAPANICOLAOU SMEAR (FOUR-QUADRANT TECHNIQUE)

This four-sample Pap smear is used to collect vaginal cell samples from females who have been exposed to DES.

- Four slides are labeled according to the area of the vagina where the specimen is collected: anterior, posterior, right lateral and left lateral.
- After placement of the speculum, excess secretions and mucus should be removed from the cervix and vaginal walls. This step is very important in proper collection.
- Cell samples are collected by gently scraping the vaginal walls starting posteriorly and drawing the spatula forward toward the introitus in each of the areas identified. Separate spatulas should be used for each sample collected.
- The specimens should be fixed immediately in 95% ethyl alcohol or sprayed with fixative and sent to the cytology laboratory for staining.
- Routine Pap smears of the ectocervix and endocervix are also collected at the same time.

## PROGESTERONE WITHDRAWAL TEST (PROGESTERONE TEST)

The progesterone withdrawal test is used in amenorrheic women to test ovarian function. After a negative serum pregnancy test, oral progesterone (medroxyprogesterone acetate [Provera] 10-20 mg) is given daily for five days or a single 100-mg, intramuscular dose of progesterone in oil may be given to determine if the amenorrheic patient will bleed.
Results:

- If amenorrhea is due to delay or failure of ovulation, the progesterone will cause the onset of bleeding in two to seven days. The patient needs to be counseled that this bleeding episode may be heavy and possibly accompanied by cramping, or that the bleeding may be light with spotting only.
- If amenorrhea is due to inadequate estrogen secretion to prime the endome-

trium or from persistent corpus luteum function, no withdrawal bleeding will occur. Lack of bleeding after progesterone is given, indicates the need for a diagnostic workup.

## RUBIN TEST

The Rubin test is used to assess the patency of the fallopian tubes. It is used primarily as a diagnostic tool for infertility. It may also be therapeutic in some patients by releasing and opening minor blockages of the tubes during the procedure.

A controlled injection of carbon dioxide is passed into the uterus and flows into the fallopian tubes. If the tubes are patent, a rush of air is heard through the end of the tube(s). It is difficult to determine if one, or both tubes are patent with this method. Referred shoulder pain, resulting from irritation of the subdiaphragmatic area when the patient stands erect, also indicates tubal patency. The Rubin test is being replaced by the hysterosalpingogram since this test provides more complete and reliable information.

Contraindications:

- Pelvic or vaginal infection
- Uterine bleeding
- Spontaneous abortion in the past two months
- Pregnancy

## SCHILLER'S TEST

Schiller's test is done to aid in the identification of suspicious areas of tissue in the cervix and vagina. The cervix and vagina are painted with a solution of iodine and potassium iodide (Shiller's or Lugol's solution). Normal squamous epithelium contains glycogen, which absorbs the iodine solution and turns the epithelium a deep mahogany color. Those areas that are nonstaining contain no glycogen, indicating abnormal epithelium and constituting a positive Schiller's test.

*Note:* The squamocolumnar junction should be identified if possible before interpreting the results. Columnar epithelium does not stain with Schiller's solution, and if ectopy exists, no staining will occur in this area. This may be a variation of normal.

Schiller's test is not diagnostic of malignancy but reveals nonstaining areas where biopsy should be directed.

## SHAKE TEST (RAPID SURFACTANT TEST)

The shake test is a qualitative measurement of the amount of pulmonary surfactant contained in the amniotic fluid. The advantage of this functional test over the L/S ratio is that it can be performed easily by a physician or technician and its results are highly reliable. The amniotic fluid specimen is centrifuged, 95% ethanol is added, and the specimen is shaken for 15 seconds. A ring of bubbles around the meniscus at 15 minutes is a positive test result, meaning that the fetal lungs are mature. A dilutional table is available from which determination can be made of the various stages of lung maturity.

## THERMOGRAPHY

Thermography is used to diagnose abnormalities of the breast by detection of "hot spots." Special heat sensors are used, which translate hot areas of the breast into a photographic image. Benign, as well as malignant lesions, may be associated with increased heat in the tissue. Therefore, an identified "hot spot" may not be specifically diagnostic of malignancy. However, thermography does have advantages over other methods because the patient is not exposed to radiation, and the test may reveal lesions not detected by other means. A hot thermogram indicates the need for further investigation and also serves as a baseline for comparison of future thermograms. (The NIH in its guidelines for breast screening has stated that thermography should not be used.)

## ULTRASONOGRAPHY

Ultrasonography is a scanning procedure that uses sound waves to display two-dimensional echo images of the area under examination. A simple procedure, it causes no discomfort to the patient and does not expose her to radiation.

Indications:

- Pregnancy (intrauterine or ectopic, fetal age, placental localization, fetal size and position, anomalies, hydramnios, multiple pregnancies)
- Ovarian cysts
- Hydatidiform mole
- Ascites
- Lost or misplaced IUD

The real-time gray-scale B-scanner is the latest ultrasound device, which in addition to image detail, shows fetal movements in utero. The B-scan can demonstrate a gestational sac as early as five weeks after the last menstrual period (LMP). By the ninth week (LMP), the placenta can be identified, and by the fourteenth week the fetal head is identifiable.

At this time understanding of tissue effects of ultrasound is incomplete. Thus, prudent use of the Doppler for picking up fetal heart tones and limited use of ultrasonography whenever possible during the first trimester seems well advised.

Instructions to the patient before sonography:

- Urinate one hour before the test is to be performed, do not urinate again until the test is completed.
- Drink 16 oz (two glasses) of clear fluid (no milk).
- The test will take 30-60 minutes and causes no discomfort except possible feelings of urgency from pressure on the bladder.

## VESICLE NECK ELEVATION TEST

The vesicle neck elevation test may be performed as one measure of clinical evaluation of stress incontinence. The patient, with a full bladder, is placed in the lithotomy position (as for a pelvic examination) and is asked to cough. The strain of the cough will produce a spurt of urine from the urethra in a patient with stress incontinence. The examiner then places an index and middle finger into the vagina on either side of the urethra, with the fingertips at the base of the bladder, and exerts upward pressure. If a strong cough by the patient does not produce urine leakage, it is likely that stress incontinence is the diagnosis. This maneuver temporarily restores the posterior vesicourethral angle, which will control urine leakage.

## XEROMAMMOGRAPHY OR XEROGRAPHY

Xeromammography is a soft tissue x-ray and is a variation of mammography. A charged selenium plate is used with the image of the breast projected on paper instead of on film. The exposure to rads is similar to that of mammography (2 rads when both breasts are examined). The use of either technique depends on the preference of the radiologist. Some mammographers feel that microcalcifications are better detected on the xerox plate, while masses are better detected on the film mammography. This method of breast screening is currently being refined, and in the future may become a more utilized diagnostic form for breast screening.

## NORMAL LABORATORY VALUES

Depending on the methods and equipment used to obtain data, laboratory values differ from one institution to another. The following laboratory values were drawn from current sources and were not intended to replace those of the laboratory used by your setting.

See *Blood Chemistry Values* on pages 375-381.

## REFERENCES

Barber H, Fields D, Daugman S: *Quick Reference to OB-GYN Procedures,* ed 2. Philadelphia, JB Lippincott Co, 1979, p 6.

Bibbo M: Screening of individuals exposed to diethylstilbestrol. *Clin Obstet Gynecol* 22:689, 1979.

Culleton B: Mammography controversy: NIH's entry into evaluating technology. *Science* 198:171, 1977.

Elstein M: The cervix and its mucus. *Clinics in Obstet Gynecol* 1:353, 1974.

Evertson L, Gauthier R, and Collea J: Fetal demise following negative contraction stress test. *Obstet Gynecol* 51:671, 1978.

Gorringe R, Lee M, Voda A: The mammography controversy a case for breast self-examination. *JOGN Nursing* 7:7, 1978.

Green T: *Gynecology Essentials of Clinical Practice,* ed 3. Boston, Little, Brown and Company, 1977, p 17.

Kaufman R, Strama T: Two sophisticated therapeutic weapons; the cryoprobe and the laser. *Contemp Obstet Gynecol* 14:83, 1979.

Kolstad P, Stafl A: *Atlas of Colposcopy.* Baltimore, University Park Press, 1972, p 13.

Marchant D: Laboratory values and diagnostic tests. *Clin Obstet Gynecol* 21: 937, 1979.

McQyarrie H: Commercial diagnostic tests for office use. *Contemp Obstet Gynecol* 14:39, 1979.

Ott W: Antepartum biophysical evaluation of the fetus. *Perinatology–Neonatality* 2:11, 1978.

Ozenberger J: Uses of cryosurgery part 2: Dermatology, gynecology and other specialties. *The Female Patient* 4:39, 1979.

Pfeffer W, Wallach E: When tubal factors cause infertility. *Contemp Obstet Gynec* 15:133, 1980.

Speroff, Glass R, Kase N: *Clinical Gynecologic Endocrinology and Infertility.* Baltimore, Williams & Wilkins Company, 1978, p 399.

Strax P: Breast cancer diagnosis: mammography, thermography, xerography, a commentary. *J Reprod Med* 14:265, 1975.

Wallach J: *Interpretation of Diagnostic Tests.* ed 3. Boston, Little, Brown and Company, 1978, p 9.

Blood Chemistry Values

| Test | Nonpregnant | Pregnant |
|---|---|---|
| Albumin (g/dl) | 3.5-5.0 | |
| Alkaline phosphatase (IU/liter) | 23-71 | 80 (≤350 IU in some) |
| Beta-hCG (mIU) | Not detectable in nonpregnant females: values > 5 may reflect cross-reaction with high LH | |
| Bicarbonate, serum (mEq/liter) | 23.2-24 | 20.5-26 |
| Bilirubin, total (mg/dl) | 0.3-1.5 | .03-1.0 |
| BUN (mg/dl) | 10-20 | Decreased |
| Calcium (mEq/liter) | 4.7-4.9 | 4.15-5.05 |
| Chloride (mEq/liter) | 102.7-107 | 98-108 |
| Cholesterol, total (mg/dl) | 130-220 | 243-305 |
| Creatinine (mg/dl) | 0.8-1.4 | 0.9-2.0 |
| Estradiol | | |
| Follicular phase (pg/ml) | 25-75 | |
| Midcycle peak (pg/ml) | 200-600 | |
| Luteal phase (pg/ml) | 100-300 | |
| Pregnancy, first trimester (ng/ml) | | 1-5 |
| second trimester (ng/ml) | | 5-15 |
| third trimester (ng/ml) | | 10-40 |
| Estriol (ng/ml) | | Week |
| | | 25   3.5-10.0 |
| | | 28   4.0-12.5 |
| | | 30   4.5-14.0 |
| | | 32   5.0-16.0 |
| | | 34   5.5-18.5 |
| | | 35   6.0-21.0 |
| | | 36   7.0-2.5.0 |

Blood Chemistry Values *(continued)*

| Test | Nonpregnant | Pregnant |
|---|---|---|
| Follicle-stimulating hormone (FSH) (mIU/ml) Increases twofold at midcycle ovulatory peak | 5–30 | |
| Leuteinizing hormone (LH) (mIU/ml) Increases threefold at midcycle ovulatory peak | 5–20 | |
| Folic acid (ng/ml) | 5–20 | 4.5–20 |
| Glucose-6-phosphate dehydrogenase (G-6-PD) (IU/g hemoglobin) | 4–8 | |
| Glucose, fasting (mg/dl) | 71.5 ± 8.5 | 77.2 ± 7.2 |
| Hemoglobin $A_2$ electrophoresis (% of total hemoglobin) | < 3.9% | |
| Hemoglobin F (alkali denaturation test) (% of total hemoglobin) | < 2% | |

| | | Week | |
|---|---|---|---|
| | | 37 | 8.0–28.0 |
| | | 38 | 9.0–32.0 |
| | | 39 | 10.0–43.0 |
| | | 40 | 10.5–25.0 |
| | | 41 | 10.5–25.0 |

| Human placental lactogen (µg/ml) | | Week | |
|---|---|---|---|
| | | 28 | 2.5–5.5 |
| | | 30 | 2.8–6.5 |
| | | 34 | 3.5–8.0 |
| | | 36 | 3.6–8.5 |
| | | 40 | 3.6–9.5 |
| | | 42 | 3.6–9.5 |

| | | |
|---|---|---|
| Immunoglobulin A (IgA) (mg/dl) | 80–350 | |
| Immunoglobulin G (IgG) (mg/dl) | 875–2,020 | |
| Immunoglobulin M (IgM) (mg/dl) | 40–275 | |
| Iron (μg/dl) | 55–200 | Decreased |
| TIBC (μg/dl) | 250–400 | 300–450 |
| Lactate dehydrogenase (LDH) (units/ml) | 244 ± 11.9 | 234.9 ± 67 |
| Lactic acid (mg/dl) | 5–18 | |
| Lecithin/sphingomyelin ratio | | Immature: 1.0–1.4 |
| | | Transitional: 1.5–1.9 |
| | | Mature: > 2.0 |
| Magnesium (mg/dl) | 1.7–2.7 | |
| Nonprotein nitrogen (NPN) (mg/dl) | 25–40 | |
| Phosphorus (mg/dl) | 2.5–4.5 | |
| Potassium (mEq/dl) | 3.5–5.3 | |
| Progesterone | | |
| Follicular Phase (ng/ml) | <1 | |
| Luteal phase (ng/ml) | 5–20 | |
| Pregnancy, first trimester (ng/ml) | | 20–30 |
| second trimester (ng/ml) | | 50–100 |
| third trimester (ng/ml) | | 100–4000 |
| Prolactin (ng/ml) | 6–8 | 200 at term |
| Protein (gm/dl) | | |
| SGOT (units/ml) | 15.2 ± 1 | 15.8 ± 8.14 |
| SGPT (units/ml) | 17.2 ± 5.7 | 13.0 ± 7.3 |
| SMA 12/6 | | |
| Protein (g/dl) | 6.0–8.0 | |
| Albumin (g/dl) | 3.5–5.0 | |
| Calcium (mg/dl) | 8.5–10.5 | |
| Cholesterol (mg/dl) | 150–300 | |
| Glucose (mg/dl) | 65–110 | |

Blood Chemistry Values (continued)

| Test | Nonpregnant | Pregnant |
|---|---|---|
| Bun (mg/dl) | 10–20 | |
| Uric Acid (mg/dl) | 2.5–8.0 | |
| Creatinine (mg/dl) | 0.7–1.4 | |
| Total Bilirubin (mg/dl) | 0.1–1.0 | |
| Alkaline phosphatase (IU/liter) | 23–71 | |
| LDH (IU/liter) | 52–149 | |
| SGOT (IU/liter) | 7–26 | |
| Sodium (mEq/liter) | 137–142 | 132.5–143 |
| $T_3$ (RIA) (ng/dl) | 100–200 | |
| $T_3$ Uptake (RT3u) (%) | 24–35 | Decreased |
| $T_4$ (D) (µg/dl) | 5.3–14.5 | Increased |
| Testosterone | | |
| Follicular phase (ng/ml) | 0.2–0.8 | |
| Midcycle peak (ng/ml) | 0.2–0.8 | |
| Luteal phase (ng/ml) | 0.2–0.8 | |
| Triglycerides (mg/100 ml) | | |
| Years | | |
| 1–19 | 10–140 | |
| 20–29 | 10–140 | |
| 30–39 | 10–150 | |
| 40–49 | 10–160 | |
| 50–59 | 10–190 | |
| Urea nitrogen (mg/dl) | 10–20 | Decreased |
| Uric acid (mg/dl) | 2.5–7.0 | Increased |
| Vitamin $B_{12}$ (pg/ml) | 160–880 | |

Hematologic Values

| Test | Nonpregnant | Pregnant |
|---|---|---|
| Bleeding time (Ivy) (minutes) | 2–9 | |
| Blood volume (total ml/kg body wt) | 3,573–3,991 | 4,946–5,346 |
| Fribrinogen (mg/100ml) | 200–450 | Increased |
| Hematocrit (%) | 35.1–46.3 | 28.6–38.4 |
| Hemoglobin (mg/dl) | 11.5–16.0 | 11.2–15.0 |
| Indices | | |
| MCV (Hct/RBC) (fl) | 82–100 | |
| MCH (Hgb/RBC) (pg) | 27–32 | |
| MCHC (Hgb/Hct) (%) | 31–35 | |
| Platelets (cu mm) | 140,000–450,000 | |
| Prothrombin time (seconds) | 100% / 11–12 | |
| Red blood cell count (RBC) (cu mm) | 4,000,000–5,000,000 | Increased |
| Reticulocytes (%) | 0.5–1.5 | |
| Sedimentation rate (mm/hr) | 0–15 | |
| White blood count (cu mm) | 5,000–10,000 | |

Serology Values

| Test | Nonpregnant | Pregnant |
|---|---|---|
| Anti-nuclear IgG (ANA) | < 1:10 | |
| Cold agglutinin | < 1:80 | |
| Rhematoid RA | < 1:40 | |
| Rubella HAI | < 1:8 = negative | |

Urine Values *(continued)*

| Test | Nonprgenant | Pregnant |
|---|---|---|
| Acetone | Negative | Negative |
| Albumin (protein) (qualitative) | Negative | Negative |
|  |  | < 100 mg |
| Bilirubin (qualitative) | Negative | Negative |
| Calcium (mg/24 hr) | 100-300 |  |
| Chloride (mEq/24 hr) | 170-250 |  |
| Creatinine (g/24 hr) | 1.0-1.8 |  |
| Estriol, placental (mg/24 hr) |  | Slight elevation Elevated 3-40 (depending on week of gestation) |
| Estrogen (total urinary) |  |  |
| Prepubertal (µg/24 hrs | 0-5 |  |
| Follicular phase (µg/24 hrs) | 10-25 |  |
| Midcycle peak (µg/24 hrs) | 35-100 |  |
| Luteal phase (µg/24 hrs) | 25-75 |  |
| Postmenopausal (µg/24 hrs) | 5-15 |  |
| Glucose (mg) | 120 |  |
| Human chorionic gonadotropin (hCG) (IU/liter) (placenta) peaks at 10 wks gestation declines and remains at lower level after 12-14 weeks gestation |  | 100,000 20,000 |
| 17-Ketosteroids (Zimmerman) (mg/24 hr) | 7-20 |  |
| Magnesium (mg/24 hr) | 15-300 |  |
| Pregnanediol |  |  |
| Follicular phase (mg/24 hr) | <1 |  |
| Luteal phase (mg/24 hr) | 2-5 |  |

| | |
|---|---|
| Pregnancy, 20 weeks (mg/24 hr) | 40 |
| 30 weeks (mg/24 hr) | 80 |
| 40 weeks (mg/24 hr) | 100 |
| Phosphorus (g/24 hr) | 1.1 (approx.) |
| Potassium (mEq/24 hr) | 40–65 |
| Protein (mg/24 hr) | <100 |
| Specific gravity | 1.015–1.025 |
| Sodium (mEq/24 hr) | 130–200 |
| Urea nitrogen (g/24 hr) | 10 (approx.) |
| Uric acid (mg/24 hr) | 300–900 |
| Urobilinogen (mg/24 hr) | 0–4 |
| Volume (ml/24 hr) | 600–1,600 |
| | 800–2,000 |

# Index

Abdominal pregnancy, 36
Abortion: inevitable, 29, 30, 32
  missed, 29, 30, 31, 33
  septic, diagnosis of, 188
  spontaneous, 28-34
    complete, 29, 30, 31, 33
    diagnosis of, 31, 37
    in incompetent cervix, 34
    incomplete, 29, 30, 32
  therapeutic: in beta-thalassemia minor, 83, 84
    laminaria in, 362
  threatened, 29, 30, 32
    diagnosis of, 41
Abruptio placenta, 49-54
  diagnosis of, 46, 51-52, 86
Abscess, 152, 193
Acidophilus tablets, in candidiasis of vagina, 133
Aci-Jel Therapeutic Vaginal Jelly: in candidiasis, 133
  in cervicitis, 160
  in trichomoniasis, 137
Acne rosacea, in menopause, 332
Adenitis, Bartholin, 150-152
Adenomyosis uteri, 226, 227, 282
Adenosis: diagnosis of, 274
  from diethylstilbestrol exposure in utero, 267-277
Adhesions, pelvic, diagnosis of, 119, 163, 237
Adrenal disorders: diagnosis of, 299
  and dysfunctional uterine bleeding, 221
Age: and breast cancer, 242
  and dysfunctional uterine bleeding, 219
  and fibroadenoma of breast, 250
  and fibrocystic breast disease, 244
  and hydatidiform mole, 40
  and hypertension, 69
  and intraductal papillomas of breast, 248
  and osteoporosis, 334
  and placenta previa, 45
  and premenstrual syndrome, 229
  and prolonged pregnancy, 106
  and vaginal infections, 130
Alcohol ingestion, and intrauterine growth retardation, 92
Aldosterone levels, in premenstrual syndrome, 230
Allergic reactions: and candidiasis of vagina, 131
  diagnosis of, 156, 165, 171
  and pruritus vulvae, 146
Altitude, and intrauterine growth retardation, 92
Amenorrhea, 212-219
  diagnosis in, 214
  progesterone withdrawal test in, 369-370
Amniocentesis, 349-350
  in beta-thalassemia minor, 82-83
  for lecithin-sphingomyelin ratio, 363
  in postdates pregnancy, 109
Amnioscopy, in postdates pregnancy, 109
Amniotic fluid: lecithin-sphingomyelin ratio, 363-364
  shake test of, 371
Ampicillin: in cystitis, 261
  in gonorrhea, 185
  in pelvic inflammatory disease, 189
  in pyelonephritis, 87, 265

# INDEX

Anemia in pregnancy, 75-84
 beta-thalassemia minor, 80-84
 Cooley's, 83
 iron-deficiency, 75-80. *See also* Iron
 sideroblastic, diagnosis of, 77
Anorexia nervosa, amenorrhea in, 214
Anovulation, and dysfunctional uterine bleeding, 219-220
Antibiotics: and candidiasis of vagina, 131
 in cervicitis, 160
 in chlamydiosis, 178
 in cystitis, 261
 in endometritis, 163
 in gonorrhea, 181, 184-185
 in granuloma inguinale, 205
 in *Hemophilus* vaginitis, 140
 in lymphogranuloma venereum, 209
 in pelvic inflammatory disease, 189, 192
 in postpartum mastitis, 123
 in pyelonephritis, 87, 265
 in subinvolution of uterus, 120
 in syphilis, 197-198
 and vaginal flora changes, 130
Appendicitis, diagnosis of, 37, 86, 187, 192, 237, 265
Arborization of cervical mucus, 359
Arias-Stella phenomenon, in ectopic pregnancy, 35
Asherman's syndrome: amenorrhea in, 218
 dysfunctional uterine bleeding in, 221
Aspirin: in dysmenorrhea, 226
 in endometriosis, 238
 in herpes genitalis, 172
Atrophic vaginitis, 142-145, 326
 diagnosis of, 143, 340
 and postmenopausal bleeding, 341

Backache: in cystocele, 315
 in follicular cysts of ovary, 287
 in osteoporosis, 336
 in prolapse of uterus, 311
 in pyelonephritis, 264
Bacteriuria: asymptomatic, in pregnancy, 85-88
 in recurrent urinary tract infections, 263-264
 and sexual intercourse, 262-263
Bartholinitis, 150-152
Bed rest: in cervicitis, 160
 in endometritis, 163, 164
 in gonorrhea, 181, 184
 in threatened abortion, 32
*Bedsonia*, see Chlamydial infection
Benzyl benzoate ointment, in scabies, 168
Biopsy, 351-353

 cervical, 351-352
 cone, 356-357
 endometrial, 352-353
 in menopause, 327, 329, 330
Bladder: changes in pregnancy, 13
 cystitis, 258-262
 in pregnancy, 85-88
 cystocele, 314-317
 disorders with urinary stress incontinence, 307, 308
 vesical neck elevation test, 372
Bleeding disorders: postmenopausal, 339-342
 in pregnancy, 28-56
Blood: chemistry values, 375-378
 flow in pregnancy: peripheral, 12
 renal, 14
 uterine, 11
 stasis in lower extremities, in pregnancy, 12, 24
 volume in pregnancy, 10
Blood pressure, in pregnancy, 12
 hypertension, 59-73
 hypotension, supine, 12, 22, 23
Bloody show, diagnosis of, 51
Bone loss, in osteoporosis, 334-338
Brain-sparing syndrome, fetal, 91, 94
Breast: cancer of, 242-244, 245
 diagnosis of, 246, 251, 253
 and screening of DES-exposed mothers, 276-277
 fat necrosis of, 245, 254
 diagnosis of, 246, 251, 253
 fibroadenoma of, 245, 250-252
 fibrocystic disease of, 244-248, 251
 graphic stress telethermometry of, 361
 intraductal papilloma of, 245, 248-250
 mammary duct ectasia in, 245, 252-254
 mammography of, 277, 364
 postpartum mastitis of, 121-125
 thermography of, 371
 xeromammography of, 373
Breastfeeding, care of breasts, 124-125
Bubo formation, in chancroid, 201
Buccal smear, 354
Burow's solution, in herpes genitalis, 172

Calcium balance, in osteoporosis, 335
Calcium carbonate, in osteoporosis, 337
Candidiasis of vagina, 130-134
 diagnosis of, 132, 156
 in molluscum contagiosum, 154
Carcinoma: of breast, 242-244, 245
 diagnosis of, 246, 251, 253

screening of DES-exposed mothers, 276-277
cervical, diagnosis of, 159, 177
after diethylstilbestrol exposure in utero, 273
Cardiac output, in pregnancy, 10-11
Cardiovascular system, in pregnancy, 10-13
Caries, dental, in pregnancy, 16
Cellulitis, in endometritis, 164
Cephalexin, in *Hemophilus* vaginitis, 140
Cervicitis, 158-161
 atrophic, diagnosis of, 143
 diagnosis of, 31, 46, 51, 86, 132, 136, 139, 159, 171, 183, 259
Cervix uteri: biopsy of, 351-352
 carcinoma of, diagnosis of, 159, 177
 changes from diethylstilbestrol exposure in utero, 267-277
 chlamydiosis of, 176-179
 conization of, 356-357
 fern test of mucus, 359
 incompetent, 34
 Papanicolaou smear, 171, 367-369
 papilloma of, 270
 polyps of, 277-280
  diagnosis of, 46, 51, 278, 340
 pregnancy in, 36
 smears on Thayer-Martin or Transgrow transport medium, 184
Cesarean section, and subinvolution of uterus, 119
Chancre, syphilitic, 194
 diagnosis of, 154
Chancroid, 200-203
 diagnosis of, 159, 177, 196, 202, 205, 208
Chiari-Frommel syndrome, amenorrhea in, 214
Chlamydial infection: cervical chlamydiosis, 176-179
 diagnosis of, 159
 and lymphogranuloma venereum, 206
Chocolate cysts of ovary, 296
Cholecystitis, diagnosis of, 86, 188
Cholestasis, in pregnancy, 16
Choriocarcinoma, 43-44
Chorionic gonadotropin, human: influences in pregnancy, 7
 secretion in amenorrhea, 217
 serum levels in hydatidiform mole, 42-43
 therapy in polycystic ovary syndrome, 300
Chorionic somatomammotropin, human, 8-9
Circulation in pregnancy: peripheral, 12
 renal, 14
 uterine, 11
Climacteric, 323. *See also* Menopause
Clomiphene citrate, in polycystic ovary syndrome, 300
Clotrimazole: in candidiasis of vagina, 133
 in tinea cruris, 156-157
Coagulation, disseminated intravascular, in abruptio placenta, 50
Colposcopy, 355-356
Colpotomy, 356
Condylomata: acuminata, 174-176
 lata, 195
Cone biopsy, 356-357
Constipation: in pregnancy, 15, 16, 20
 in rectocele, 318
Contraceptives, oral: and amenorrhea, 214
 and candidiasis of vagina, 131
 cervical polyps from, 278
 and chlamydiosis, 177
 contraindications to, 331
 in corpus luteum cysts, 289
 in dysfunctional uterine bleeding, 222, 223
 in dysmenorrhea, 227
 in endometriosis, 238-239
 in follicular cysts, 287
 in premenstrual syndrome, 232
 and urinary tract infections, 256
 and vaginal infections, 130
Contraction stress test, 366-367
 in intrauterine growth retardation, 95
 in postdates pregnancy, 108, 109
Convulsions, in eclampsia, 60, 63
Cooley's anemia, 83
Corpus luteum cysts, 288-289
Corticosteroid therapy, in pelvic inflammatory disease, 192
Couvelaire uterus, 50
Crab lice, 164-167
Cramps: leg, in pregnancy, 21
 menstrual, 224-228
Cryosurgery, 357
Culdocentesis, 357
Culdoscopy, 358
Culdotomy, 356
Cushing's syndrome, diagnosis of, 299, 336
Cystadenoma of ovary: mucinous, 294-295
 serous, 293-294
Cystitis, 258-262
 diagnosis of, 119, 163, 259, 265
 honeymoon, 262-263
 in pregnancy, 85-88
Cystocele, 314-317
 diagnosis of, 259, 315
Cysts: in bartholinitis, 150

fibrocystic breast disease, 244-248
of Gartner's duct, 269, 315
inclusion, vaginal, 270
nabothian, 270-271
ovarian, 285-301. *See also* Ovary, cysts of
sebaceous, 151, 269

Danocrine, in endometriosis, 239
Death, fetal: in abruptio placenta, 53, 54
counseling for grieving, 54-56
and spontaneous abortion, 28, 32
Dermatitis, contact: diagnosis of, 156
pruritus vulvae in, 146
Dermoid cyst of ovary, 291-292
Detrusor dyssynergia, and urinary incontinence, 308
Diabetes mellitus: and candidiasis of vagina, 131
and folliculitis of genital region, 148
and glucose tolerance tests, 360-361
and hypertension, 69
maternal: complications of, 102
and intrauterine growth retardation, 92
signs of, 99
uterine size in, 98
of pregnancy onset, 111-116
Diagnostic procedures, 349-373
Diaphragm, changes in pregnancy, 10, 17
Dienestrol cream: in atrophic vaginitis, 341
in menopause, 331
in urethral prolapse, 343
Diethylstilbestrol: in atrophic vaginitis, 145
exposure in utero, vaginal and cervical changes from, 267-277
in menopause, 330
in postmenopausal bleeding, 341
Dilatation and curettage: in cervical polyps, 279
in dysfunctional uterine bleeding, 222
in endometritis, 163
in leiomyoma of uterus, 284
perimenopausal, 328, 330
in postmenopausal bleeding, 340
Discharge, vaginal: in adenosis after DES exposure, 273
in cervical polyps, 278
in cystitis, 259
in *Hemophilus* vaginitis, 139
in pregnancy, 26
in pyelonephritis, 264
in trichomoniasis, 135
*see also* Leukorrhea
Diuretics: in hypertension, 71
in premenstrual syndrome, 232

Diverticulitis, diagnosis of, 187, 192, 237, 265
Dizziness, in pregnancy, 23
*Donovania granulomatis*, 204
Douching: povidone-iodine: in candidiasis of vagina, 133
in *Hemophilus* vaginitis, 141
in trichomoniasis, 137
vinegar: after polypectomy, 280
in candidiasis of vagina, 133
in *Hemophilus* vaginitis, 141
in trichomoniasis, 138
Drug ingestion: and dysfunctional uterine bleeding, 221
maternal: and diethylstilbestrol exposure in utero, 267-277
and intrauterine growth retardation, 92
and pruritus vulvae, 146
Dysmaturity syndrome, fetal, 106
Dysmenorrhea, 224-228
in cervicitis, 158
diagnosis in, 226, 231, 237
in endometriosis, 226, 236
in endometritis, 162
Dyspareunia: in adenosis after DES exposure, 273
in atrophic vaginitis, 143
in candidiasis of vagina, 131
in cervicitis, 158
in condylomata acuminata, 174
in cystitis, 259
in endometriosis, 236
in herpes genitalis, 170
in ovarian cysts, 287
in prolapse of uterus, 311
in trichomoniasis, 135
Dyspnea, in pregnancy, 17, 22

Eclampsia, 60
symptoms of, 61, 62-63, 64
Ectopic pregnancy, 34-39
diagnosis of, 31, 37, 188, 192, 237, 265, 282
Eczema marginatum, of vulva, 155-157
Edema: in pre-eclampsia, 59, 61, 62
in pregnancy, 14, 25-26
in premenstrual syndrome, 231
Endometrial biopsy, 352-353
in menopause, 327, 329, 330
Endometrioma of ovary, 296-297
Endometriosis, 235-241
diagnosis of, 188, 192, 237
dysmenorrhea in, 226, 236
Endometritis, 161-164
subinvolution of uterus, 119

Enterocele, diagnosis of, 315, 318
Epulis, 16
Ergot preparations, in subinvolution of uterus, 120
Erythroblastosis fetalis, 101, 102
Erythrocyte changes, in pregnancy, 11
Erythromycin, in syphilis, 198
*Escherichia coli*: and cystitis, 258
  and pyelonephritis, 264
Estriol levels in urine, 359
  in pregnancy, 358-359
  and fetal well-being, 94
  in postdates pregnancy, 108-109
Estrogen: deficiency of, and atrophic vaginitis, 142
  influences in pregnancy, 4-5
  secretion in menopause, 324
  serum levels of: and maturation index, 365
    in premenstrual syndrome, 230
  therapy with: in atrophic vaginitis, 144-145, 341
    contraindications to, 328-329
    in cystocele, 316
    and growth of uterine leiomyoma, 280
    in menopause, 328-331
    in osteoporosis, 337
    and postmenopausal bleeding, 339
    in urethral prolapse, 343
    in uterine prolapse, 313
  withdrawal bleeding in amenorrhea, 216

Fallopian tubes: pregnancy in, 35
  Rubin test of patency, 370
Fatigue, in pregnancy, 27
Fat necrosis of breast, 245, 254
  diagnosis of, 246, 251, 253
Feminization, testicular, amenorrhea in, 218
Fern test of cervical mucus, 359
Fetus: anomalies, intrauterine growth retardation, 92
  brain-sparing syndrome in, 91, 94
  head measurements in, 94
  postmaturity (dysmaturity) syndrome, 106
  small-for-gestational age, 90-91
Fibroadenoma of breast, 245, 250-252
Fibrocystic breast disease, 244-248
  diagnosis of, 246, 251
Fibroma: labial, 268
  of uterus, *see* Leiomyoma of uterus
Fitz-Hugh-Curtis syndrome, 190
Flatulence, in pregnancy, 21

Floraquin Vaginal Suppositories, in trichomoniasis, 137
Fluorescent antibody test, 360
Fluorescent treponemal antibody absorption test, 196
Follicle-stimulating hormone levels: in amenorrhea, 217
  in polycystic ovary syndrome, 298, 300
Follicular cysts, ovarian, 286-287
Folliculitis, genital, 147-149
  diagnosis of, 154
Foreign body, vaginal, diagnosis of, 132, 139
Fox-Fordyce disease, 146
Fractures, in osteoporosis, 335
Frei test, 208
Fungus infection of vulva, 155-157
Furunculosis, genital, 147-149

Gartner duct cyst, 269
  diagnosis of, 315
Gastrointestinal tract, in pregnancy, 15-16
Gentipax tampons, in candidiasis of vagina, 133
Glucose: serum levels in diabetes of pregnancy onset, 113-114
  tolerance test: in menopause, 328
    in pregnancy, 114, 360-361
Glycosuria: diagnosis of, 165
  in pregnancy, 113
  renal, diagnosis of, 113
Gonadal agenesis or dysgenesis: amenorrhea in, 218
  and dysfunctional uterine bleeding, 221
Gonadotropin: chorionic, *see* Chorionic gonadotropin
  human menopausal, 300
Gonorrhea, 179-186
  acute lower tract infection in, 182-186
  bartholinitis in, 150
  cervicitis in, 158
  diagnosis of, 159, 177, 196
  endometritis in, 161
  and penicillinase-producing *Neisseria gonorrhoeae*, 180-181, 186
  salpingitis in, 187-190
Granuloma: inguinale, 203-206
  diagnosis of, 205, 208
  venereum, diagnosis of, 159, 177
Grief and grieving, counseling guide for, 54-56
Griseofulvin, in tinea cruris, 157
Growth hormone, and growth of uterine leiomyoma, 281
Growth retardation, intrauterine, 90-97

diagnosis of, 93

Hair, genital: follicle infection, 147-149
  parasitic infestation of, 164-167
Head, fetal, measurements of, 94
Headache, in pregnancy, 24
Heart: changes in pregnancy, 10-11
  cyanotic disease, and intrauterine growth retardation, 92
Heartburn, in pregnancy, 75-76
Hematologic values, 379
Hemoglobin, 376
  in anemia, 75
  in beta-thalassemia minor, 82
Hemolytic disease, fetal, 101
*Hemophilus: ducreyi*, 201
  vaginitis, 138-142
Hemorrhoids: in postmenopausal bleeding, 339
  in pregnancy, 15, 25
  and pruritus vulvae, 146
  in rectocele, 318
Herpes genitalis, 169-173
Herpes zoster, diagnosis of, 171
Herpes virus infections, diagnosis of, 154, 159, 177, 195
Hidradenoma of vulva, 268
Hirsutism, in polycystic ovary syndrome, 299
Hormonal influences in pregnancy, 4-9
Hot flashes, in menopause, 326
Hydatidiform mole, 40-44
  diagnosis of, 31, 41
  uterine size in, 98
Hydramnios: complications of, 102
  management of, 101
  signs of, 99
Hydrocephalus, fetal: complications of, 103
  management of, 101
  signs of, 99
  uterine size in, 98
Hydrosalpinx, 193
hygiene practices, poor: and candidiasis of vagina, 131
  and pediculosis pubis, 165
  and pruritus vulvae, 146
  and urinary tract infections, 256
Hyperemesis gravidarum, diagnosis of, 41
Hypertension, 59-73
  essential, pregnancy with, 68-73
    diagnosis of, 64, 70
  pregnancy-induced, 59-68
    and abruptio placenta, 50
    diagnosis of, 64

  and intrauterine growth retardation, 91-92
Hyperventilation, in pregnancy, 17, 23
Hypochromia: in alpha-thalassemia minor, 82
  in beta-thalassemia minor, 81
  in iron-deficiency anemia, 77
Hypoglycemia, and premenstrual syndrome, 230
Hypoparathyroidism, and candidiasis of vagina, 131
Hypotension, supine, 12, 22, 23
Hypothalamic disorders, diagnosis of, 299
Hysterectomy: in endometrioma of ovary, 297
  in leiomyoma of uterus, 284
  in mucinous cystadenoma of ovary, 295
  in serous cystadenoma of ovary, 294
Hysterosalpingogram, 361-362

Ibuprofen, in dysmenorrhea, 227
Impetigo, diagnosis of, 148, 168
Inclusion cyst, vaginal, 270
Incompetent cervix, 34
Incontinence, urinary, 304-310
  diagnosis of, 307-308
Indomethacin, in dysmenorrhea, 227
Infections: chronic, hypochromic anemia in, 77, 82
  gynecologic, 129-210
  sexually transmitted, 169-182, 193-210
  urinary tract, 256-266
    in pregnancy, 85-89
  vaginal, 129-145
  vulvar, 145-157
Infertility: in adenosis from DES exposure, 275
  in cervicitis, 160
  in endometriosis, 236
  in endometritis, 162
  in leiomyoma of uterus, 282
  in pelvic inflammatory disease, 191, 192
  in polycystic ovary syndrome, 301
Insect bites, diagnosis of, 148, 168
Insomnia, 26-27
Intertrigo, 268
Intrauterine contraceptive device, and endometritis, 162
Involution of uterus, 118
  subinvolution, 118-121
Iron: deficiency of: diagnosis of, 77, 81
  in endometritis, 163
  in pregnancy, 75-80
  and pruritus vulvae, 146
  requirements in pregnancy, 11, 76

# INDEX

Kegel exercises, 320-321
  in cystocele, 316
  in menopause, 334
  in rectocele, 319
  in urinary stress incontinence, 309, 310
Kidney: function in pregnancy, 13-15
  pyelonephritis, 264-266
  in pregnancy, 85-88
Kwell: in pediculosis pubis, 166
  in scabies, 168

Laboratory values, 375-381
Lactogen, human placental, 376
  influences in pregnancy, 8-9
Laminaria use, 362
Laparoscopy, 362-363
Lecithin-sphingomyelin ratio, in amniotic fluid, 363-364
Le Fort operation, in prolapse of uterus, 313
Leg cramps, in pregnancy, 21
Leiomyoma of uterus: diagnosis of, 237, 282
  in pregnancy: management of, 101
  size of uterus in, 98, 99
  and subinvolution of uterus, 119
Leukorrhea: in candidiasis of vagina, 131
  in cervical polyps, 278
  in cervicitis, 158
  in *Hemophilus* vaginitis, 139
  in herpes genitalis, 170
  in trichomoniasis, 135
Lice, 164-167
Lichen planus, 168
Lie of fetus, transverse, 93
Lordosis, in pregnancy, 18, 23
Luteal cysts, 288-289
Luteinizing hormone levels: in amenorrhea, 217
  in polycystic ovary syndrome, 298, 300
Lymphogranuloma venereum, 206-210
  diagnosis of, 196, 205, 208
Lysine therapy, in herpes genitalis, 172

McDonald operation, in cervical incompetence, 34
Macrosomia, fetal, 106
Magnesium sulfate, as anticonvulsant, 66
Malignancies: diagnosis of, 31, 46, 119, 143, 151, 163, 196, 282
  and hydatidiform mole, 43-44
Mammography, 364
  in screening of DES-exposed mothers, 277
  xeromammography, 373

Manchester-Fothergill operation, in prolapse of uterus, 313
Mastitis: chronic cystic, 244-248
  postpartum, 121-125
  diagnosis of, 123
  epidemic, 121, 123, 124
  sporadic, 121-122, 123
Maturation index, for estrogen status, 365
Medroxyprogesterone acetate, in menopause, 329, 330
Melanoma, diagnosis of, 175
Menopausal gonadotropin, human, in polycystic ovary syndrome, 300
Menopause, 323-324
  artificial, 324
  diagnosis of, 327
  management and treatment, 328-332
  osteoporosis in, 334-338
  and postmenopausal bleeding, 339-342
  premature, 324
    diagnosis of, 299
    dysfunctional uterine bleeding in, 221
  symptoms and signs of, 326-327
  and urethral prolapse, 342-344
Menstrual calendar, use of, 228, 232
Menstrual disorders, 212-233
  amenorrhea, 212-219
  in corpus luteum cysts, 288
  dysfunctional uterine bleeding, 219-224
  dysmenorrhea, 224-228
  in follicular cysts, 287
  premenstrual syndrome, 229-233
Menstruation, and vaginal infections, 130
Metronidazole: and candidiasis of vagina, 131
  in *Hemophilus* vaginitis, 130
  side effects of, 138
  in trichomoniasis, 137
Miconazole nitrate cream, in candidiasis of vagina, 133
Mite infestations, 167-169
Molar pregnancy, *see* Hydatidiform mole
Molluscum contagiosum, 153-155
  diagnosis of, 148, 154
Moniliasis of vagina, *see* Candidiasis of vagina
Mononucleosis, infectious, diagnosis of, 196
Monsel's solution, in molluscum contagiosum, 154
Mullerian anomalies, amenorrhea in, 218
Multiple pregnancy: after clomiphene therapy, 301
  complications of, 102
  diagnosis of, 41, 113
  and intrauterine growth retardation, 92
  iron deficiency in, 76

management and treatment of, 100-101
  signs of, 99
  uterine size in, 98
Murmurs, cardiac, in pregnancy, 10
Musculoskeletal system, in pregnancy, 17-18
Mycolog cream: in candidiasis of vagina, 133
  in trichomoniasis, 137
Myoma, see Leiomyoma of uterus
Myomectomy, 283-284

Nabothian cyst, 270-271
Naprosyn: in dysmenorrhea, 227
  in endometriosis, 238
Nausea and vomiting, in pregnancy, 19
Neisseria gonorrhoeae, 179
  penicillinase-producing, 180-181, 186
Neurectomy, presacral, in dysmenorrhea, 228
Nitrofurantoin, in urinary tract infections, 87
Nitrofurazone, in Hemophilus vaginitis, 141
Nocturia: in cystitis, 259
  in pregnancy, 15, 22
  in stress incontinence, 307
Nonstress test in pregnancy, 365-366
  in intrauterine growth retardation, 95
  in postdates pregnancy, 108
Nutrition: carbohydrate intake affecting vaginal environment, 131
  in diabetes of pregnancy onset, 114
  and intrauterine growth retardation, 91, 92
  iron deficiency in, 75-80
  in postmenopausal bleeding, 342
Nystatin: in candidiasis of vagina, 133
  in Hemophilus vaginitis, 141

Obesity: amenorrhea in, 219
  and candidiasis of vagina, 131
  dysfunctional uterine bleeding in, 221
  and gestational diabetes, 113
  and hypertension, 69
  uterine size in, 98
Oligohydramnios: diagnosis of, 93
  in postdates pregnancy, 109
Orange-peel skin: in breast cancer, 244
  in mammary duct ectasia, 253
Osteoporosis, 334-338
Ovary: cysts of, 285-301
  chocolate, 296
  corpus luteum, 288-289
  dermoid, 291-292
  diagnosis of, 37, 119, 188, 192
  dysmenorrhea in, 226

  follicular, 286-287
  mucinous cystadenoma, 294-295
  parovarian, 290-291
  serous, 293-294
  theca-lutein, 289-290
  endometrioma of, 296-297
  polycystic syndrome, 298-301
    amenorrhea in, 214
    diagnosis of, 299
    dysfunctional uterine bleeding in, 221
    pregnancy in, 36
Oxytetracycline, in granuloma inguinale, 205
Oxytocin: challenge test, 366-367
  in intrauterine growth retardation, 95
  in postdates pregnancy, 108, 109
  influences in pregnancy, 6-7

Pain: abdominal: in cervicitis, 158
  in dysmenorrhea, 225
  in endometritis, 162
  in back, see Backache
  suprapubic, in ovarian cysts, 289, 293
Pancreatitis, diagnosis of, 188
Papanicolaou smear, 367-369
  four-quadrant technique, 369
  in herpes genitalis, 171
Papilloma: cervical, 270
  intraductal, of breast, 245, 248-250
  squamous, diagnosis of, 175
Parametritis, diagnosis of, 159, 177
Parasitic infestation, with pediculosis, 164-167
Peau d'orange: in breast cancer, 244
  in mammary duct ectasia, 253
Pediculosis: corporis, diagnosis of, 168
  pubis, 164-167
  folliculitis in, 148
Pelvic adhesions, diagnosis of, 119, 163, 237
Pelvic inflammatory disease: acute, 187-190
  chronic, 190-193
  diagnosis of, 37, 265, 282
Pelvic masses, benign, 267-301
Pelvic relaxation, 303-321
Penicillin: in gonorrhea, 181, 184
  in syphilis, 197-198
Penicillinase-producing Neisseria gonorrhoeae, 180-181, 186
Pessary: in cystocele, 316
  in prolapse of uterus, 313
pH of vagina, 129-130
  in atrophic vaginitis, 143
  in candidiasis, 132
  in Hemophilus vaginitis, 139
  in trichomoniasis, 136

# INDEX 391

Pharyngeal smears, on Thayer-Martin or Transgrow transport medium, 184
Phenazopyridine, in cystitis, 261
Pica, in pregnancy, 16, 21
   and iron-deficiency anemia, 76, 79
Pinworms, diagnosis of, 132
Pituitary lesions: amenorrhea in, 214, 218
   diagnosis of, 299, 327
Placenta: abruption of, see Abruptio placenta
   accreta, 45
   anomalies, and intrauterine growth retardation, 92
   previa, 45-49
      diagnosis of, 46, 52
Pneumonia, diagnosis of, 41
Podophyllin, in condylomata acuminata, 175
Polycystic ovary syndrome, 298-301
Polyhydramnios: diagnosis of, 113
   and gestational diabetes, 113
Polyps, cervical, 277-280
   diagnosis of, 46, 51, 278, 340
Postdates pregnancy, 105-111
   diagnosis of, 107-108
Postmaturity syndrome, fetal, 106
Postpartum complications, 118-125
Postural changes in pregnancy, 18, 23
Povidone-iodine douche: in candidiasis of vagina, 133
   in *Hemophilus* vaginitis, 141
   in trichomoniasis, 137
Pragmatar ointment, in tinea cruris, 157
Pre-eclampsia, 59-68
Pregnancy: abortion of, spontaneous, 28-34
   amniocentesis in, 349-350
   anemia in, 75-84
   cardiovascular changes in, 10-13
   common complaints of, 19-27
   diabetes in, 111-116
   ectopic, 34-39
   estriol measurement in, 358-359
   gastrointestinal changes in, 15-16
   glucose tolerance tests in, 360-361
   hormonal influences in, 4-9
   hypertension in, 59-73
   laboratory values in, 375-381
   and lecithin-sphingomyelin ratio in amniotic fluid, 363-364
   loss in, and grief counseling, 54-56
   molar, 40-44
   multiple, see Multiple pregnancy
   musculoskeletal changes in, 17-18
   nonstress test in, 95, 108, 365-366
   oxytocin challenge test in, 95, 108, 109, 366-367
   placental disorders in, 45-54
   postdates, 105-111
   and postpartum com?lications, 118-125
   respiratory changes in, 16-17
   urinary changes in, 13-15
   urinary tract infection in, 85-89
   variations in uterine growth patterns, 90-104
Premarin: in atrophic vaginitis, 144, 341
   in candidiasis, 133
   in menopause, 329, 331
   in osteoporosis, 337
   in urethral prolapse, 343
Premenstrual syndrome, 229-233
Procidentia, 311-314
Progesterone: influences in pregnancy, 5-6
   serum levels in premenstrual syndrome, 229, 230
   withdrawal test, 369-370
   in amenorrhea, 214-216
   in menopause, 328
   in postmenopausal bleeding, 342
Prolactin, influences in pregnancy, 8
Prolapse: of bladder wall, 314-317
   urethral, 342-344
   of uterus, 311-314
      diagnosis of, 312
Prostaglandins: and dysmenorrhea, 225
   influences in pregnancy, 7
   inhibitors of: in dysmenorrhea, 227
   in endometriosis, 238
Proteinuria, in pre-eclampsia, 59, 61, 62
Pruritus: in atrophic vaginitis, 142
   in candidiasis of vagina, 131
   in *Hemophilus* vaginitis, 139
   in herpes genitalis, 170
   in pediculosis pubis, 165
   in scabies, 167
   in tinea cruris, 155
   in trichomoniasis, 135
   vulvae, 145-147
Pseudomyoma peritonei, and mucinous cystadenoma of ovary, 294
Psoriasis, diagnosis of, 156
Psychogenic problems: and amenorrhea, 214
   and candidiasis of vagina, 131
   diagnosis of, 156
   and dysfunctional uterine bleeding, 220
   and dysmenorrhea, 226
   in menopause, 325-326, 327
   and premenstrual syndrome, 229

and pruritus vulvae, 146
and urinary stress incontinence, 307, 308
Ptyalism, in pregnancy, 16
Pubococcygeus muscle, voluntary control of, 320-321
Puerperium, complications in, 118-125
Pyelitis, diagnosis of, 265
Pyelonephritis, 264-266
  diagnosis of, 86, 259, 265
  in pregnancy, 85-88
Pyosalpinx, 193
Pyrinate A-200, in pediculosis pubis, 166

Radiation exposure: and intrauterine growth retardation, 92
  and pruritus vulvae, 146
Rash, in syphilis, 195
Rectocele, 317-320
  diagnosis of, 318
Relaxation, pelvic, 303-321
Respiratory tract, in pregnancy, 16-17
Rho-GAM immunization, 39
  after spontaneous abortion, 33
Rib cage changes, in pregnancy, 17
Ringworm of vulva, 155-157
Round ligament pain, 18, 22-23
Rubin test, for fallopian tube patency, 370

Salpingitis, 187-190
  diagnosis of, 37, 159, 177, 259
Scabies, 167-169
Scheuermann's disease, diagnosis of, 336
Schiller's test, 370-371
Sclerocystic ovarian disease, 298-301
Sebaceous cyst, 269
  diagnosis of, 151
Serology values, 379
Sexual activity: cystitis associated with, 262-263
  dyspareunia in, see Dyspareunia
  in menopause, 334
  and urinary tract infections, 256
  and vaginal infections, 130
Sexually transmitted diseases: chancroid, 200-203
  chlamydiosis, 176-179
  condylomata acuminata, 174-176
  diagnosis of, 132, 136, 139, 143, 148, 171
  gonorrhea, 179-182
  granuloma inguinale, 203-206
  *Hemophilus* vaginitis, 139
  herpes genitalis, 169-173
  lymphogranuloma venereum, 206-210
  molluscum contagiosum, 153

  pediculosis pubis, 165
  syphilis, 193-200
  trichomoniasis, 135
Shake test of amniotic fluid, 371
Shirodkar procedure, in cervical incompetence, 34
Sideroblastic anemia, diagnosis of, 77
Skin diseases: molluscum contagiosum, 153-155
  scabies, 167-169
  tinea cruris, 155-157
Smallpox vaccine, in herpes genitalis, 172
Smears: buccal, 354
  cervical, on Thayer-Martin or Transgrow transport medium, 184
  Papanicolaou, 367-369
    in herpes genitalis, 171
  pharyngeal, on Thayer-Martin or Transgrow transport medium, 184
Smith-Hodge pessary, in prolapse of uterus, 313
Smoking in pregnancy: and hypertension, 69
  and intrauterine growth retardation, 92
Somatomammotropin, human chorionic, 8-9
Spectinomycin, in gonorrhea, 180, 185
Sphingomyelin, ratio to lecithin, in amniotic fluid, 363-364
Spirochetal infection, 193-200
Staphylococcal infections: and bartholinitis, 150
  and endometritis, 161
  and folliculitis of genital region, 148
  and postpartum mastitis, 122
Stein-Leventhal syndrome, 298-301
Stomach, changes in pregnancy, 15-16
Streptomycin, in granuloma inguinale, 205
Stress incontinence, urinary, 304-310
Subinvolution of uterus, 118-121
Sulfa cream, in *Hemophilus* vaginitis, 140-141
Sulfisoxazole: in cystitis, 261
  in lymphogranuloma venereum, 209
  in urinary tract infections, 87
Surgery: in cervical incompetence, 34
  in cystocele, 316
  in dysmenorrhea, 228
  in endometrioma of ovary, 296-297
  in endometriosis, 239-240
  in leiomyoma of uterus, 283-284
  in mammary duct ectasia, 253
  in ovarian cysts, 291, 292, 294, 295
  in pelvic inflammatory disease, 192
  in prolapse of uterus, 313

in rectocele, 319
in urinary stress incontinence, 309
Syphilis, 193-200
    chance in, diagnosis of, 154, 159, 195-196, 205, 208
    congenital, 198-199

Tabes dorsalis, 200
Telethermometry, graphic stress, 361
Temperature, basal body, 232, 351
Testicular feminization, amenorrhea in, 218
Tetracycline: in chlamydiosis, 178
    in cystitis, 261
    in gonorrhea, 185
    in lymphogranuloma venereum, 209
    in pelvic inflammatory disease, 189
    in syphilis, 198
Thalassemia: alpha-thalassemia minor, 82, 83
    beta-thalassemia minor, 80-84
    differential diagnosis of, 77, 81-82
    major, 83
Theca-lutein cysts, 289-290
Thermography of breast, 371
Thiazide diuretics, in hypertension, 71
Thyroid disorders: diagnosis of, 299, 327
    dysfunctional uterine bleeding in, 221
Thyroxine, influences in pregnancy, 8
Tinea cruris, 155-157
Tolnaftate, in tinea cruris, 156
Trachelitis, 158
Tranquilizers, in menopause, 332
Transverse fetal lie, diagnosis of, 93
Treponemal immobilization test, 197
*Treponema pallidum*, 193
Trichloroacetic acid, in condylomata acuminata, 175
Trichomoniasis, 135-138
Trichophytosis vulvae, 155-157
TRIC organisms, 176-179, 206
Trophoblastic disease, gestational, 119
Trophoblastic tumors, and theca-lutein cysts, 289
Tubal conditions, see Fallopain tubes
Tums, in osteoporosis, 337
Turner's syndrome, amenorrhea in, 218
Twin pregnancy, see Multiple pregnancy
Tzank test, in herpes genitalis, 171

Ulcus molle, 200
Ultrasonography, 371-372
Urethral prolapse, 315, 342-344
Urethritis: in gonorrhea, 182
    nonspecific, in males, 177

Urethrocystogram, chain, 354
Urethrovesical angle, posterior, 305
Urinary frequency: in cystitis, 259
    in pregnancy, 13, 22
    in stress incontinence, 307
Urinary stress incontinence, 304-310
    diagnosis of, 307-308
Urinary tract: changes in pregnancy, 13-15
    infections of, 256-266
        cystitis, 258-262
        diagnosis of, 86, 136
        fluorescent antibody test in, 360
        in pregnancy, 85-89
        pyelonephritis, 264-266
        recurrent, 263-264
Urine: collection of specimens, 257
    estriol levels in pregnancy, 358-359
    evaluation of specimens, 258
    laboratory values for, 380-381
Uterus: blood flow in pregnancy, 11
    cervicitis, 158-161. See also Cervix uteri
    Couvelaire, 50
    dilatation and curettage of, see Dilatation and curettage
    endometritis, 161-164
    leiomyoma of, 280-285
    postpartum infection of, 86
    prolapse of, 311-314
    rupture of, differential diagnosis of, 52
    size and dates of pregnancy, 97-104
    subinvolution of, 118-121
        diagnosis of, 119, 282
        in endometritis, 164

Vagina: candidiasis of, 130-134
    changes from diethylstilbestrol exposure in utero, 266-267
    discharge from, see Discharge, vaginal
    inclusion cyst of, 270
    infections of, 129-145
    maturation index, 365
    pH of, 129-130
    in rectocele, 317
    trichomoniasis of, 135-138
Vaginal bleeding, see Bleeding disorders
Vaginitis: atrophic, 142-145, 326
    diagnosis of, 143, 340
    and postmenopausal bleeding, 341
    diagnosis of, 86, 159, 177, 259
    *Hemophilus*, 138-142
    and pruritus vulvae, 146
Varicosities, in pregnancy, 15, 24-25
VDRL test for syphilis, 196
Venereal disease, see Sexually transmitted diseases

Verruca acuminata, 174
Vesical neck elevation test, 372
Vinegar douches:
  in candidiasis of vagina, 133
  in *Hemophilus* vaginitis, 141
  after polypectomy, 280
  in trichomoniasis, 138
Virus diseases: condylomata acuminata, 174-176
  herpes genitalis, 169-173
  molluscum contagiosum, 153-155
Vitamin D therapy, in osteoporosis, 337
Vomiting, in pregnancy, 19
Vulva: in bartholinitis, 150-152
  folliculitis or furunculosis of, 147-149
  infections of, 145-157
  molluscum contagiosum of, 153-155
  parasitic infestations of, 164-167
  tinea cruris of, 155-157

Warts, venereal, 174-176
Weight gain: in pre-eclampsia, 61, 62
  in premenstrual syndrome, 231
Whitfield's ointment, in tinea cruris, 157

Xeromammography, 373

Yogurt ingestion: in candidiasis of vagina, 133
  in gonorrhea, 181
  in *Hemophilus* vaginitis, 142
  in trichomoniasis, 138